THE CULTURE OF M.
PSYCHIATRIC PRACTICE IN AFRICA

THE
CULTURE OF MENTAL ILLNESS
AND
PSYCHIATRIC PRACTICE
IN AFRICA

EDITED BY
EMMANUEL AKYEAMPONG, ALLAN G. HILL,
AND ARTHUR KLEINMAN

Indiana University Press

Bloomington and Indianapolis

This book is a publication of

INDIANA UNIVERSITY PRESS
Office of Scholarly Publishing
Herman B Wells Library 350
1320 East 10th Street
Bloomington, Indiana 47405 USA

iupress.indiana.edu

♾ The paper used in this publication meets the minimum requirements of the American National Standard for Information Sciences—
Permanence of Paper for Printed Library Materials, ANSI Z39.48–1992.

Manufactured in the United States of America

Library of Congress Cataloging-in-Publication Data

The culture of mental illness and psychiatric practice in Africa / edited
by Emmanuel Akyeampong, Allan G. Hill, and Arthur Kleinman.
    p. ; cm.
  Includes bibliographical references and index.
  ISBN 978-0-253-01286-9 (cl : alk. paper) — ISBN 978-0-253-01293-7
(pb : alk. paper) — ISBN 978-0-253-01304-0 (eb)
  I. Akyeampong, Emmanuel Kwaku, editor. II. Hill, Allan G., editor.
III. Kleinman, Arthur, editor.
  [DNLM: 1. Mental Disorders—Africa. 2. Cultural Characteristics—
Africa. 3. Health Care Reform—methods—Africa. 4. Socioeconomic
Factors—Africa. WM 140]
  RC451.A43
  362.196890096—dc23
                                                    2014047048

1 2 3 4 5 20 19 18 17 16 15

To all those who suffer from mental illness in Africa and their caregivers (professionals and families)

CONTENTS

ACKNOWLEDGMENTS

THE EDITORS ACKNOWLEDGE with gratitude sponsorship from the Committee on African Studies at Harvard University and the Michael Crichton Fund of the Harvard Medical School, which funded the December 2006 international workshop on African psychiatry. The following provided invaluable assistance in the preparation of the manuscript: Olufolakemi Alalade, Marty Alexander, Marilyn Goodrich, Bridget Hanna, Emily Harrison, Richard Landrigan, Maria Stalford, and Liang "Moses" Xu.

THE CULTURE OF MENTAL ILLNESS AND PSYCHIATRIC PRACTICE IN AFRICA

INTRODUCTION

Culture, Mental Illness, and Psychiatric Practice in Africa

EMMANUEL AKYEAMPONG, ALLAN G. HILL,

AND ARTHUR KLEINMAN

THIS VOLUME ORIGINATED in a working group at Harvard University on "Health, Healing and Ritual Practice," which was part of an interdisciplinary and interschool research project of the Committee on African Studies called the "Africa Initiative." The working group's members were scholars with training in public health, demography, medical science, anthropology, linguistics, ethnomusicology, and history, and their deliberations on health and healing brought to light revealing interdisciplinary perspectives. John Mugane, the linguist, was interested in medical diagnosis in African languages. Kay Shelemay, the ethnomusicologist, had worked for many years on Ethiopian church music and its interface with healing. The demographer, Allan Hill, was part of a multiyear research project on women's health in urban Africa. Wafaie Fawzi, the epidemiologist, worked on HIV/AIDS. Majid Ezzati, a public health expert on environmental health, had worked in East and West Africa, examining different kinds of domestic fuels used for cooking and their impact on health and the environment. Emmanuel Akyeampong, the historian, had worked on the history of addiction and on disease and urbanization in West Africa. Arthur Kleinman, a psychiatrist and medical anthropologist, has published extensively on mental illness and psychiatry in non-Western contexts, with a particular focus on China. Akyeampong and Kleinman jointly offered a course on "Violence, Substances, and Mental Illness: African Perspectives," in the fall of 2006 (and again in 2011), and the working group hosted a workshop on psychiatry in Africa in December 2006. The interest that this generated encouraged the editors to compile a select number of papers in what, we hope, is a coherent volume.

This volume thus emerged out of conversations between a psychiatrist and nonpsychiatrists about the history, culture, and practice of psychiatry in Africa.

The conversation highlighted the changing social terrain for the practice of psychiatry and psychology in Africa, and why both disciplines are attracting the interest of nonspecialists in African studies. This book is not intended to be a comprehensive volume on psychiatry in sub-Saharan Africa. Its significance lies in the ways in which psychiatry or mental health can provide a lens for our understanding of African worldviews, lifestyles, and social processes, while African ideologies and lived realities can provide an important critique of psychiatry. Africa has figured prominently in contemporary global health planning and policy, particularly regarding HIV/AIDS, tuberculosis, malaria, and other infectious diseases. It has figured less centrally in thinking about mental illness and the sequelae of social suffering. This has not always been the case.

To the extent that these have been the subjects of inquiry, the West regarded Africa and Africans in the nineteenth and twentieth centuries through lenses tinted by psychiatry and presumptions of African inferiority (Fabian 2000). Medical science—in particular, psychiatry—was an important medium for the construction of knowledge about the African "other" in the colonial period (Carothers 1953; McCulloch 1995). Studies have revealed similar processes in the case of colonial India (Arnold, 1993; Mills 2000). Works by historians have examined the social construction of medical knowledge, and how Western medical science in the colonial era framed the production of knowledge about the African (Hunt 1999; Lyons 1992; Vaughan 1991; Wylie 2001). Africans, however, have gazed back, their therapeutic practices resilient even in an era of colonialism, and their innovative eclecticism in the realm of medical pluralism a reflection of a confident rather than a diffident spirit (Abdalla 1997; Flint 2008; Luedke and West 2006; Taylor 1992). These nuances inform the growing interest by psychiatrists in African studies, as well as their interest in the history, practice, and culture of psychiatry and psychology. Africans seem to score quite favorably compared to European and North American populations on scales used worldwide to assess mental disorders (de Menil et al., 2012). The possibility that schizophrenic patients in the developing world may have better outcomes than those in the developed world—according to the International Pilot Study of Schizophrenia, which included Ibadan, Nigeria—has raised questions about the matrix of African social structures and relations and how they may provide a more supportive social environment (Odejide, Oyewunmi, and Ohaeri 1989, 710–11). This possibility potentially revises our understanding of schizophrenia as a progressively deteriorating condition that is frequently irreversible, thereby illustrating how Africa and African studies can influence psychiatry.

This introductory chapter provides a historical and social context for mental health in twentieth-century Africa and for changing psychiatric practices, with the objective of shedding light on social dynamics in colonial and independent

Africa and the challenges these throw up in terms of mental health—or, more precisely, the approach to the care and treatment of the mentally ill. This discussion situates the subsequent chapters in this volume, as we review the history of psychiatry in Africa; common mental disorders in community and primary care treatment; psychosis; violence and its aftermath; HIV/AIDS and mental health; and the infrastructure of psychiatric treatment, including alternative healing systems. The chapters that follow address key issues that lie at the center of psychiatry's intersection with African studies, and the growing appreciation of mental health in postcolonial Africa. These include how medical science—in particular, psychiatry—informed the production of knowledge about Africa and Africans; the common incidence of mental illness in Africa; the interface between destitution and mental illness; the training of Africans in psychiatry at African medical institutions and the Africanization of a Western science; specialties within psychiatric practice in Africa; mental health and rehabilitation in postconflict societies; the changing face of depression, especially with the advent of HIV/AIDS; and the long history of mental health care by indigenous healers.

SOCIAL CHANGE AND MENTAL HEALTH IN AFRICA, 1930s–1960s

Early psychiatric practice in colonial Africa had the goal of documenting difference. It sought insights into African mentalities that would, among other outcomes, aid colonial governments to understand, govern, and control their subjects. Inspired by anthropological ideologies about cultural diffusion and imbued by scientific racism, methods such as craniology sought correlations between the size of the brain and social development (or civilization). It was assumed that non-Western peoples would have smaller brain sizes, thus providing scientific support for Western racial assumptions. The East African school in the 1930s—H. L. Gordon, F. W. Vint, and others—sought to scientifically demonstrate this correlation. John C. Carothers emerged from this East African school and drew on the work of Gordon and Vint in support of his theories about African biological inferiority (Vaughan 1991, 110–11). In the early twentieth century it was difficult for even liberal-minded psychiatrists to escape the racist biases of that era or the racial framing of psychiatric inquiry in Africa (Sachs 1937; Simmons 1958). The line of thinking that linked race and mental capacity reached its climax with the Mau Mau Emergency in Kenya in the 1950s, when the Kenyan government invited Carothers to provide a psychological explanation of the Mau Mau and the presumed African mental depravity of its members (Carothers 1954).

During these early years a number of stereotypical views emerged from colonial psychiatry. One compared the mental development of the African adult to that of a European child; a second assumed that mental illness was more a phenomenon of urban Africa, especially among Africans caught in the process of acculturation, sometimes called detribalized Africans; and a third was the misperception that depression was rare among Africans because they had an undeveloped sense of individuality.

The appointment of trained anthropologists to the British colonial service, as well as the penchant for colonial medical personnel to dabble in amateur anthropology, underpinned the growth of ethnopsychiatry and the emergence of some pioneering work like that of Margaret Field in colonial Ghana. A trained ethnographer who was appointed a colonial anthropologist (along with others such as Robert Rattray in the Gold Coast and Charles Meek in Nigeria), Field conducted research in the Gold Coast that shed light on religion and medicine among the Ga on the coast of Accra (Field 1937) and on witchcraft, depression, and healing (Field 1955). She wrote about the search for psychosocial security in a rapidly changing Gold Coast, where the rise of the cocoa industry, a boom in trade, and growing urbanization beginning in the 1930s had resulted in the proliferation of wealth, a weakening of kinship ties, and increased accusations and fears of witchcraft during a period of heightened political activity (Field 1960).

As urbanization accelerated in late colonial and early independent Africa, exerting new pressures on kinship, and as new social classes emerged in the urban context and first-generation urbanites struggled to raise children in city environments, numerous anthropologists, sociologists, demographers, historians, and psychiatrists examined these momentous transitions and their impact on life and health (Caldwell 1968; Lambo 1967; Little 1973, 1974a, 1974b). Among the topics of interest, sociologists studied the new social elites and the first generation of university-educated graduates; social anthropologists looked at hometown associations as institutions of urban socialization; and psychiatrists examined the impact on child upbringing of frequent transfers in the postings of a new generation of African civil servants, and the incidence of "brain fag" (short for brain fatigue) among first-generation university students under severe social pressure to excel academically (Prince 1960a). The recreational use of cannabis and synthetic drugs was noted beginning in the 1950s and 1960s (Lambo 1965), as was the growing visibility of alcohol abuse (Adomako 1976). Drug abuse and anxieties about urban life were connected in several important studies. Historians and anthropologists also contributed to the growing body of works on drinking and alcoholism in Africa (Akyeampong 1996; Ambler 1991; Karp, 1980; La Hausse 1988; Parkin 1972; Willis 2002).

These studies, though strongly marked by the colonial context, suggest that mental health interventions cannot be simply overlain on existing health structures; rather, we must consider a cluster of interventions particular to local mental health problems and their social context. Even primary care for mental health needs to be rethought as community service. The need for such multifaceted approaches becomes clear throughout this book's chapters.

ECONOMIC DECLINE AND POLITICAL INSTABILITY IN INDEPENDENT AFRICA

Nationalism in Africa has been described as an omnibus movement, an amalgamation of disparate interests united only in their common desire to overthrow alien rule (Daddieh 2006). Indeed, Mahmood Mamdani (1996) has argued that so focused were Africans on overthrowing European rule that the political transformation of colonial Africa ended prematurely with the exit of the former colonial masters, with no root-and-branch review of the structures left in place by the departing rulers. In short, decolonization was—and remains—incomplete. The economic prosperity of the 1940s and 1950s papered over the cracks in the nationalist movement and reinforced the false sense of unity. As world prices for Africa's primary exports began to decline in the 1950s, and nationalist governments were compelled to redefine priorities in the face of shrinking resources, centrifugal forces were unleashed in African societies with various interest groups lobbying for state resources. This was the context of patrimonialism and clientelist politics. The first to be sidelined were peasants and rural dwellers. Over time, even more favored groups came under threat, including the military. In the mid-1960s Africa experienced its first military coups (Assensoh and Alex-Assensoh 2001; Austin and Luckham 1975; Hutchful and Bathily 1998).

The first generation of African psychiatrists trained in the Western tradition began practicing in the early years of African independence. The overlap of advances in psychotherapy and psychotropic medications with a turning away from the institutionalization of the mentally ill in the West freed African psychiatrists from the racist biases that had prejudiced colonial psychiatry. The focus on Africanization by new African governments encouraged the new generation of African and Africanist psychiatrists to engage in dialogue with indigenous healers who had long dealt with mental illness. Psychiatrists and ethnopsychiatrists examined the interface between mental illness and witchcraft (Field 1955) and explored spirit possession and local herbs as mediums for healing (Baasher 1975; Prince 1960b). Out of this dialogue between Western-trained and indigenous healers came the novel experiment at Aro Village, in southern Nigeria, in which Thomas Lambo, the first trained Nigerian psychiatrist, tested the provision of community mental health care in a village setting under the auspices of the University of Ibadan's medical school. Lambo worked closely with indigenous healers, who had a deep understanding of African cultures and psychologies. The patients were placed with families in Aro Village because that familiar social environment was considered more conducive to recovery than the sterile and impersonal nature of the hospital ward (Asuni 1967; Jegede 1981; Lambo 1966). In Dakar in the 1960s and 1970s, Henri Collomb and the Dakar school at Fann Hospital also set up what they called "psychiatric villages," inspired by Collomb's interactions with indigenous therapeutic communities, the Aro example, and a genuine desire to come to terms with indigenous understandings of mental disorder (Collignon 1995–96, and in this volume). But the young profession of African psychiatry was overwhelmed by Africa's numerous problems in the period following the 1960s.

Africa's first civil wars occurred in the 1960s in what is now the Democratic Republic of the Congo and Nigeria (the Biafran war). Both started with military coups and degenerated into civil conflict along ethnic and regional lines. These conflicts were the subject of various disciplinary studies, including psychiatry (Lamontague 1971). These early studies served as the prelude for later studies in the 1990s and after that have examined post-traumatic stress disorder in conflict zones like the Portuguese colonies of Angola and Mozambique in their wars of liberation and subsequent civil wars; the liberation struggle in Zimbabwe; and the long-drawn-out civil wars in Uganda, Sudan, Liberia, and Sierra Leone. Economic decline in Africa in the 1970s and 1980s—the 1980s has been referred to as Africa's lost decade—reinforced state decay, and compounded the continent's lack of preparation for the health challenges of the period following the 1980s. Declines in public services, including health care, further undermined the legitimacy of various African states.

Two major shocks to African economic systems in the 1960s and 1970s were the pronounced Sahelian drought, between 1967 and 1975, and the petroleum crisis after 1973. Debts mounted for most African economies, with the exception of the few oil-rich nations, and several sought relief from the World Bank and the International Monetary Fund (IMF) in the late 1970s and early 1980s. Even what had been called the Ivorian Miracle unraveled as the Côte d'Ivoire's spectacular economic growth came to a halt in the 1980s. Industrialization declined in Africa, and the continent's share of world trade fell from 3 percent in the 1950s to less than 2 percent in the 1990s. Structural adjustment programs were imposed by the World Bank and the IMF on African countries that had essentially gone into economic receivership.[1] African governments needed help to meet their foreign debt burdens, and the World Bank and the IMF instructed them to retrench as part of the process of trimming down bloated bureaucracies. As a result, government subsidies were removed in vital sectors such as health care, currencies were devalued, and economies opened up to the market and free trade. Massive layoffs caused further social dislocation. Several scholars have noted the adverse effects of structural adjustment programs on health in Africa and the developing world (Kanji, Kanji, and Manji 1991; Loewenson 1993; Peabody 1996; Pfeiffer and Chapman 2010). These programs have been associated with decreasing food security and undernutrition, as well as a rise in poor health and decreased access to health care services for the poor, who form two-thirds of Africa's population (Loewenson 1993). The very rationale of structural adjustment—the need for present pain, or socioeconomic sacrifices through fiscal austerity, for the sake of future gain, or economic growth and prosperity—has been seen as inapplicable to health, where "present suffering cannot always be offset by future improvements" (Peabody 1996, 823). The World Bank's (1987) prescription for the financing of health services in developing countries in the 1980s and 1990s weakened government health services at a time when sub-Saharan Africa was ravaged by the AIDS crisis and civil wars, with unfortunate implications for mental health. The World Bank recommended the privatization of health services along the following lines: the introduction of user fees for government facilities, the introduction of private health insurance, making nongovernmental bodies central to health delivery, and the decentralization of health services. James Pfeiffer and Rachel Chapman reflect on how the World Bank, with its 1993 publication of *World Development Report: Investing in Health,* effectively "superseded the WHO [World Health Organization] as the primary driver of global health policy" (2010, 151).

The end of the Cold War and the emergence of a unipolar world motivated the World Bank to impose uniform lending policies on Africa, and to require democratization as one of the preconditions for financial assistance. Dictatorial regimes were pressured, and civil societies became more vocal and critical. The era of people's power had dawned in Africa (Cooper 2002; Manning 1998). Liberia, courted during the Cold War, was allowed to degenerate into violence when a coup removed Samuel Doe as president in 1989. The bloody civil war that followed lasted for over a decade (Ellis 1999). Liberia's conflict spilled over into Sierra Leone through the proxy Revolutionary United Front, and Sierra Leone descended into a decade of civil war itself (Abdullah 2004; Richards 1996). Ironically, more diamonds and timber would be exported annually from Liberia and Sierra Leone during their civil wars than previously. Conflict diamonds (also called blood diamonds) would fuel conflicts in West Africa and Angola (Hirsch 2001). And conflict would extend to Guinea and the Côte d'Ivoire, further destabilizing West Africa. After the 1980s the Horn of Africa, Uganda and Sudan, and the Great Lakes region also became sites of violence and instability. Genocidal conflict has flared episodically in Rwanda and Burundi since independence, though it was the Rwandan genocide of 1994 that riveted international attention. Civil war in Uganda with the Lord's Resistance Army has dragged on for over three decades, so long that this ongoing conflict has become "normalized" and the world has forgotten about it. The end of the Cold War, however, also helped bring a resolution to proxy wars in Angola and Mozambique (Stockwell 1978).

The psychological impact of long-term states of violence and repression such as the one that persisted in South Africa for almost half a century under apartheid; the maiming of many people through land mines in Mozambique and Angola; the creation through numerous conflicts of large groups of physically disabled people; the phenomenon of child soldiers in conflicts in Uganda, Liberia, and Sierra Leone, and the challenges of their rehabilitation; as well as multiple generations of traumatized war victims have preoccupied psychiatrists and others with an interest in mental health. The mental health implications of children caught up in war as victims and perpetrators have received attention by various authors (Barnett 1999; West 2000; Wilson 2001). These problems have been contrasted with episodic traumatic events such as the bombing of the American embassies in Kenya and Tanzania (Carlos and Njenga 2006). Key works of scholarship have examined refugee life, the violence that persists even in these camps, and the health conditions of refugees (Malkki 1995; Sommers 2001). How refugees deal with death in their displaced existence and the need to broaden existing understandings of humanitarian intervention has received sensitive treatment by Harri Englund (1998). The psychiatric condition of refugees in Sierra Leone has been examined in Steven Fox and S. S. Tang (2000). New methods of reconciliation in postviolence societies are being explored, and several African countries are taking lessons from the Truth and Reconciliation Commission in South Africa (Borneman 2002; Minow 1998; Wilson 2001). And novel systems of justice are being experimented with in postgenocide societies, including the Gacaca courts in Rwanda.

The collapse of states, conflicts, streams of refugees across borders, and the use of rape as an instrument of war have all coincided with and exacerbated the HIV/AIDS pandemic in Africa since the 1980s. The timing of the pandemic in Africa could have not been more disastrous (Iliffe 2006). The tenuousness of life and reduced life expectancy, overwhelmed extended family networks, AIDS orphans, teenager-headed households, and the rise in opportunistic infections have all added to the mental illness load. Depression rates have spiked in connection with HIV/AIDS. Uganda, one of the early hotspots of HIV infection and home to a distinguished school of medicine at Makerere University, has provided some of the pioneering studies analyzing the mental health effects of HIV/AIDS on patients and AIDS orphans (Antwine, Cantor-Graae, and Banjunirwe 2005; Wilk and Bolton 2002). Studies have also examined how AIDS patients deal with stigma (Kalichman and Simbayi 2004). The opportunistic diseases that AIDS facilitates, such as tuberculosis and depression, often all manifest themselves in the same patient, an overlaying of three diseases associated with stigma. And the burden of providing care to AIDS patients has posed key challenges to the mental health of doctors and nurses in regions like East Africa (Raviola, this volume). Triple stigma and displacement related to the combination of conflict and marginality highlight the importance of sustaining links between human rights and mental health interventions. A human rights approach to AIDS proved to be instrumental in securing treatment for AIDS patients in Africa. It may take a similar human rights–based movement to prioritize patients with mental illness as deserving recipients of available treatment options.

The growing interest in psychiatry in Africa by non-African psychiatrists and nonpsychiatrists alike must be placed in the contexts examined above. The dire need for psychiatric services has come at a time when some African countries are not equipped to deal with this pressure. Sierra Leone has only one trained psychiatrist, Edward Nahim. He has recounted how the warring sides in the Sierra Leonean civil war were very circumspect in their treatment of the country's sole psychiatrist, because all sides needed him alive.[2] Such wartime practicality makes the dearth of psychiatric care and the existing burden on the health infrastructure in some regions of Africa chillingly clear. In postconflict, postcolonial settings where economies are drained and health infrastructure is lacking, myths that mental health care is neither important nor feasible are particularly damaging. On the contrary, mental health must be prioritized. Mental illness accounts for about 15 percent of the total global burden of disease, and depression is a leading cause of disability with about 350 million people around the world suffering from depression according to the World Health Organization (2012). Coupled with myths of inconsequentiality are myths of the resistance of mental illness to treatment. In fact, the treatment of depression has the same success rate as that of hypertension. Many demonstration projects have shown that early and appropriate pharmaceutical intervention and therapy by paraprofessionals can be effective, but few of these projects have been scaled up. Contributions to this volume make it clear that mental health care in contexts with limited resources is both necessary and feasible.

The growing interest during the last two decades in psychiatry by Africanists who are not psychiatrists has also been promoted by postmodernist turns in humanistic studies, which have underscored the subjectivity of knowledge and the multiplicity of texts. The works of Michel Foucault and Edward Said have underpinned a generation of scholarship on difference or the "other" within societies (such as the poor, the ill, and the physically disabled), as well as across cultures. As a "soft" medical science, psychiatry may be the discipline that most lent itself to manipulation and contestation in colonial Africa. Carothers demonstrated the utility of psychiatry to colonial ideology and hegemony as he sought to ground European rule in the psychological superiority of the colonizers. But the racist

ideas in colonial psychiatry did not go uncontested, and even in the colonial period there were European psychiatrists who dissented from the racial interpretations of the African mind or explored African understandings of mental illness
(Sachs 1937; Simmons, 1958). The very fact that the definition of mental disorder
is caught up in layers of interpretation strengthened the relevance of alternative paradigms and therapies in Africa. Richard Keller notes that "as psychiatry
occupies a unique space between the social and natural sciences, the discipline
constitutes a crucial locus for study of the relationship between knowledge and
power" (2001, 296).

OVERVIEW OF THE BOOK

This volume contains thirteen chapters whose authors are from the fields of
history, anthropology, psychiatry, social psychology, demography, and public
health. Emmanuel Akyeampong (chapter 1) provides an overview of psychiatry
in Africa, examining key shifts in psychiatric thought and practice from the colonial period to the present. He situates his analysis within changing political,
economic, and social dynamics to provide a better understanding of the political
economy of mental health, examining landmark events such as the French initiative in psychiatry in colonial Algeria, the experiment in community psychiatric
care at Aro Village in Nigeria, and the major innovations in psychiatry in Senegal by Collomb and his circle at Fann Hospital in Dakar. Akyeampong notes
how current developments such as the HIV/AIDS pandemic and casualties from
Africa's numerous civil wars are shaping the contours of mental illness and care.
He also provides an original case study of the perceived social and medical links
between cannabis use and madness in Ghana and Nigeria.

Vikram Patel and Dan Stein (chapter 2) explore the concept of common
mental disorders (CMDs), which include depression, anxiety, and the presentation of these and other mental health problems through somatization. Although
each of the component conditions may have different risk factors and treatments,
Patel and Stein argue for the utility of the umbrella term of CMD in both the
clinical setting and public health planning because of the very high comorbidity
of these conditions. The authors show that nearly 25 percent of adult patients presenting for primary care services have CMDs, constituting the largest burden of
disease and cause of disabilities globally. Patel and Stein point out that although
the symptoms of CMDs are essentially shared worldwide, they are expressed and
characterized in diverse ways across different settings. Although CMDs often
present through somatization of symptoms, acknowledgment of mental health
issues by the patient often occurs after the condition becomes chronic. Multiple
explanatory models are deployed by patients with CMDs, but supernatural expla-

nations are especially prominent in Africa. Drawing on extensive research and data from Zimbabwe, Patel and Stein show that marginalization and lack of life choices are risk factors for CMDs and that, in the African context, this particularly applies to women.

One of the most significant challenges facing medical professionals in Africa is finding ways to incorporate cross-cultural understandings of mental illness into psychiatric evaluations of patients. Psychiatric models of symptomatology are based largely on European and North American behavioral norms and are not necessarily applicable in other cultures. Care for individuals with schizophrenia and psychosis in general continues to be hindered by language and cultural barriers between caregivers and patients, the scarcity of psychiatric professionals and antipsychotic drugs, and the lack of governmental support and infrastructure. In chapter 3, Ursula Read, Victor Doku, and Ama de-Graft Aikins focus on the challenges of psychiatric care in West Africa. They describe how individuals suffering from schizophrenia and psychosis, along with the caregivers and communities trying to support them, are affected not only by these disorders, but also by the current medical establishment's inability to provide relief. This is due to both poor economic conditions and cultural miscommunication. Even when those suffering from mental illness can be accurately identified, determining the causes of their symptoms requires an intimate knowledge of local culture and practice. The gulf between modern psychiatric models and traditional belief systems obstructs a clear understanding of the nature of psychosis on both sides of the cultural divide, leading to confusion and disagreements over how best to treat patients.

The authors highlight the dearth of multidisciplinary data on mental illness and argue that current funding for such research remains starkly inadequate. They call for anthropological, sociological, and psychological perspectives to be added to the current literature so that the lived experiences of people suffering from mental illness, as well as of their family members and friends who may be serving as their primary caregivers, can be observed and understood. The authors argue that such research, together with a partnership with traditional healers, would aid West African medical professionals in developing responsive and culturally appropriate services that reflect local realities rather than attempting to replicate North American and European models.

In chapter 4, on "Mental Illness and Destitution in Ghana: A Social-Psychological Perspective," de-Graft Aikins examines four key aspects of the relationship between mental illness and destitution in Ghana. First, she seeks to identify which groups of mentally ill persons are most vulnerable to destitution. Second, she explores the factors that mediate the relationship between mental illness and destitution. Third, she probes the experiences of actual and potentially ill destitute people for lessons on preventing destitution or minimizing its impact on the mentally ill. And fourth, she examines the state of current interventions for the mentally ill and future challenges to their successful treatment. Merging the concepts of the individual-society interface and biographical disruption, de-Graft Aikins examines the relationship between mental illness and destitution at four levels: the intrasubjective (an individual's perceptions of his or her own illness); intersubjective (relations between the patient, family, and caregivers); social (the ideas of the community and the larger society about mental illness and how the ill individual responds to these); and the structural context of mental illness and destitution, such as family poverty and the absence of job skills. In training her lens on the mentally ill destitute, de-Graft Aikins demonstrates the broad range of mental conditions outside of psychosis that can result in both mental illness and destitution, how people can become vagrants or destitute without being mentally ill, and how mental illness and destitution can be mutually reinforcing. The profiles and experiences of vagrants and revolving-door patients at the Accra Psychiatric Hospital demonstrate these dynamics and underscore the complex relationship between structural poverty, mental illness, and destitution. De-Graft Aikins shows how the gender and geographical profiles of the mentally ill destitute have changed in the fifty years since Ghana became independent, with an increase in the female and Ghanaian (as distinct from foreign) destitute population. The chapter highlights three forms of interventions with the mentally ill destitute, aside from being kept in psychiatric hospitals: village settlements (a traditional approach, with shrine villages as the settlements' precursors); Christian outreach interventions (especially Pentecostal prayer camps); and humanitarian and rights-based interventions, particularly with the advent of mental health nongovermental organizations such as BasicNeeds and Mind Freedom. This last category offers a more patient-centered, rights-based intervention that is more in line with the present orientation of mental health care worldwide, though the chapter highlights the limits of current initiatives as well.

Chapter 5, by Alan Flisher and coauthors, focuses on the current status, policy, and plans for child and adolescent mental health care in South Africa. The authors report the prevalence of child and adolescent psychiatric disorders in the country to be estimated at 17 percent, although they highlight the dearth of comprehensive epidemiological studies of mental health in South Africa. The rate estimated for South Africa is higher than that for other developing countries. The authors believe that this can be explained by the higher level of economic inequality in South Africa, given that such inequality is a well-established risk factor for mental illness. In 2003 and 2004 the South African government released policy guidelines for child and adolescent mental health care, and Flisher and coauthors draw on these guidelines to create a model for child and adolescent mental health services in the country. First, the authors discuss the core features of care, focusing on the provision of mental health services in primary care settings and triaging the children most in need of services. Second, they address the need for evidence and service planning, which would allow for regular assessments of mental health programs and bolster the ability to revise program strategies and services as needed. Third, they examine the range of staffing and facilities that are needed to provide services and effectively refer children to the most appropriate treatment program. Flisher and coauthors develop a detailed model for South African child and adolescent mental health services, including numbers of required staff members based on the government's policy guidelines, and they contrast this with current norms of assessment and treatment. They conclude with the observation that their model addresses only the current needs of the population and urge that resources be allocated for the prevention of mental illness in children and adolescents.

In chapter 6, René Collignon provides insights into the school of psychiatry founded by Collomb at the Fann Hospital in Senegal in the 1960s, its research activities and training initiatives, and its legacy in French West Africa more broadly. Examining developments in social psychiatry, psychoanalysis, and medical anthropology, Collignon explores the broader context that enabled the charting of a new direction away from the precepts or presumptions of colonial psychiatry, and that permitted a serious engagement with indigenous understandings of mental illness among peoples like the Lebu and the Wolof. The chapter examines the place of culture in the practice of psychiatry, whether the psychiatrist is from the same or a different culture. Thus, among the Lebu and the Wolof, psychosensory experiences such as auditory or visual representations (for example, the hearing of voices) are not deemed abnormal in a world suffused by spirits and are seen as normal in the community. This raises the question of when the patient, the family, and the community determine that these experiences have become pathological and require the attention of a healer or psychiatrist. This also makes it challenging for the psychiatrist to distinguish between delusion and hallucination, as the division between reason and unreason established in classical Western psychiatry becomes blurred. These were some of the issues the Fann therapists under Collomb's leadership engaged. Consequently, their receptive attitude to indigenous belief systems pleasantly surprised Senegalese families. The chapter reviews the challenges that faced psychiatry in Senegal from the 1980s on, including those associated with the departure of Collomb, the Africanization of medical personnel in the country, and the withdrawal of French help for development in mental health. The broader context of economic decline beginning in the 1980s, and the introduction of structural adjustment programs, with their cutbacks in areas such as health care, sharpen these challenges and help explain the current disrepair of hospital structures and low morale among health personnel. Some of the innovations of Collomb's circle at the Fann Hospital have suffered setbacks in this climate; yet the tradition of pioneering psychiatry lives on not just in Senegal, but also in French West Africa, as graduates of Fann Hospital have founded training and research programs in Mali, Niger, Benin, and Burkina Faso.

Allan Hill and Victoria de Menil (chapter 7) explore women's mental health in Accra based on a 2003 health survey of 3,200 adult women across a broad age range. The survey asked several direct questions about mental health, providing one of the earliest comprehensive sources of information on the prevalence of mental disorders in a large urban population in Africa. The authors provide a useful discussion of the development of instruments for measuring health—cross-cultural and cross-country surveys, often under the auspices of the World Health Organization—and what we can learn about health in comparative perspective by measuring the burden of disease across countries. These survey instruments include the World Health Organization's Multi-Country Survey Study in 2000–2001, the 2002 World Health Survey, the World Health Organization's Study on Global Ageing and Adult Health, and the ongoing World Mental Health Survey, sponsored by the World Health Organization. These surveys reveal the prevalence and severity of mental health conditions worldwide. Epidemiological studies on mental health in Ghana are few, with the available studies mostly based on data from the Accra Psychiatric Hospital.

This is what makes the 2003 Women's Health Survey of Accra invaluable. It used the Short Form 36 instrument and included some questions on mental health, home interviews, and contextual cultural and country-relevant information. An analysis of the results of this survey does not indicate any notable differences across ethnic groups. The more significant variables are socioeconomic differentials such as education, and employment or income levels. Thus better education seems to protect against mental illness, and the best mental health was seen among those with formal or regular employment. Assessing severity in mental illness revealed an intriguing U-shaped pattern, with severity of mental health conditions manifesting themselves in women younger than twenty-five or older than fifty. Severe depression among young women seemed to be more pronounced among those who were better educated and who had high but unfulfilled expectations about job prospects. High levels of depression among young women, Hill and de Menil argue, may be an unforeseen side effect of the rising age at marriage and at the birth of a woman's first child. This chapter shows that standard instruments developed elsewhere that have known psychometric properties can be used in contexts such as Ghana to detect age patterns and differentials in mental illness, suggesting the universality of socioeconomic gradients seen elsewhere.

People living with HIV/AIDS have higher rates of mental illness than the general population, and this is exacerbated by lack of economic, health care, and social support opportunities available to many of the afflicted in Africa. Recent scholarship has highlighted the compelling issues of the mental health of health care professionals who must deal with the HIV/AIDS epidemic with scant resources, as well as the stigma sometimes imposed on patients by health care providers. The disjuncture between the theory of medical science as taught in African medical schools that share basic texts with Western medical schools and the practice of the medical profession in a resource-poor continent can prove demoralizing, with significant mental health implications (Quigley 2009; Wendland 2010).

In chapter 8, Pamela Collins evaluates the outcomes of a 1994 reorganization of the South African health care system, which integrated mental health care with primary care. In South Africa, the ratio of trained psychiatric staff to the population is very low. In efforts to remedy this situation, legislation has forced health care providers who lack the proper training to try to treat mentally disabled patients. Further compounding the problem, over half of the trained psychiatrists in South Africa work in private practice, serving only the wealthy. As a result, psychopharmacology remains the predominant form of treatment. This situation has been worsened by the serious scale of the AIDS epidemic in South Africa. In 1998, 23 percent of women attending antenatal clinics were infected, a 34 percent increase over the previous year. Collins argues that solving this problem requires frank and open discussion of preventive measures. Improving the attitudes and knowledge of mental health care workers is a critical factor in achieving this goal. However, South Africans typically hold conservative views about sex; secrecy is the norm. In 2002 a new Mental Health Care Act recognized that sexuality is part of the lives of people in the mental health care system, breaking with past legislation that reinforced social stigma of those with mental illness. This becomes a double-edged sword, given the connections between positive HIV status and depression and other mental illnesses. Collins and her colleagues, in collaboration with the South African Mental Health Directorate and a South African research team, conducted pilot workshops in psychiatric wards in several of that country's hospitals, involving both clinicians and administrators, in an attempt to help break down barriers resulting from culturally embedded stereotypes and give caregivers the skills they need to better serve their communities. Disagreements arose, particularly regarding condom distribution, the efficacy of indigenous methods versus Western medicine in treating HIV/AIDS, and providers' responsibilities to patients and patients' families. The collaborating teams talked about the origins of and ways to combat stigma, approaches to discussing sex and HIV/AIDS with mental health patients, and educating communities about prevention. The results were improved attitudes and knowledge, laying a foundation for further progress.

Continuing the theme of professional development and training, Giuseppe Raviola addresses the issue of caregiver burnout in chapter 9. Professional caregivers in Africa experience a greater number of intense stressors than their Western counterparts do, leading to higher rates of fatigue and demoralization and reducing their ability to perform their duties adequately. Burnout is an intangible, yet ever-present and hazardous psychological side effect of medical practice, particularly in developing countries. Raviola examines this issue from a biosocial viewpoint, arguing that this phenomenon has its roots in the changing nature of health care worldwide, local cultures and practices of medicine, resource shortages, working conditions, and the impotency of measures designed to combat AIDS. Studies of provider stress in Western nations have found that individuals' perception of stressors plays a role in burnout. The use of internal or external coping strategies is a good indicator of the likelihood of burnout, with internal strategies predicting much lower levels of exhaustion. Most studies in Africa and other resource-poor settings have tended to focus more on occupational concerns such as needle sticks and contacts with bodily fluids of HIV-positive people; knowledge, attitudes, and practices; and parameters of burnout. African medical culture itself has been identified as a source of stress and burnout. Overcrowding and underfunding of hospitals, negative relationships with senior staff members, and the bioethical dimensions of the explosion of AIDS cases have all been identified as sources of stress for trainees. Largely missing, in Raviola's view, are studies of the emotional and affective conditions of professional caregivers. Difficult decisions on how to allocate too few resources among too many patients cause a great deal of mental anguish. The increasing political and economic pressures worldwide to privatize mental health makes an already stressful situation more difficult. Although health care professionals have clearly been attracted to private practice for financial reasons, Raviola argues that the "basic psychological necessity" of working in a less stressful environment has also been a major factor. He urges that further research on the mental health of psychiatrists and other health professionals is necessary to more fully understand the impact of working in underfunded medical systems with a high prevalence of HIV/AIDS in order to improve working conditions, and he also encourages African mental health professionals to engage with policymakers to find solutions and work toward their implementation.

The next two chapters review the infrastructure of psychiatric treatment. They complement several of the contributions in this volume, with Elialilia Okello and Seggane Musisi (chapter 10) focusing on traditional healers in mental health care in Africa, and Shoba Raja, Sarah Wood, and Michael Reich (chapter 11) discussing the pharmaceutical industry and mental health. Medical pluralism is a reality of African therapy, particularly in the realm of mental health care. Traditional, Muslim, and Christian healers represent real alternatives to Western psychiatry. Okello and Musisi underscore the facts that approximately 80 percent of Africans use traditional healers, and that traditional medicine is patronized by more than 66 percent of the world's population. The authors draw on their own work on Uganda and refer to other published sources to provide a thoughtful discussion of the training and services of traditional healers to African communities in the realm of mental health. The poor development and funding of mental health in Africa, as well as theories of causality that often ascribe religious or spiritual causes to mental illness, lead the authors to stress the continued relevance of traditional healers in psychiatric care and the need to incorporate them into formal structures of health care. They examine how community explanatory models, the convenient services that traditional healers provide, and the unsatisfactory present state of health care systems explain the continued demand for traditional healers. They advocate a genuine integration of Western and traditional medicine by according traditional medicine legal recognition, funding it, and facilitating a meaningful collaboration between the two types of medicine.

Using four studies from 2007 conducted by BasicNeeds, Raja, Wood, and Reich examine the provision and adequacy of pharmaceutical drugs to psychiatric institutions in Ghana, Uganda, Kenya, and Tanzania. These were part of a larger study by BasicNeeds, an international mental health organization that works mostly with governments in selected African and Asian countries to provide essential medicines for the poor. Raja and Wood work for BasicNeeds and collaborate in this chapter with Reich, a professor of public health at Harvard University with a long-standing interest in global pharmaceuticals. Founded in 2000, BasicNeeds responded to a World Health Organization recommendation in 2001 advocating the combination of psychosocial and pharmacological approaches in treating mental illness. The success of this strategy presupposes the availability of essential medicines for mental illness, and BasicNeeds's 2007 study on access to such medicines enables the authors to test this presupposition in this chapter. The authors compare the 2007 *WHO Model List of Essential Medicines* with the national lists for Ghana, Uganda, Kenya, and Tanzania to determine how current the national lists are. Some of the newer drugs are missing from the national lists, as African countries—with their limited budgets for medicines—are not key markets for global pharmaceutical companies. Moreover, the appearance of medicines on a national list does not mean they are available in the country. The authors remind us that older generations of essential medicines are not necessarily less efficacious than newer ones, but the perception among government leaders that they lack adequate knowledge of current medicines and alternative psychiatric treatments informs the low priority assigned to psychiatric medicines in health budgets. Uganda, Kenya, and Tanzania have adopted what is called a push system, whereby they acquire standardized kits of essential medicines and distribute these periodically to local districts irrespective of specific demands on the ground based on the local prevalence of various mental disorders. Ghana is dependent on donor funds for all imported medicines, an unreliable way to meet essential needs in medicine. The lack of essential medicines in public health facilities places a premium on the services of private pharmacies.

Having adequate means of health care delivery is just as crucial as a supply of the essential medicines. In low- and middle-income countries, community-based mental health care through the primary health care system has proven appropriate and cost-effective. But at this level the lack of trained personnel in psychiatry works against the distribution of essential medicines. In the four countries surveyed in the chapter, psychotropic drugs are not distributed to primary health care centers as there are too few psychiatrists to prescribe the medicines or monitor their use. The chapters by Okello and Musisi on traditional healers and Raja, Wood, and Reich on psychiatric medicine in Africa together provide a more comprehensive understanding of the provision of medicines for psychiatric treatment. The role of diviners as distinct from herbalists makes it difficult to quantify the provision of herbal medicines for psychiatric treatment, and thus to ascertain how well traditional and Western medicine together are meeting mental health needs. The meaningful integration of these two spheres, as advocated by Okello and Musisi, would be an important step toward evaluating the complementarity of herbal and Western medicines and their ability to adequately provide psychiatric care in Africa.

The final two chapters in this volume deal with violence and its consequences for mental health. William Murphy (chapter 12) pays close attention to the structural or institutional arrangements within a society that can predispose the population to particular risks. His analysis of the recruitment and demobilization of child soldiers in Sierra Leone forcefully demonstrates how long-standing patrimonial relationships in a society expose its members to exploitation. Such well-established dependencies may have long-term ill effects; in the short term in Sierra Leone, they were used to institutionalize the recruitment and discipline of young boys into militias. Murphy makes the important point that in many societies such patrimonial relationships may not be benign, let alone an established part of local traditions. The discovery of the underlying logic of the recruitment of young boys, and later of amputations, reveals how organizational arrangements can permit gangsterism and inhuman practices when underlying power structures are perverted or allowed to rule unchecked. The integration process after the war therefore required not just individual reconciliation but also adjustments to the patrimonial arrangements that had produced the militias.

Theresa Betancourt (chapter 13) deals with children affected by war and describes the challenge of measuring the effects of war on children's health with a range of different instruments. Her main point, illustrated with reference to the Ugandan experience, is that the methods chosen can have a major impact on which conditions are identified. In contrast to the classic, clinically based assessment tools, added measures from social anthropology and social psychiatry are capable of revealing new mental health problems and contextualizing them in new ways. Both chapters alert us to the risks to mental health in every population, even those not directly touched by war or civil strife. The authors collectively raise the interesting possibility that although wars and civil strife certainly have a dramatic impact on mental health, the origins of the stressful situations in which individuals find themselves may well be in the normal processes of social interaction arising from structural and power inequalities within society.

By virtue of being interdisciplinary and via its focus on the historical, social, and cultural contexts of mental illness and psychiatric practice in Africa, this volume is designed for both health care professionals and those in the social sciences and the humanities. A number of observations stand out. The first is how political economy frames health, and the mental health infrastructure in pre- and postapartheid South Africa reflects this reality. The second is the low priority accorded to mental health in policies, programs, and funding across sub-Saharan Africa and the developing world. The third is the growing burden of mental illness in Africa, a burden unappreciated in official health policies and underserved by the mental health infrastructure. Africa's numerous conflicts and the ravages of HIV/AIDS have added to the continent's mental health burden. Major categories of mental diseases manifest themselves globally, as indicated in world mental health surveys, but symptomatology and the social course of the illness experience reflect cultural and social influences. The implementation of mental health care interventions is as powerfully affected by political, economic, and institutional processes as are the implementations of interventions for AIDS, tuberculosis, and malaria. And the stigma affecting both patients and family caregivers suggests that social and cultural determinants are as powerful for mental health care as for mental illnesses. Africa teaches local and regional lessons about psychiatry and psychology. Africa also stands to benefit from informing itself about global trends and approaches to mental health and adopting best practices. The scientific case for implementation of mental health interventions is being made, as chapters in this book illustrate. It is the moral and political case that now needs to be advanced, if general essential programs for mental health are to be funded in the future. Hence, the study of psychiatry and mental health in Africa contributes to improved understanding of African history and societies and of global changes, knowledge of mental health problems, and the reform and strengthening of health care systems. It is a subject whose time has come.

NOTES

1. For a good review of structural adjustment in Africa, see Monga (2006).
2. Emmanuel Akyeampong interview with E. A. Nahim, Freetown, Sierra Leone, July 18, 2002.

REFERENCES

Abdalla, I. H. 1997. *Islam, Medicine and Practitioners in Northern Nigeria*. Lewiston, ME: Edwin Mellen.

Abdullah, I., ed. 2004. *Between Democracy and Terror: The Sierra Leone Civil War*. Dakar: Council for the Development of Social Science Research in Africa.

Adomako, C. C. 1976. "Alcoholism: The African Scene." *Annals of the New York Academy of Science* 273 (1): 39–46.

Akyeampong, E. 1996. "What's in a Drink? Class Struggle, Popular Culture, and the Politics of Akpeteshie (Local Gin) in Ghana, 1940–1967." *Journal of African History* 37 (2): 215–36.

Ambler, C. 1991. "Drunks, Brewers and Chiefs: Alcohol Regulation in Colonial Kenya, 1900–1939." In *Drinking: Behavior and Belief in Modern History*, edited by S. Barrows and R. Room, 165–83. Berkeley: University of California Press.

Antwine, B., E. Cantor-Graae, and F. Banjunirwe. 2005. "Psychological Distress among AIDS Orphans in Rural Uganda." *Social Science and Medicine* 61 (3): 555–64.

Arnold, D.. 1993. *Colonizing the Body: State Medicine and Epidemic Disease in Nineteenth-Century India*. Berkeley: University of California Press.Assensoh, A. B., and Y. Alex-Assensoh. 2001. *African Military History and Politics*. New York: Palgrave.

Asuni, T. 1967. "Aro Hospital in Perspective." *American Journal of Psychiatry* 124 (6): 763–77.

Austin, D., and R. Luckham, eds. 1975. *Politicians and Soldiers in Ghana, 1966–1972*. London: Frank Cass.

Baasher, T. A. 1975. "Traditional Treatment of Psychiatric Disorders in Africa." *African Journal of Psychiatry* 1 (1): 77–85.

Barnett, L. 1999. "Children and War." *Medicine, Conflict, and Survival* 15 (4): 315–27.

Borneman, J. 2002. "Reconciliation after Ethnic Cleansing: Listening, Retribution, Affiliation." *Public Culture* 14 (2): 281–304.

Caldwell, J. C. 1968. *Population Growth and Family Change in Africa: The New Urban Elite in Ghana*. Canberra: Australian National University Press.

Carlos, J. O., and F. G. Njenga. 2006. "Lessons in Post-Traumatic Stress Disorder from the Past Venezuelan Floods and Nairobi Bombing." *Journal of Clinical Psychiatry* 67 (Suppl. 2): 56–63.

Carothers, J. C. 1953. *The African Mind in Health and Disease*. Geneva: WHO.

———. 1954. *The Psychology of Mau Mau*. Nairobi: Government Printer.

Collignon, R. 1995–96. "Some Reflections on the History of Psychiatry in French Speaking West Africa: The Example of Senegal." *Psychopathologie africaine* 27 (1): 37–51.

Cooper, F. 2002. *Africa since 1940: The Past of the Present.* Cambridge: Cambridge University Press.

Daddieh, C. K. 2006. "Ethnicity, Conflict and the State in Contemporary West Africa." In *Themes in West Africa's History,* edited by E. Akyeampong, 265–84. Oxford: James Currey.

De Menil, V., A. Osei, N. Douptcheva, A. G. Hill, P. Yaro, and A. de-Graft Aikins. 2012. "Predictors of Women's Mental Health in Accra, Ghana." *Ghana Medical Journal* 46 (2): 17–24.

Ellis, S. 1999. *Mask of Anarchy: The Destruction of Liberia and the Religious Dimension of an African Civil War.* New York: New York University Press.

Englund, H. 1998. "Death, Trauma and Ritual: Mozambican Refugees in Malawi." *Social Science and Medicine* 46 (9): 1165–74.

Fabian, J. 2000. *Out of Our Mind: Reason and Madness in the Exploration of Central Africa.* Berkeley: University of California Press.

Field, M. J. 1937. *Religion and Medicine of the Ga People.* London: Oxford University Press.

———. 1955. "Witchcraft as a Primitive Interpretation of Mental Disorder." *Journal of Mental Science* 101 (425): 826–33.

———. 1960. *Search for Security: An Ethno-Psychiatric Study of Rural Ghana.* London: Faber and Faber.

Flint, K. E. 2008. *Healing Traditions: African Medicine, Cultural Exchange, and Competition in South Africa, 1820–1948.* Athens: Ohio University Press.

Fox, S. H., and S. S. Tang. 2000. "The Sierra Leonean Refugee Experience: Traumatic Events and Psychiatric Sequelae." *Journal of Nervous and Mental Disease* 188 (8): 490–95.

Hirsch, J. 2001. *Sierra Leone: Diamonds and the Struggle for Democracy.* Boulder, CO: Lynne Rienner.

Hunt, N. R. 1999. *A Colonial Lexicon of Birth Ritual, Medicalization, and Mobility in the Congo.* Durham, NC: Duke University Press.Hutchful, E., and A. Bathily, eds. 1998. *The Military and Militarism in Africa.* Dakar: Council for the Development of Social Science Research in Africa.

Iliffe, J. 2006. *The African AIDS Epidemic: A History.* Athens: Ohio University Press.

Jegede, R. O. 1981. "Aro Village System of Community Psychiatry in Perspective." *Canadian Journal of Psychiatry* 26 (3): 173–77.

Kalichman, S. C., and L. Simbayi. 2004. "Traditional Beliefs about the Cause of AIDS and AIDS-Related Stigma in South Africa." *AIDS Care* 16 (5): 572–80.

Kanji, N., N. Kanji, and F. Manji. 1991. "From Development to Sustained Crisis: Structural Adjustment, Equity and Health." *Social Science and Medicine* 33 (9): 985–93.

Karp, I. 1980. "Beer Drinking and Social Experience in an African Society: An Essay in Formal Sociology." In *Explorations in African Systems of Thought,* edited by I. Karp and C. S. Bird, 83–120. Bloomington: Indiana University Press.

Keller, R. 2001. "Madness and Colonization: Psychiatry in the British and French Empires, 1800–1962." *Journal of Social History* 35 (2): 295–326.

———. 2007. *Colonial Madness: Psychiatry in French North Africa.* Chicago: University of Chicago Press.

La Hausse, P. 1988. *Brewers, Beerhalls and Boycotts: A History of Liquor in South Africa.* Johannesburg: Ravan.

Lambo, T. A. 1965. "Medical and Social Problems of Drug Addiction in West Africa (with Special Emphasis on Psychiatric Aspects)." *West African Medical Journal* 14 (6): 236–54.

———. 1966. "The Village of Aro." In *Medical Care in Developing Countries,* edited by M. King, n.p. Nairobi: Oxford University Press.

———. 1967. "Adolescents Transplanted from their Traditional Environment: Problems and Lessons out of Africa." *Clinical Pediatrics* 6 (7): 438–44.

Lamontague, Y. 1971. "Psychological Problems of Biafran Children." *Psychopathologie africaine* 7:225–33.

Little, K. 1973. *African Women in Towns.* London: Cambridge University Press.

———. 1974a. *Urbanization as Social Process.* London: Routledge and Kegan Paul.

———. 1974b. *Urbanization, Migration and the African Family.* Reading, MA: Addison-Wesley.

Loewenson, R. 1993. "Structural Adjustment and Health Policy in Africa." *International Journal of Health Services* 23 (4): 717–30.

Luedke, T. K., and H. G. West, eds. 2006. *Borders and Healers: Brokering Therapeutic Resources in Southeast Africa.* Bloomington: Indiana University Press.

Lyons, M. 1992. *The Colonial Disease: A Social History of Sleeping Sickness in Northern Zaire, 1800–1940.* Cambridge: Cambridge University Press.

Malkki, L. 1995. *Purity and Exile: Violence, Memory, and National Cosmology among Hutu Refugees in Tanzania.* Chicago: University of Chicago Press.

Mamdani, Mahmood. 1996. *Citizen and Subject.* Princeton, NJ: Princeton University Press.

Manning, P. 1998. *Francophone Sub-Saharan Africa 1880–1995.* Cambridge: Cambridge University Press.

McCulloch, J. 1995. *Colonial Psychiatry and "The African Mind."* Cambridge: Cambridge University Press.

Mills, J. H. 2000. *Madness, Cannabis and Colonialism: The "Native-Only" Lunatic Asylums of British India, 1857–1900.* London: Macmillan.

Minow, M. 1998. *Between Vengeance and Forgiveness: Facing History after Genocide and Mass Violence.* Boston: Beacon.

Monga, C. 2006. "Commodities, Mercedes-Benz & Structural Adjustment: An Episode in West African Economic History." In *Themes in West Africa's History,* edited by E. Akyeampong, 227–63. Oxford: James Currey.

Odejide, A. O., L. K. Oyewunmi, and J. U. Ohaeri. 1989. "Psychiatry in Africa: An Overview." *American Journal of Psychiatry* 146 (6): 708–16.

Parkin, D. J. 1972. *Palms, Wine, and Witnesses: Public Spirit and Private Gain in an African Community.* Prospect Heights, IL: Waveland Press.

Peabody, J. W. 1996. "Economic Reform and Health Sector Policy: Lessons from Structural Adjustment Programs." *Social Science and Medicine* 43 (5): 823–35.

Pfeiffer, J., and R. Chapman. 2010. "Anthropological Perspectives on Structural Adjustment and Public Health." *Annual Review of Anthropology* 39 (1): 149–65.

Prince, R. 1960a. "The 'Brain Fag' Syndrome in Nigerian Students." *British Journal of Psychiatry* 106: 559–70.

———. 1960b. "The Use of Rauwolfia by Nigerian Native Doctors." *American Journal of Psychiatry* 118 (2): 147–49.

Quigley, F. 2009. *Walking Together, Walking Far: How a U.S. and African Medical School Partnership Is Winning the Fight against HIV/AIDS.* Bloomington: Indiana University Press.

Richards, P. 1996. *Fighting for the Rainforest: War, Youth and Resources in Sierra Leone.* Oxford: James Currey.

Sachs, Wulf. 1937. *Black Hamlet: The Mind of an African Negro Revealed by Psychoanalysis.* London: G. Bles.

Sadowsky, J. 1999. *Bedlam: Institutions of Colonial Madness in Southwest Nigeria.* Berkeley: University of California Press.

Simmons, H. J. 1958. "Mental Disease in Africans: Racial Determinism." *Journal of Mental Science* 104 (435): 377–88.

Sommers, M. 2001. *Fear in Bongoland: Burundi Refugees in Urban Tanzania.* New York: Berghahn.

Stockwell, J. 1978. *In Search of Enemies: A CIA Story.* New York: Norton.

Taylor, C. 1992. *Milk, Honey and Money: Changing Concepts in Rwandan Healing.* Washington: Smithsonian Institution Press.

Vaughan, M. 1991. *Curing Their Ills: Colonial Power and African Illness.* Oxford: Polity.

Wendland, Claire L. 2010. *A Heart for the Work: Journeys through an African Medical School.* Chicago: University of Chicago Press.

West, H. G. 2000. "Girls with Guns: Narrating the Experience of War of Frelimo's 'Female Detachment.'" *Anthropological Quarterly* 73 (4): 189–94.

Wilk, C. M., and P. Bolton. 2002. "Local Perceptions of the Mental Health Effects of the Uganda Acquired Immunodeficiency Syndrome Epidemic." *Journal of Nervous and Mental Disease* 190 (6): 394–97.

Willis, J. 2002. *Potent Brews: A Social History of Alcohol in East Africa 1850–1999.* Oxford: James Currey.

Wilson, R. 2001. "Children and War in Sierra Leone: A West African Diary." *Anthropology Today* 17 (5): 20–22.

World Bank. 1987. *Financing Health Services in Developing Countries: An Agenda for Reform.* Washington: World Bank.

———. 1993. *World Development Report: Investing in Health.* Washington: World Bank.

World Health Organization. 2012. "Depression." October. http://www.who.int/mediacentre/factsheets/fs369/en/.

Wylie, D. 2001. *Starving on a Full Stomach: Hunger and the Triumph of Cultural Racism in Modern South Africa.* Charlottesville: University Press of Virginia.

1 A HISTORICAL OVERVIEW OF PSYCHIATRY IN AFRICA

EMMANUEL AKYEAMPONG

Mental illness is a phenomenon in all societies. The predominance of pre-literate societies in sub-Saharan Africa before the nineteenth century meant fewer written records on medical systems that could enable us to study mental illness in precolonial Africa and the efficacy of traditional African therapeutic systems. Diviners, priests, and healers (including herbalists) have a long tradition of healing in Africa, and their practice certainly predated the colonial encounter. Their skills were particularly indispensable in the case of mental illnesses, which many African societies even in the 1980s ascribed to supernatural causes such as witchcraft or offenses against the gods and ancestors (Odejide, Oyewunmi, and Ohaeri 1989, 709). It is, however, with the colonial encounter that we have our first studies of the African mind, usually by colonial psychiatrists and medical practitioners, and by extension of African healing traditions by curious Western medical men. The racial context of colonialism informed psychiatry, coloring psychiatric observations with racial prejudice and bias. Colonial psychiatry became not just a scientific interrogation of mental illness among Africans, but also an endeavor to explain the African psyche and cultures. Or, to be more precise, "African culture," since key practitioners of colonial psychiatry, such as John Carothers, assumed a common African culture that had produced a generic African individual. Consequently, sweeping statements could be made about the African psyche, such as: "The psychology of the African is essentially the psychology of the African child. The pattern of his mental development is defined by the time he reaches adolescence and little remains to be said" (Carothers 1953, 106).

Perhaps, this should not surprise us. Foucault (1988, chap. 9) reminds us of how the positivism of the nineteenth century, which cloaked psychiatry in the discourse of science, obscured the reality of psychiatry's foundations at the end of the eighteenth century in family and authority, law, and social and moral order. Colonial rule appealed to psychiatry's authoritative predisposition. By the 1980s the psychiatrist and medical anthropologist Arthur Kleinman would critique the strong turn toward biology in psychiatry and the push back against culture, as advances in psychoactive medications in the previous two decades had generated excitement in the field about finding the magic bullet for every psychiatric ailment (Kleinman 1988, 1). Colonial psychiatry in the first half of the twentieth century was caught between these two poles: struggling to account for the interactions between biology and culture, and seeking objective evidence about African psychopathology in racialist science and biology. Given that it was trapped in a European mind-set that assumed the cultural superiority of the European and the naturalness of European rule in Africa, this was not an easy undertaking. The contradictions in these positions would call for a psychological, rather than a sociopolitical, analysis of the Mau Mau movement in Kenya in the 1950s and the strong British denial of its nationalist roots (Carothers 1954). In its preoccupation with social and moral order, colonial psychiatry became a handmaiden of colonial hegemony. Psychiatry's investment in social and moral order has continued into the postcolonial period, leading to intriguing overlaps in lay and psychiatric opinions on major social issues.

The psychiatric literature about Africa changed significantly with the continent's independence in the 1950s and 1960s, as trained African and Western psychiatrists began to practice and conduct research in an entirely different political environment. It quickly became evident that psychiatric disorders (both neurotic and psychotic) were as common in Africa as they were in the West across age, gender, and rural-urban divides (Diop et al. 1980; Giel and Van Lujik, 1969; Giel et al. 1981; Leighton et al. 1963). Several comparative studies removed the artificial divide in conceptualizations of mental illness between those in Africa and those in the West. In some newly independent African countries like Ghana, attempts were made to incorporate indigenous healers into the formal health system (Warren et al. 1982), a trend that has been pursued more systematically in southern African countries like Mozambique and Zimbabwe (Luedke and West 2006). Such attempts built on insights from colonial ethnopsychiatrists like Margaret Field in Ghana, who presented a sympathetic evaluation of indigenous therapeutic practices in psychiatric conditions such as depression (Field 1955). Thomas Lambo in Nigeria in the 1950s pioneered community-based psychiatry at the Aro Village system in Abeokuta, housing psychiatric patients and their attending relatives in collaborating villages and partnering with indigenous healers. The wisdom in these initiatives is underscored by Jerome Frank's observations that "part of the efficacy of psychotherapeutic methods lies in the shared belief of participants that these methods will work" and that these methods would vary across historical time and space (1974, 3).

The 1970s and 1980s witnessed foundational works on ethnopsychiatry and the history and culture of Western psychiatry in Africa (Janzen 1978; Sow 1980; Yoder 1982). Some were written by trained psychiatrists, who sought to situate their training in Western psychiatry within African cognitive frameworks and cultural practices (Sow, 1980). Works by historians and anthropologists have examined the social construction of medical knowledge, and how Western medical science in the colonial era framed the production of knowledge about the African (Hunt 1999; Lyons 1992; Vaughan 1991; Wylie 2001). A few works are beginning to provide an African perspective on the encounter with Western medicine during colonial rule (Flint 2008).

The growth in the interest in psychiatry in the last two decades has been obvious, as postmodernism underscored the subjectivity of knowledge and the multiplicity of texts and has placed a premium on African agency and autonomy, even in the colonial period. Foucault has been instrumental to this interest, as his works have shaped our understanding of the technologies of rule through seminal studies on the birth of the asylum, the clinic, and the prison. As a "soft" medical science, psychiatry may have lent itself more than any other discipline to manipulation and contestation in colonial Africa. Colonial psychiatry was not an uncontested field, for the efficiency that germ theory and the discovery of vaccines lent biomedicine in the treatment of physical diseases was absent in the realm of colonial psychiatry (Keller 2007; Sadowsky 1999). The very fact that the definition of mental disorder is conceptual and not empirical (Cooper 2005) strengthened the relevance of alternative paradigms and therapies in Africa, and some Western-trained psychiatrists conceded the viability of African psychotherapeutic practices even during colonialism (Sachs 1937).

The remainder of this chapter will examine the provision of psychiatric institutions and changing therapeutic practices in Africa in the nineteenth and twentieth centuries. It does not claim to be an exhaustive review, as it would be impossible to provide adequate continental coverage. It intends to set out some of the key developments in the thinking and practice of psychiatry in Africa, which will serve as historical context for the essays in this volume and an introduction to readers who may want to read further in this area. It begins with the colonial period and the provision of lunatic asylums to confine the mentally insane. As many studies have emphasized, there was no great confinement of the mentally ill in Africa as happened in nineteenth-century Europe (Foucault 1988), and asylums did not constitute an arm of colonial social control (Sadowsky 1999; Vaughan 1991). In many cases, colonial asylums were designed to remove the insane from public places, since they were more of a nuisance than a danger to the public. The role of the asylums was primarily custodial. The provision of care and a commitment to curing in the 1940s and 1950s due to advances in chemotherapy and a growing resort to electroconvulsive therapy coincided with decolonization and African independence and ushered in a new era of African psychiatry.

The context was then set for the first Western-trained African psychiatrists to turn the practice of psychiatry in Africa in new directions. Pioneers included Tigani El Mahi in the Sudan (the first Western-trained African psychiatrist) and Lambo of Nigeria, two psychiatrists who were keenly aware of how social contexts and relations framed both the experience of mental illness and its treatment. Through the Aro Village system, later attached to the University of Ibadan, Lambo sought to provide a conducive and familiar African environment for the treatment of mental illness. Thus in Africa a precedent was set for community care in mental health before this direction became evident in the West. Another important site of innovation was the Dakar school at Fann Hospital, led by Henri Collomb, which took a multidisciplinary approach to the study of mental illness in Senegal and was commited to understanding local representations of mental disorder, as well as indigenous forms of control and socialization (Collignon 1995–96, and this volume).

The focus of this chapter is more on Western psychiatry as introduced in the colonial era and practiced in the postcolonial period, though some reference is made to African, Muslim, and Christian healing practices. I examine the introduction of psychiatric institutions in the colonial era, the rationale for their creation and their place within technologies of colonial rule, the initial custodial nature of psychiatric institutions, and the gradual shift to effective therapy and cure beginning in the 1950s, which coincidentally was also the period of African nationalism and independence. New drugs and a new mind-set would underpin a new practice of psychiatry in independent Africa, where some of the most innovative developments in psychiatry occurred until the economic and political challenges of the 1970s and 1980s undermined the infrastructure of psychiatric practice, ironically just when the need for psychiatry was increasing. The review ends with the 1990s and the birth of the new millennium, when civil wars ravaged Africa and created waves of traumatized refugees, and soaring rates of HIV/AIDS led to depression among sick adults. The impact of mental illness on AIDS orphans, the growing ranks of destitute youth, and teenager-headed households has yet to be studied in any detail. In line with the earlier statement about psychiatry's preoccupation with social and moral order in the colonial period, a short case study on cannabis and madness in postcolonial West Africa ends this chapter, to underscore the overlap of lay and psychiatric opinions and the fact that—as Kleinman recently put it—psychiatric diagnosis is "an interpretation of an interpretation" (personal communication, February 2, 2011). Kleinman observes that "culture and profession contribute significantly, if more or less tacitly, to the construction of mental illness" (Kleinman 1988, 73).

COLONIAL ASYLUMS

The imposition of colonial rule was accompanied by the establishment of asylums, not necessarily as an instrument of social control, as I have mentioned above, but as part of the infrastructure of colonial rule. In this regard, asylums—together with hospitals, public works, and censuses—were part of the making of the colonial order. The earliest asylum in sub-Saharan Africa was opened by the British in Freetown, Sierra Leone, one of West Africa's oldest colonies. This was the Kissy Lunatic Asylum, a facility that was used for all types of dependent people, including the mentally and physically ill, starting in the 1820s. It was designated a colonial hospital in 1844 (Bell 1991, 44). In the nineteenth century it received mental patients from the Gambia, the Gold Coast, and Nigeria, other British territories in West Africa (ibid., 16). In colonial Nigeria specialist asylums for the mentally insane were built in Lagos in 1903 (Yaba Asylum) and in southeastern Nigeria in 1904 (Calabar Asylum) (Sadowsky 1999). The Gold Coast gained its first asylum in Victoriaborg in 1888, and a new asylum was opened in Accra in 1907 (Forster 1962), which is the site of the Accra Psychiatric Hospital today, in a suburb now known as Asylum Down. In 1868 the government of the Colony of Natal passed southern Africa's first legislation authorizing the detention of the "dangerously insane" or those "of unsound mind" (Parle 2007, 4). Natal Government Asylum became the first asylum in the subregion to be constructed specifically for the insane. In Southern Rhodesia (now Zimbabwe) Ingutsheni Hospital was opened in 1908. Zomba Asylum was built in Nyasaland in 1910, and in the same year Mathari Mental Hospital was constructed in Kenya. Femi Oyebode points out correctly that "many of these asylums were extensions of the local prisons and often complemented other designated areas in prisons and annexes that functioned as prisons" (2006, 321). The objective was to remove the disorderly, the destitute, and the dangerous from public view. The impetus for the establishment of asylums was more complicated in settler colonies with their more conspicuous politics of racial superiority, and more elaborate psychiatry services characterized areas where European populations were largest (Keller 2007; Parle 2007; Swartz 1998).

It follows, then, that the process of committing a mentally insane person was political (Akyeampong 2006), as chiefs and colonial officials mediated the diagnosis of insanity. At a time when asylums were largely custodial and not curative, trained psychiatrists were rare in colonial Africa, and physicians doubled as psychiatrists when needed. In the 1930s Yaba Asylum shifted from its strictly custodial role and began to provide treatment for its patients, a pattern that become noticeable all over colonial Africa (Oyebode 2006). The 1930s had seen the introduction of electroconvulsive therapy, and a better understanding of neurology had created some optimism that intervention in mental illness was possible. This shift was underpinned in Britain by the passage of the Mental Treatment Act of 1930, which sought to "encourage voluntary treatment and to promote psychiatry as a curative rather than a custodial discipline" (McCulloch 1995, 9). Prior to this a pamphlet written in 1928 by the secretary for the British National Council for Mental Hygiene, J. R. Lord, had proposed measures that would encourage voluntary admission and advocated a change of name from "asylum" to "mental hospital" and from "lunatic" to "mentally ill person." Lord stressed the need for medical personnel with psychiatric experience in mental hospitals, underscoring a transition from a custodial to a therapeutic agenda (Bell 1991, 58).

An important landmark in the history of psychiatry in sub-Saharan Africa was a survey conducted on psychiatric care in colonial Nigeria by Robert Cunynham Brown, a doctor, in 1936. He found much that was commendable about the care traditional healers provided for the insane, and he assessed their role in a very sympathetic light. However, he found many government asylums in Nigeria to be inadequate, with prisons often doubling as asylums, and he recommended the use of a village system of care that would combine a familiar social environment with modern medical care (Asuni 1967; McCulloch 1995, chap. 3).[1] This challenge would be taken up in the 1950s, when Lambo returned to Nigeria from England in 1953 to work at the Neuropsychiatric Hospital in Aro, Abeokuta and established the Aro Village system.

In Lusophone Africa, an asylum for the criminally insane was opened in Lourenço Marques in Mozambique in 1930, and in Luanda, Angola, a neuropsychiatric unit was attached to the main hospital in 1946. The late establishment of institutions for the mentally ill in Mozambique and Angola is striking, considering that these were among the earliest European colonies in Africa. In German East Africa (present-day Tanzania), colonial attention in the 1890s was drawn to mentally ill porters in the Swahili caravan trade to the interior, who were abandoned in Dar es Salaam when the caravans returned to the coast. Mentally ill and destitute, they soon crowded the cells of the native prison set aside for native lunatics (Diefenbacher 1995–96). These developments led to an official recommendation to establish a lunatic asylum in German East Africa, a recommendation welcomed by colonial officials on the coast who were struggling with the phenomenon of homeless lunatics. German colonial officers in the interior were less enthusiastic. When a lunatic asylum was finally opened in German East Africa in Lutindi in 1905, which could accommodate fifteen patients, it was at the initiative of a missionary body, the Evangelical Africa Society (Evangelischer Afrika

Verein), with the encouragement of the governor of German East Africa (Diefen-bacher 1995–96). For the first two years the institution remained virtually empty, as local communities refused to send their mentally ill to it. The governor's inter-vention was required to change this situation, leading to the asylum being at full capacity for the first time, in 1907. The continued growth in admissions thereafter required an almost yearly expansion of the physical infrastructure of Lutindi, until the outbreak of World War I in 1914. Under the capable management of deacons who received some psychiatric training in the Bodelschwinghian insti-tutes, the staff at Lutindi began quite early to view it not as a custodial institution, though therapy was chiefly through moral management (a regimen of work). In many ways the asylum in Lutindi was ahead of its time, as it was not until decolo-nization that the shift from custodial care to therapy would take place in other African colonies. The work regimen could be likened to occupational therapy that would become important in the treatment of the mentally ill.[2]

In the French colonies the mentally ill—both French citizens and colonial subjects—were initially evacuated to mental asylums in France. Algeria had ar-rangements with asylums in France beginning in the 1840s. This was to save the colonizing power the embarrassment of having insane Frenchmen tarnish the French image in the colonies, and also because of the late development of mental asylums in the colonies. So in French North Africa, "colonial authorities shipped [French] civilians and even indigenous Algerians who posed a significant dan-ger to public safety to asylums in Marseille, Montpellier, and Aix-en-Provence" (Keller 2007, 41). In 1897 the colony of Senegal signed a nine-year agreement with the asylum of the department of Bouches-du-Rhône, arranging for insane pa-tients to be transferred to Marseille (Collignon 1995–96, 39). This situation proved unsatisfactory, and mortality was high among African mental patients in France, who not only endured the alienation of being relocated far from their homes but also suffered high mortality rates from tuberculosis and exposure (Keller 2007, 41). French policy toward the insane in colonial Africa was thus driven by concerns for public order, not unlike British preoccupations. The insane who remained in the colonies in the absence of specialized clinics were kept in abject conditions. Knowledge of this situation informed a reform movement in France at the beginning of the twentieth century, particularly among the students of the French psychiatrist Emmanuel Régis, a professor at the school of medicine at Bordeaux. The situation in the French colonies gained international attention at the Twenty-Second Congress of French and Francophone Alienists and Neurolo-gists, held in Tunis in 1912.

World War I intervened to defer any action in the French colonies. But the war itself heightened awareness of mental health, with a large number of soldiers having mental problems, and the 1920s witnessed a resumption of efforts to establish specialized psychiatric clinics in Africa. There was a national consensus that the French law of 1838 regulating care of the insane, premised on the incurability of insanity, was outmoded. The new spirit was to treat the insane person as a patient and not as a dangerous individual or a nuisance. A distinction was drawn between chronic and acute cases and the establishment of open services was advocated to shift the emphasis from confinement and its attendant stigma. The important settler colony of Algeria would be the site of one major initiative, the creation of North Africa's largest psychiatric hospital in the late 1920s, the Hôpital Psychiatrique de Blida-Joinville in the city of Blida (Keller 2007). While metropolitan France debated these developments, North Africa came to represent the cutting edge of French psychiatric medicine beginning in the 1930s. French psychiatrists in North Africa took the hospital and not the asylum as their model, and they viewed the absence of an infrastructure of mental health care as an opportunity to innovate.

Though the principle of psychiatric reform was embraced in French West Africa, nothing much happened beyond the passage of a law in 1918 by the governor general of French West Africa mandating that insane people were to be confined to their home village and made the responsibility of the local chief. This was a political and not a medical response. It was not until the political and economic reforms in the aftermath of the Brazzaville Conference of 1944—a conference made possible because the Free French Government led by General Charles de Gaulle was then based on African soil, and the Free French army was essentially an African force—that money from the Funds for Investment and Social and Economic Development enabled the birth of neuropsychiatry at the Fann Hospital in Dakar in 1956 (Collignon 1995–96, 44). The psychiatry department at Fann Hospital would go on to chalk up notable successes in the training of Africans from French West Africa and in the pioneering of innovative and culturally sensitive ways of dealing with the mentally insane.

Any discussion of psychiatry in colonial Africa would be incomplete without a mention of Frantz Fanon, important both for his contributions to psychiatric thought and practice and for his influence on nationalist and political thought in general. Born in Martinique in 1925, Fanon fought with the Free French forces during World War II and then attended medical school in Lyon, France, specializing in psychiatry. In 1953 he accepted a position in Blida, Algeria, the most prominent psychiatric institution in French North Africa. Fanon and other physicians at Blida were apparently frustrated at the conditions at the hospital for patients and staff members. Fanon and four other physicians wrote a critical report on the state of health care at the hospital in 1955, noting severe overcrowding that rendered serious attempts to treat patients ineffective. Once Blida's capacity had been exceeded, new patients could be admitted only when old patients died or were discharged, creating a backlog of psychiatric patients at general hospitals who were awaiting admission to Blida (McCulloch 1995, 35–36).

Fanon's later writings would direct attention to the political assumptions and foundations underpinning psychiatry in Africa. A major transition in his life happened when he quit psychiatric practice at Blida to join the National Liberation Front, which had launched a war of liberation against French colonialism in Algeria. Fanon seems to have left a greater legacy on political thought in the developing world than in psychiatry, though his political writings were inspired by psychiatric theory (McCulloch 1995, 122). He sought to investigate the claims of African inferiority that were rife in colonial psychiatry, to understand the psychology of colonial violence and the creation of a colonial personality, and to examine the impact of colonialism on African cultures (Fanon 1963, 1965). An astute student of the negative impact of European colonialism on the African psyche, Fanon became an advocate of the use of revolutionary violence in overthrowing colonial rule, arguing that violence was the only language the colonizer understood. He and Walter Rodney (1972) may be the most widely read authors on the phenomenon of neocolonialism in Africa.

INDEPENDENCE AND INNOVATION:
ARO VILLAGE AND OTHER SITES

The period after World War II saw a broadening of the range of disorders seen at psychiatric institutions in Africa. In Sierra Leone, Leland Bell (1991) notes a shift from most patients being institutionalized for mental disorders before 1945 to an increasing proportion of patients being institutionalized for social disorders—including alcoholism, drug addiction, crime, divorce, unemployment, and homelessness—after 1945. Nigeria was one of the important sites of innovation in psychiatry starting in the 1950s, and it remains the only black African country with a relatively advanced infrastructure for psychiatric care. It pioneered community psychiatric care in the 1950s through the Aro Village and hospital system, and its huge population, petroleum wealth, and broadening educational and industrial base from the 1960s and 1970s on supported a number of psychiatric units established in general hospitals and university medical schools at Ibadan, Ife, Lagos, Benin, and Ahmadu Bello. The Anambra State Psychiatric Hospital was opened in Enugu in 1970 to deal with the psychiatric casualties of the Biafran civil war (Bell 1991, 17).

Aro Hospital was conceived of in the late 1940s, when the colonial authorities approved the establishment of a mental hospital just outside Abeokuta, where the Lantoro Asylum had been opened in 1944. From its inception, Aro was seen as a mental hospital and not a custodial asylum. Set on three hundred acres of land, the hospital was designed to accommodate two hundred patients at first, and there were plans to expand its capacity to five hundred patients. At the planning stage, Samuel Manuwa, later Nigeria's director of medical services, encouraged Lambo to acquire specialist training in psychiatry. Lambo later returned from training in England in 1953 and assumed charge of Lantoro and Aro, which was still under construction. He combined his extensive networks and knowledge of Abeokuta and its environment as a local resident with lessons he had learned from visiting El Mahi's outpatient service in Sudan to create what became the village system (Asuni 1967; Sadowsky 1999, 46). While the hospital was under construction, Lambo entered into arrangements with residents of neighboring villages to lodge patients there who came to the hospital for treatment. Patients had to be accompanied by a relative, and their mental disorder could not have lasted for more than two years—regulations designed to ensure that they would benefit from treatment and perhaps to avoid the dumping of chronic patients that had characterized colonial asylums. Aro Village was a cross between outpatient and inpatient services. Residing in the village provided rural patients with a familiar social environment for treatment and convalescence. The villagers received income from the hospital for lodging patients and an increased understanding of and tolerance for mental disorders. The involvement of patients in the village's social and economic activities constituted a form of occupational therapy. Violent patients and those who did not come from a rural background were not placed in the villages but referred to wards in Aro or Lantoro (Asuni 1967; Lambo 1966).

Lambo's work was in response to colonial psychiatrists who had privileged race in explaining differences between Africans and Europeans. For Lambo the operative factor in explaining group differences was culture, not race. Hence, urbanized psychiatric patients were not placed in Aro Village. Lambo conducted collaborative research with international teams on mental illness in western Nigeria and among the Yoruba. One such collaboration with a Canadian team established that there were no major differences in mental illness between rural and urban Africans in western Nigeria, or between Africans and Canadians (Leighton et al. 1963). In Nigeria the establishment of Aro brought to official attention a range of mental illnesses that were less severe than the psychotic cases that dominated public understanding of madness. Under Lambo, patients at Aro in the 1950s were treated with electroconvulsive therapy, insulin coma, psychotropic drugs, occupational therapy, and group psychotherapy (Asuni 1967, 769; McCulloch 1995, 33).

Lambo learned from indigenous healers and sought their collaboration when he ran Aro in the 1950s. He discovered in one head count of mentally ill patients in Abeokuta that there were eight times as many patients in the compounds of traditional healers than at Aro. After he moved to the University of Ibadan's medical school to take the chair in psychiatry in 1963, Lambo was replaced as medical superintendent of Aro by Tolani Asuni. It is evident that Asuni was more skeptical than Lambo about the efficacy of traditional healers in the treatment of mental illness, in cases of both psychoses and neuroses (Asuni 1967, 767–68). By the 1970s, traditional healers were no longer formally involved in the Aro Village system, and Aro Hospital was supervised by the Department of Psychiatry at the University of Ibadan (Jegede 1981). Rapid urbanization and the weakening of kinship ties in the trend toward nuclear families posed the greatest threat to the continuing viability of the Aro Village system.

Collomb may have taken a cue from Lambo's Aro Village system and been inspired in his encounter with the therapeutic communities of traditional healers. In any case, he conceived of psychiatric villages as a step in the regionalization of care in Senegal in the 1960s and 1970s (Collignon, this volume). In these villages medical presence took a back seat to the therapeutic action of nurses and organizers. Patients were accompanied by relatives into Collomb's therapeutic communities, a situation that minimized the patient's sense of alienation. Consultations in the psychiatric village allowed patients to articulate their subjective drama in their own words. In Aro in the 1960s, relatives accompanying patients were relied on to assist in providing an objective account of a case (Asuni 1967), perhaps deprivileging the voices of patients. Unfortunately, the condition of the psychiatric villages in Senegal and the care they offered, much like the situation with Aro, deteriorated once their founders left the psychiatric scene (Collignon 1983). But Senegalese trained at Fann Hospital by Collomb and his team—who created psychiatric internships in Dakar, a diploma in psychiatry, and a diploma of initiation into psychopathology for nurses and health technicians—have carried on the work in the regionalization of care, forming partnerships with nongovernmental organizations and other bodies to provide mental health care outside Dakar (Collignon, this volume). Fann's networks and infrastructure remain in place, including the only remaining psychiatry journal published in sub-Saharan Africa, *Psychopathologie africaine,* founded by Collomb and his circle.

THE POLITICAL ECONOMY OF MENTAL HEALTH
IN CONTEMPORARY AFRICA

Severe reverses in African economies from the 1970s on undermined African countries' ability to create and support solid infrastructures to deliver psychiatric care. Droughts in the 1970s in West Africa and the oil crisis of that decade—created by the oil embargo declared by Arab countries in the Organization of the Petroleum Exporting Countries in 1973—effectively checked economic growth in most African countries, and in the 1980s many African countries experienced reverses in their fledgling industrial sectors and saw their economies shrink. The accumulation of heavy external debts ushered in structural adjustment programs under the auspices of the World Bank and the International Monetary Fund (see the introduction to this volume for a discussion of those programs' tenets and health consequences). This period of economic uncertainty coincided with the end of French cooperation and the provision of aid for development in the field of mental health. The departure of French medical personnel like Collomb affected the indigenization of the health care profession (Collignon, this volume). With indigenization it has become challenging for Africans trained in a Western psychiatry forged on the basis of racial and cultural difference to practice in their own societies and cultures. This process has sparked an introspective and critical reevaluation of the profession (Sow 1980). Parallel to this is the continued influence of Western paradigms in psychiatric practice, as evidenced in the worldwide adoption and distribution of the *Diagnostic and Statistical Manual of Mental Disorders* (DSM) in the last two to three decades. Now in its fifth edition, the DSM is the official classification system of the American Psychiatric Association, and it has become extremely influential in global mental health care. The manual has also grown enormously in length and weight, describing a few dozen conditions in the 1950s and covering more than 400 today. Although the DSM covers conditions that have a universal presence—delirium associated with infections, psychosis, dementia, depressive disorders, anxiety disorders, alcohol intoxication and addiction, and so on—the evidence for cultural construction of the categories is substantial (for example, eating disorders, bereavement, and the slippery slopes of spectrum disorders such as autism. The fourth edition of the DSM even contains an appendix with so-called culture-bound disorders like *nervios* (*ataque de nervios;* an attack of nerves) among Latino Americans; *shenjingshuairuo* (neurasthenia) among Chinese; and brain fag (mental exhaustion brought about by extreme external pressure on the young to excel in school) in West Africa and *zar* (spirit possession) in Ethiopia, Somalia, and Sudan.

Kleinman (1988, 14–17), among others, critiqued this classificatory jumble as an example of "category fallacy" because it failed to adequately account for cultural influences on universal syndromes; failed to present local idioms of distress and illness experience as real diseases; and insisted on using data from Euro-American populations, which make up less than 20 percent of the global population, as its evidence base. Like Kleinman, Young (1997) and others criticized DSM categories like post-traumatic stress disorder, arguing that they were the result of political, economic, and sociocultural constraints on scientific methods and interpretations. Nonetheless, even most psychiatric anthropologists and cultural psychiatrists today accept the view that a relatively small number of serious psychiatric disorders occur in Africa as well as in America, Asia, Europe, and Latin America. These include schizophrenia, bipolar disorder, depression, anxiety disorders, autism, dementia, and various forms of substance abuse. As presently understood, these conditions appear to be biosocially constructed, with important differences based on genetic, geographic, ethnic, gendered, and age-related processes that contribute to the development of pathology, experience of symptoms, course of disease, and response to treatment. The global popularity of the DSM, including in Africa, can lead to conflicts with the World Health Organization's *International Classification of Diseases* system as well as with local professional, folk, and popular religious interpretations. It is widely recognized now that there is a politics and a sociology of mental illness classifications that is increasingly affected by globalization, local moral worlds, and the role of states, the United Nations, and nongovernmental organizations. Not insignificant is the financial interest of the pharmaceutical industry. The huge influence of medical science on everyday life in the twentieth century, particularly in the United States, has led to two important developments of our time: the pathologization of social problems and moral experience (Canguilhem 1991; Horwitz and Wakefield 2007; Foucault 2003), which has led to the pharmaceuticalization of populations (Dumit 2012); and the normalization of experiences of the body and the self, which brings psychiatry more fully into the nominative disciplining and policing of societies. However, in the global health perspective, a third development seems most significant for mental illness and mental health care in Africa. Among the world's poor, treatable psychiatric conditions are, unfortunately, not commonly diagnosed and do not receive the professional biomedical treatments that have been found to be useful in more affluent societies. There is evidence that this treatment gap contributes to disability and stigma. Hence, the use of the DSM in Africa and African studies needs to be viewed in this broad context.

Practices initiated by Collomb and his colleagues at Fann have continued to shape health care in Senegal in positive ways. For example, relatives still accompany patients on admission, a local practice that predated the innovations of Collomb and his group. This has assumed a practical value in the era of structural adjustment and the removal of hospital subsidies, and relatives have become essential in the delivery of health care in understaffed hospitals all across Africa. But also significant are recent advances in psychiatric practice in Francophone West Africa, spawned by the legacy of Collomb and his circle. A notable example is the growth in child psychiatry since the 1980s in Benin and Burkina Faso. René Gualbert Ahyi and Thérèse Agossou in Benin are among the psychiatrists who trained at Fann, and they have set up a center in Cotonou to train other personnel from Francophone countries in psychiatry. Arouna Ouedraogo in Burkina Faso is another leading figure who was trained at Fann. Since the 1980s psychiatrists in Mali have pursued major collaborations with healers, reflected on the place of culture in psychiatry, and entered into partnerships with international psychiatry research groups (Collignon, this volume).

Psychiatric services in most African countries today cannot be described as satisfactory. Nigeria has fewer than a hundred psychiatrists for its present population of close to 140 million. Zambia has the Chainama Hill Psychiatric Hospital with over four hundred beds, but only a few psychiatrists. In addition to its sole psychiatric hospital, two psychiatric units have been attached to general hospitals and mental health units have been attached to the remaining six provincial hospitals in Zambia (Rwegellera 1980). Ghana has three main psychiatric hospitals—in Accra, Pantang (just outside Accra), and Ankaful, in Cape Coast—with psychiatric units attached to main hospitals. The number of trained psychiatrists in Ghana remains insignificant compared to the demand for psychiatric care. Except for Senegal, Francophone African countries in the last two to three decades have had a paucity of facilities and trained psychiatrists (Bell 1991, 19). In 2001 Kenya's 30 million people had thirty psychiatrists. Tanzania had ten psychiatrists serving a population of 35 million. Rwanda, Burundi, Chad, Mozambique, and Sierra Leone—all countries that have undergone serious civil strife in recent decades—have one psychiatrist each. In contrast, South Africa has witnessed rapid growth in its infrastructure for mental health care since World War I (Bell 1991; Parle, 2007; Swartz 1998). Funds and trained personnel were available in South Africa to put its mental health institutions on a different level from the rest of Africa. By 2001 it had the largest number of trained psychiatrists in Africa, 474 serving a population of 43 million. It must be mentioned, moreover, that medical missionary work continues in Africa, a phenomenon that dates back to the early colonial years. An article in the *Lancet* on March 7, 2009, commented on the upsurge of medical missionaries from the United States to Africa Loewenberg 2009). Medical missionaries augment the capacity of health professionals in African countries in significant ways. Partnerships between European and North American medical schools and African ones also have the potential to expand training opportunities in psychiatry (Quigley 2009).

Economic crises have reinforced the continuing relevance of indigenous healers where mental illness is concerned, even in contemporary urban Africa (Okello and Musisi, this volume). The retrenchment in civil services that accompanied structural adjustment and the removal of subsidies for the provision of health care has led to a recent popularity of herbal medicines in urban Africa (Osseo-Asare 2005). In the mid-1970s a group of Nigerian psychiatrists studied the practice of fifty-three traditional healers in Ibadan who regularly treated patients with mental illness (Odejide et al. 1977). This collaborative research had been motivated by the psychiatrists' awareness of the heavy patronage of the treatment centers of these traditional healers. Bell studied the practice of an "herbalist magician" in Freetown in the 1980s, who claimed to have practiced his art of healing in over forty-two countries (1991, 168). This healer recognized four categories of mental disorder: epileptic fits, hypomania, depression, and mental illness brought on by accident or brain injury. He emphasized his ability to assist victims of sorcery and witchcraft. And a short distance from Kissy Mental Hospital, a Muslim herbalist who comes from a family of herbalists also operates a healing compound. This healer also recognized four types of mental disorder: "Each is identified with a color, a model styled from concepts of the ancient world. Black signifies depression; yellow represents a laughing disorder, or schizophrenia; red is mania, and is best typified by a violent person who wants to attack someone; and pink denotes a phobia, an irrational fear, or perhaps a borderline psychosis" (Bell 1991, 170).

The Muslim healer places great importance on the healing power of rest and sleep, administering herbal prescriptions that induce drowsiness and reduce anxiety. This healer also utilizes "Koranic medicine," writing appropriate verses from the Qur'an on a slate and washing the slate with water that he pours into a receptacle and gives to the patient to drink (Bell 1991, 173). Amulets are also made that contain appropriate Qur'anic verses and that the patient wears on his or her body. For many Sierra Leoneans, the social etiology of mental disorders makes treatment by healers rather than Western-trained psychiatrists more appropriate.

This conviction, perhaps, also explains the attractiveness of prayer camps, run by charismatic and Pentecostal Christian churches that specialize in spiritual healing. Alexander Boroffka has commented on the role of Christian healing sects in Nigeria: "Of greater importance for our subject was the establishment of Christian sects, like Cherubim and Seraphim, some concentrating on the treatment of [the] mentally disturbed by providing blessed oil to drink or to pour on the head, accompanied by communal praying, singing, and hand clapping, sometimes to possession states mainly of the participants and less often of the patient, to drive away bad spirits or counteract curses or other influences of black magic" (1995–96, 30).

With the growth of Islamism and Pentecostalism (Larkin and Meyer 2006) and the little-noted resurgence in African indigenous religions (Akyeampong and Owusu-Ansah 2009), traditional and faith healing will remain integral parts of the landscape of healing in Africa. Clarifying the relation between them and Western psychiatry remains one of the ongoing challenges in mental health care in Africa.

CANNABIS AND MADNESS IN INDEPENDENT GHANA AND NIGERIA

This chapter began with a discussion of colonial psychiatry and its preoccupation with social and moral order, noting the interaction of culture and the psychiatric profession in the diagnosis of mental illness. It ends with a short case study of cannabis and madness in postcolonial Ghana and Nigeria, highlighting the persistence of social and moral concerns in psychiatric practice. In both countries, psychiatric opinion is firm about the connection between cannabis use and madness. The common belief is that West African soldiers who fought in Asia in World War II introduced cannabis smoking to Ghana and Nigeria on their return. The common name for cannabis in the two countries, Indian hemp, suggests this Asian provenance. Cannabis was illegal from the time it was introduced into Nigeria and Ghana, and its introduction by colonial soldiers (the West African Frontier Force was not exactly an icon of respectability) and the association of the military with a life of violence—all of which gave cannabis a reputation that connected it immediately with social and moral disorder (Lambo 1965). It is striking how quickly cannabis joined ranks with illicitly distilled gin (*akpeteshie* in Ghana) in the colonial period: both were illegal, had the same patrons, and were supported by the same popular culture. Initially used by servicemen and certain occupational groups associated with arduous or dangerous work—stevedores, night-soil collectors, fishermen, farmers, prostitutes, and criminals—cannabis had much in common with *akpeteshie,* and both fed into a counterculture that rationalized what were criminal activities (Akyeampong 1996).

There is another account of the spread of cannabis in West Africa that is less well known and that refers to a tradition of its nonviolent use, connected to arduous labor such as farming and fishing. Sierra Leone apparently cultivated cannabis (locally called *diamba*) long before other West African countries, and at least as early as the colonial period, indigenous midwives were using cannabis as anesthesia during difficult childbirth.[3] Fishermen used it to help them do their hard work; by the 1920s, when statistics for arrests for cannabis possession become available for Sierra Leone, most of the arrested were fishermen.[4] In 1920 cannabis was added to the list of narcotic drugs prohibited under Sierra Leone's 1913 Opium Ordinance, making the production, possession, and consumption of cannabis all punishable offenses. Beginning in the 1930s, Sierra Leoneans began to explore the market for cannabis in other British West African colonies. Capitalizing on Freetown's importance as a major port, the presence of Sierra Leoneans as sailors on many ships and as stevedores in other West African ports, and a larger Krio diaspora[5] in the service of British colonialism in West Africa, Sierra Leoneans began to sell cannabis in other West African colonies. The colonial governments in the Gambia and the Gold Coast insisted that the government in Sierra Leone help them curtail this trade.[6]

What popularized the use of cannabis in West Africa among young people was the global spread of reggae music and the Rastafarian movement in the 1970s. In Senegal the Baye Faal branch of the Mouride Islamic brotherhood is characterized by dreadlocks, colorful patchwork clothes, the sacred and secular use of cannabis, and the perception of the lion as a sacred symbol. Neil Savishinsky, who has worked on the Baye Faal movement and the global spread of Jamaican popular culture, notes that the smoking of cannabis among the Baye Faal is a recent practice, strongly related to the increasing popularity of reggae and Rastafarianism in Senegal (Savishinsky 1994a, 1994b). The complex, layered social context of the drug in Nigeria and Ghana included the phenomenon of students in secondary schools and universities using cannabis.

Both lay people and medical professionals in West Africa readily associated cannabis and madness. In his mid-1980s study of 226 patients at the Lantoro Annex of the Aro Neuropsychiatric Hospital in Abeokuta, Olabisi Odejide (1985) found that in 21 of the 37 patients clinically diagnosed with organic psychoses, their condition was attributed to gross abuse of cannabis. Indeed, a diagnosis of cannabis psychosis emerged in the United Kingdom in the 1980s, as psychiatrists without much medical proof assumed that cases of psychoses among the African Caribbean population in the United Kingdom had to be connected to the group's chronic use of cannabis. A detailed review of the literature on psychosis among that population concluded that the evidence connecting psychosis to cannabis use was confusing at best (Sharpley et al. 2001). One of the few psychiatric studies in West Africa that compared psychosis in an experimental group of chronic cannabis users in a Nigerian psychiatric hospital against a control group that did not use cannabis also concluded that the findings did not support the category of cannabis psychosis, since "the symptoms of psychopathology that they [the experimental group] experienced were similar in terms and outcome, to the control group that had not used cannabis" (Nnaji et al. 1998–99, 212).

West African youth were attracted to cannabis use not just because of their participation in Rastafarian culture. Many seemed to believe, erroneously, that drugs such as cannabis enhanced their learning capacity. This belief draws on the tradition that associated cannabis use with hard work. Many students at secondary schools and universities in the region in the 1960s and 1970s were first-generation urbanites and often the first in their families to enter secondary and tertiary institutions of education. As a result, they may not have been unfamiliar with the association of cannabis and hard work, and the pressure to do well in school might have turned them to the use of cannabis. Student users seemed not to have distinguished physical from intellectual work. An editorial in the

Table 1.1. Cannabis-Related Admissions at the Accra Psychiatric Hospital, 1983–93

		CANNABIS ABUSER ADMISSIONS							
	ALL		% OF ALL						
YEAR	ADMISSIONS	NUMBER	ADMISSIONS	AGE 16–29		AGE 30–39		AGE 40+	
				M	F	M	F	M	F
1983	614	72	11.7	64	0	8	0	0	0
1985	1,156	258	22.3	207	0	41	2	7	1
1987	2,494	392	15.7	306	6	72	1	7	1
1989	3,121	463	14.8	450	0	13	0	0	0
1991	3,048	266	8.2	187	18	40	5	13	3
1993	2,810	190	6.8	148	8	30	1	3	3

Ghanaian *Daily Graphic* in April 1994 reported that a survey had been conducted among girls and boys in secondary school, which sought to understand the significant differences in academic performance between boys and girls. It notes that: "A survey, reportedly undertaken by the Ghana Education Service recently, has established that [pupils in] girls' schools are performing academically better than [those in] the boys' schools, and the phenomena might not be unrelated to drug abuse" ("Checking Drug Abuse," 1994).

The evidence was not just anecdotal, as statistics on age, gender, and cannabis use by patients admitted to the Accra Psychiatric Hospital from 1983 became available. Though the statistics do not indicate the occupations of the patients, the predominance of young people in school is clear. Table 1.1 provides figures for admissions of cannabis-related cases at the Accra Psychiatric Hospital between 1983 and 1993.

It is clear from the table that the number of cannabis-related cases were quite high in the 1980s, on average accounting for about 16 per cent of all psychiatric cases admitted to the hospital. Most of the cannabis users were male and between sixteen and twenty-nine. By 1999 the National Union of Ghana Students, the university students' association, had added its voice to the campaign against drug use among students at secondary schools and universities. The union noted that many students were enticed to drug use because they believed it would boost their academic performance. Instead, they ended up being "confused" or mentally unhinged ("Campuses Full of Student Junkies," 1999).

The social history of cannabis use is thus a story of the social image of the military; of intergenerational tensions between youth and elders about social identity and acceptable behavior; of how lay opinion can shape a medical diagnosis of addiction; and of the multiple sides to the social life of a substance simultaneously associated with quiet and hard physical labor on the one hand and cognitive disruption, violence, and madness on the other hand. In short, the link between cannabis use and madness is not direct, in spite of the belief that it is by lay and medical people alike in Ghana and Nigeria. Jerome Frank reminds us that "psychotherapy, like psychiatric diagnoses, cannot be divorced from cultural influences and moral judgments" (1974, 10). With the recent entry of cocaine and heroin into countries like Nigeria and Ghana, the social costs of addiction are becoming rapidly evident in West African psychiatric hospitals and communities. These new developments will probably reinforce the associations among cannabis, violence, and madness.

VIOLENCE AND MENTAL HEALTH

The discussion of cannabis and madness and the images of cannabis-smoking, gun-toting youth in Africa's recent civil wars necessitates some reflection—albeit brief—on violence and mental health in contemporary Africa, as I close this chapter (see the detailed studies by Murphy and Betancourt in this volume). As African economies declined, beginning in the 1970s, and unemployment escalated even among university graduates, frustrated urban and rural youth have expressed their disillusionment and anger in violence (Bay and Donham 2006). Youth have been fodder in violence and civil wars in Uganda, Rwanda, the Democratic Republic of the Congo, Liberia, Sierra Leone, and the Côte d'Ivoire, with drugs fueling the violence in disturbing ways. The use of drugs—cannabis, cocaine, and heroine—in the civil wars in Liberia and Sierra Leone has been documented in important studies (Abdullah 1998; Ellis 1999; Richards 1996). The depredation of child soldiers has been attributed to the drugs fed them by their military superiors and older adults, as illustrated in the memoirs of a boy soldier from Sierra Leone (Beah 2007). The Sierra Leonean civil war was notorious for the amputation of the limbs of civilians by the Revolutionary United Front (RUF). A disturbing component of these civil wars has been sexual violence, against both civilians and forcibly conscripted girl soldiers. In Sierra Leone girl soldiers were not just represented in the ranks of the RUF but were also found in the Armed Forces Revolutionary Council, the Sierra Leone Army, and the Civil Defense Forces, each reportedly having about two thousand girl soldiers. The RUF had about four times this number (Mazurana, McKay, and Carlson 2003, 13). During the Rwandan genocide of 1994, an estimated 250,000 to 500,000 women were raped, often in front of their family members (Baines 2003, 489; Twagiramariya and Trushen 1998, 102).

Civil war and state collapse have prompted the involvement in Africa of international bodies such as the United Nations and nongovernmental organizations in the sphere of mental health, which has been defined as an important component in humanitarian intervention and community reconstruction. The weak mental health infrastructure outlined above in this chapter has, in crisis situations, opened the door to hundreds of nongovernmental organizations that have sought "to heal individual and collective trauma by conducting psychosocial interventions, treating post-traumatic stress disorder (PTSD), anxiety and depression, as well as facilitating the social integration of displaced groups" (Abramowitz and Kleinman 2008, 220). Cultural and diagnostic fallacies have abounded in this environment, as foreign experts prescribed talk therapy among cultures with nondiscursive ways of dealing with trauma and misdiagnosed clinical PTSD among people for whom the concept lacked meaning or relevance (Abramowitz and Kleinman 2008; Englund 1998). This criticism of the approaches used does not undermine the reality of the huge mental illness burden and the need for meaningful, successful interventions.

In the wake of criticisms that followed internationally driven mental health and psychosocial support projects, the Inter-Agency Standing Committee published the IASC *Guidelines on Mental Health and Psychosocial Support in Emergency Settings* in 2007. Though this initiative has itself been criticized, its recognition of the need to foreground mental health humanitarian interventions in the cultural and local experiences of suffering represents an important advance. Thus we have moved from the earlier presumption of experts and donors that "everyone who had been exposed to war suffered debilitating trauma and required psychotherapeutic interventions, and gave little attention to individual and cultural resilience" (Abramowitz and Kleinman 2008, 220) to more-nuanced understandings of the social context of conflicts and culturally appropriate interventions, reflected in the contributions by William Murphy and Theresa Betancourt to this volume.

This chapter has provided a historical overview of the history of psychiatry and psychiatric practice in Africa. Though its focus has been on Western psychiatry in Africa, the chapter sought to include indigenous, Islamic, and Christian therapeutic alternatives as well. Studies across the continent have revealed the stigma attached to mental illness. A Yoruba saying is that "my child is dead is preferable to my child is mad."[7] Bell notes that across Sierra Leone great stigma is attached to mental illness, which is viewed as a curse or a "manifestation of evil" (1991, 159). In Ghana insanity in families is one of the key issues that people investigate before allowing their children to marry. This continuing stigma attached to mental illness in Africa must be put in the context of studies from the 1950s and 1960s that demonstrated there are no striking differences between the range and incidence of mental illness in Africans and nonAfricans, and between rural and urban Africans. Recent World Health Organization reports and other studies identify mental illness as one of the leading causes of morbidity globally, including in Africa (Desjarlais et al. 1995; World Health Organization 2005). We must also consider developments in Africa's political economy: the acute economic decline in the 1970s and 1980s and the resulting massive unemployment and underemployment, civil wars and the widespread phenomenon of refugees and displaced persons, casualties of war and a new generation of physically handicapped people (Betancourt, this volume; Bolton, Neugebauer, and Ndogoni 2002; Englund, 1998; Fox and Tang 2000; Murphy, this volume), the toll of HIV/AIDS on mental health (Antwine, Cantor-Graae, and Banjunirwe 2005; Collins, this volume; Raviola, this volume; Wilk and Bolton 2002), and the growing incidence of drug use and addiction (Affinih 1999; Bryceson 2002; Parry, Pluddermann, and Myers 2005).

Yet mental health is a low priority on national medical agendas and in ministries of health. Mental health care is underfunded and poorly staffed across Africa. Within the medical profession, psychiatry as a specialization continues to attract few health care providers in Africa. This presents us with desperate situations such as the one in Sierra Leone, a country undergoing postviolence reconstruction with large numbers of people physically handicapped by civil war and only one trained psychiatrist. There is an urgent need to move psychiatric care to the foreground of the delivery of health services in Africa. The World Health Organization's declaration at Alma-Ata in 1978, advocating for the integration of mental health care into primary health care centers and the training of community nurses in mental health, is one major response. Considering the importance of traditional healers to mental health care, and the social etiology of mental illness that privileges cultural and religious factors, the call of Olokayode Jegede (1981), a Nigerian psychiatrist, for a return to collaboration with traditional healers—a suggestion reminiscent of the Aro experiment in the 1950s and Collomb's psychiatric villages in the 1960s and 1970s—is worth considering. Moving mental health care up in the priorities of ministries of health would be a step in the right direction.

NOTES

1. Subsequent reviews of mental illness and psychiatric institutions would be conducted by Carothers in Nigeria in 1955 and Geoffrey Tooth in the Gold Coast in 1949. Tooth's was part of a larger study of mental illness, and his focus was on the links between trypanosomiasis (sleeping sickness) and mental abnormalities. McCulloch (1995, chap. 3) provides a useful review of their reports.

2. The Bodelschwinghian Bethel Institute was founded in 1867 in Bielefeld, Germany, as a Protestant institute of healing and care for epileptics. It expanded consider-

ably from the 1870s to care for the poor in general under the leadership of one of its early directors, Pastor Friedrich von Bodelschwingh Sr.

3. Emmanuel Akyeampong interview with E. A. Nahim, Freetown, Sierra Leone, July 18, 2002.

4. "Annual Report on Traffic in Opium and Dangerous Drugs, 1924–29, CSO 2/13/39, National Archives of Sierra Leone, Fourah Bay College, Freetown.

5. The Krio are a linguistic and cultural group that emerged from the mixing of returned Africans and liberated slaves in the nineteenth century.

6. Governor H. R. Palmer of Gambia, letter to Governor Arnold Hodson of Sierra Leone, February 13, 1933; and Colonial Secretary of the Gold Coast, letter to Colonial Secretary of Sierra Leone, May 3, 1937, CSO 1/25/13, National Archives of Sierra Leone.

7. Personal communication from Ronke Olawale, senior correspondent for the Nigerian *Guardian,* February 11, 2009.

REFERENCES

Abdullah, I. 1998. "Bush Path to Destruction: The Origin and Character of the Revolutionary United Front/Sierra Leone." *Journal of Modern African Studies* 36 (2): 203–35.

Abramowitz, S., and A. Kleinman. 2008. "Humanitarian Intervention and Cultural Translation: A Review of the *IASC Guidelines on Mental Health and Psychosocial Support in Emergency Settings*." *International Journal of Mental Health, Psychosocial Work and Counselling in Areas of Armed Conflict* 6 (3–4): 219–27.

Affinih, Y. F. 1999. "A Preliminary Study of Drug Abuse and Its Mental Health and Health Consequences among Addicts in Greater Accra, Ghana." *Journal of Psychoactive Drugs* 31 (4): 395–403.

Akyeampong, E. 1996. "What's in a Drink? Class Struggle, Popular Culture, and the Politics of Akpeteshie (Local Gin) in Ghana, 1940–1967." *Journal of African History* 37 (2): 215–36.

———. 2006. "Cannabis and Madness in Ghana." Paper presented at the Workshop on African Psychiatry, Harvard University, Cambridge, MA, December 2006.

Akyeampong, E., and D. Owusu-Ansah. 2009. "Religious Pluralism and Peaceful Co-existence: Cultivating Interfaith Tolerance in Ghana." Unpublished paper commissioned by Trust Africa, Dakar.

Antwine, B., E. Cantor-Graae, and F. Banjunirwe. 2005. "Psychological Distress among AIDS Orphans in Rural Uganda." *Social Science and Medicine* 61 (3): 555–64.

Asuni, T. 1967. "Aro Hospital in Perspective." *American Journal of Psychiatry* 124 (6): 763–77.

Baines, Erin K. 2003. "Body Politics and the Rwandan Crisis." *Third World Quarterly* 24 (3): 479–93.

Bay, E., and D. Donham, eds. 2006. *States of Violence: Politics, Youth and Memory in Contemporary Africa.* Charlottesville: University of Virginia Press.

Beah, I. 2007. *A Long Way Gone: Memoirs of a Boy Soldier.* New York: Farrar, Straus and Giroux.

Bell, L. V. 1991. *Mental and Social Disorder in Sub-Saharan Africa: The Case of Sierra Leone, 1787–1990.* New York: Greenwood.

Bolton, P., R. Neugebauer, and L. Ndogoni. 2002. "Prevalence of Depression in Rural Rwanda Based on Symptom and Functional Criteria." *Journal of Nervous and Mental Disease* 190 (9): 631–37.

Boroffka, A. 1995–96. "Psychiatric Care in Nigeria." *Psychopathologie africaine* 27 (1): 27–36.

Bryceson, D. H. 2002. "Pleasure and Pain: The Ambiguity of Alcohol in Africa." In *Alcohol in Africa: Mixing Business, Pleasure and Politics,* edited by D. F. Bryceson, 267–91. Portsmouth, NH: Heinemann.

"Campuses Full of Student Junkies. NUGS Moves to Check Menace." *Ghanaian Times,* January 16, 1999.

Canguilhem, G. 1991. *The Normal and the Pathological.* Translated by C. R. Fawcett and R. S. Cohen. New York: Zone.

Carothers, J. C. 1953. *The African Mind in Health and Disease.* Geneva: World Health Organization.

———. 1954. *The Psychology of Mau Mau.* Nairobi: Government Printer.

"Checking Drug Abuse." *Daily Graphic,* April 19, 1994.

Collignon, R. 1983. "A propos de psychiatrie communautaire en Afrique noire: les dispositifs villageois d'assistance: éléments pour un dossier." *Psychopathologie africaine* 19 (3): 287–328.

———. 1995–96. "Some Reflections on the History of Psychiatry in French Speaking West Africa: The Example of Senegal." *Psychopathologie africaine* 27 (1): 37–51.

Cooper, F. 2005. *Colonialism in Question: Theory, Knowledge, History.* Berkeley: University of California Press.

Desjarlais, R., L. Eisenberg, B. Good, and A. Kleinman. 1995. *World Mental Health: Problems and Priorities in Low-Income Countries.* Oxford: Oxford University Press.

Diefenbacher, A. 1995–96. "The Implementation of the Lunatic Asylum in Africa: The Example of the Colony of German East Africa," *Psychopathologie africaine* 27 (1): 53–65.

Diop, B., R. Collignon, M. Gueye, T. W. Harding. 1980. "Symptomatologie et diagnostic psychiatriques dans une region rurale du Senegal." *Psychopathologie africaine* 16 (1): 5–20.

Dumit, J. 2012. *Drugs for Life: How Pharmaceutical Companies Define our Health.* Durham, NC: Duke University Press.

Ellis, S. 1999. *Mask of Anarchy: The Destruction of Liberia and the Religious Dimension of an African Civil War.* New York: New York University Press.

Englund, H. 1998. "Death, Trauma and Ritual: Mozambican Refugees in Malawi." *Social Science and Medicine* 46 (9): 1165–74.

Fanon, F. 1963. *The Wretched of the Earth.* Translated by Constance Farrington. New York: Grove.

———. 1965. *A Dying Colonialism.* Translated by Haakan Chevalier. New York: Grove.

Field, M. J. 1955. "Witchcraft as a Primitive Interpretation of Mental Disorder." *Journal of Mental Science* 101 (425): 826–33.

Flint, K. E. 2008. *Healing Traditions: African Medicine, Cultural Exchange, and Competition in South Africa, 1820–1948.* Athens: Ohio University Press.

Foucault, M. 1988. *Madness and Civilization: A History of Insanity in the Age of Reason.* Translated by Richard Howard. New York: Vintage.

———. 2003. *Abnormal.*Translated by Graham Burchell. New York: Picador.

Fox, S. H., and S. S. Tang. 2000. "The Sierra Leonean Refugee Experience: Traumatic Events and Psychiatric Sequelae." *Journal of Nervous and Mental Disease* 188 (8): 490–95.

Frank, J. D. 1974. *Persuasion and Healing: A Comparative Study of Psychotherapy.* New York: Schocken.

Giel, R., M. V. de Arango, C. E. Climent, T. W. Harding, H. H. Ibrahim, L. Ladrido-Ignacio, R. S. Murthy, M. C. Salazar, N. N. Wig, and Y. O. Younis. 1981. "Childhood Mental Disorders in Primary Health Care: Results of Observations in Four Developing Countries," *Pediatrics,* 68 (5): 677–83.

Giel, R., and J. N. Van Luijk. 1969. "Psychiatric Morbidity in a Small Ethiopian Town." *British Journal of Psychiatry* 115: 149–62.

Horwitz, A. V., and J. C. Wakefield. 2007. *Loss of Sadness: How Psychiatry Transformed Normal Sorrow into Depressive Disorder.* Oxford: Oxford University Press.

Hunt, N. R. 1999. *A Colonial Lexicon of Birth Ritual, Medicalization, and Mobility in the Congo.* Durham, NC: Duke University Press.

Janzen, J. M. 1978. *The Quest for Therapy in Lower Zaire.* Berkeley: University of California Press.

Jegede, R. O. 1981. "Aro Village System of Community Psychiatry in Perspective." *Canadian Journal of Psychiatry* 26 (3): 173–77.

Keller, R. 2007. *Colonial Madness: Psychiatry in French North Africa.* Chicago: University of Chicago Press.

Kleinman, A. 1988. *Rethinking Psychiatry: From Cultural Category to Personal Experience.* New York: Free Press.

Lambo, T. A. 1965. "Medical and Social Problems of Drug Addiction in West Africa (with Special Emphasis on Psychiatric Aspects)." *West African Medical Journal* 14 (6): 236–54.

———. 1966. "The Village of Aro." In *Medical Care in Developing Countries,* edited by M. King, n.p. Nairobi: Oxford University Press.

Larkin, B., and B. Meyer. 2006. "Pentecostalism, Islam and Culture: New Religious Movements in West Africa." In *Themes in West Africa's History,* edited by E. Akyeampong, 286–312. Oxford: James Currey.

Leighton, A. H., T. A. Lambo, C. C. Hughes, D. C. Leighton, J. M. Murphy, and D. B. Macklin. 1963. "Psychiatric Disorder in West Africa." *American Journal of Psychiatry* 120 (6): 521–27.

Loewenberg, S. 2009. "Medical Missionaries Deliver Faith and Health Care in Africa." *Lancet* 373 (9666): 795–96.

Luedke, T. K., and H. G. West, eds. 2006. *Borders and Healers: Brokering Therapeutic Resources in Southeast Africa.* Bloomington: Indiana University Press.

Lyons, M. 1992. *The Colonial Disease: A Social History of Sleeping Sickness in Northern Zaire, 1800–1940.* Cambridge: Cambridge University Press.

Mazurana, D., S. McKay, and K. C. Carlson. 2003. *Girls in Fighting Forces in Northern Uganda, Sierra Leone and Mozambique: Policy and Program Recommendations.* Montreal: Child Protection Research Fund.

McCulloch, J. 1995. *Colonial Psychiatry and "The African Mind."* Cambridge: Cambridge University Press.

Nnaji, F. C., J. U. Ohaeri, R. O. Agidee, and R. O. Osahon. 1998–99. "A Follow-Up Study of Psychoses Associated with Cannabis Use at the Psychiatric Hospital of Uselu (Benin City, Nigeria)." *Psychopathologie africaine* 29 (2): 191–217.

Odejide, A. O. 1985. "Psycho-Social Features of In-Patients in Long Stay Psychiatric Hospitals: A Cross-Cultural Study." MD thesis, University of Ibadan.

Odejide, A. O., M. O. Olatawura, A. O. Sanda, and A. O. Oyeneye. 1977. "Traditional Healers and Mental Illness in the City of Ibadan." *African Journal of Psychiatry* 3 (4): 99–106.

Odejide, A. O., L. K. Oyewunmi, and J. U. Ohaeri. 1989."Psychiatry in Africa: An Overview," *American Journal of Psychiatry* 146 (6): 708–16.

Osseo-Asare, A. 2005. "Bitter Roots: African Science and the Search for Healing Plants in Ghana, 1885–2005." PhD diss., Harvard University.

Oyebode, F. 2006. "History of Psychiatry in West Africa." *International Review of Psychiatry* 18 (4): 319–25.

Parle, J. 2007. *States of Mind: Searching for Mental Health in Natal and Zululand, 1868–1918.* Scottsville, South Africa: University of KwaZulu-Natal Press.

Parry, C., A. Pluddermann, and B. J. Myers. 2005. "Heroin Treatment Demand in South Africa: Trends from Two Large Metropolitan Sites (1997–2003)." *Drug and Alcohol Review* 24 (5): 419–23.

Quigley, F. 2009.*Walking Together, Walking Far: How a U.S. and African Medical School Partnership Is Winning the Fight against HIV/AIDS.* Bloomington: Indiana University Press.

Richards, P. 1996. *Fighting for the Rainforest: War, Youth and Resources in Sierra Leone.* Oxford: James Currey.

Rodney, W. 1972. *How Europe Underdeveloped Africa.* London: Bogle-L'Ouverture.

Rwegellera, G. G.1980. "The Present State of Psychiatry in Zambia and Suggestions for Future Development." *Psychopathologie africaine* 16 (1): 21–38.

Sachs, Wulf. 1937. *Black Hamlet: The Mind of an African Negro Revealed by Psychoanalysis.* London: G. Bles.

Sadowsky, J. 1999. *Bedlam: Institutions of Colonial Madness in Southwest Nigeria.* Berkeley: University of California Press.

Savishinsky, N. J. 1994a. "The Baye Faal of Senegambia: Muslim Rastas in the Promised Land?" *Africa* 64 (2): 211–19.

———. 1994b. "Rastafari in the Promised Land: The Spread of a Jamaican Socioreligious Movement among the Youth of West Africa." *African Studies Review* 37 (3): 19–50.

Sharpley, M. S., G. Hutchinson, R. M. Murray, and K. McKenzie. 2001. "Understanding the Excess of Psychosis among the African-Caribbean Population in England." *British Journal of Psychiatry* 178 (40): s60–68.

Sow, I. 1980. *Anthropological Structures of Madness in Black Africa.* New York: International Universities Press.

Swartz, L. 1998. *Culture and Mental Health: A Southern African View.* Cape Town: Oxford University Press.

Twagiramayriya, C., and M. Turshen. 1998. "'Favours' to Give and 'Consenting' Victims: The Sexual Politics of Survival in Rwanda." In *What Women Do in Wartime: Gender and Conflict in Africa,* edited by M. Turshen and C. Twagiramariya, 101–17. London: Zed.

Vaughan, M. 1991. *Curing Their Ills: Colonial Power and African Illness.* Oxford: Polity.

Warren, D. M., G. S. Bora, M. A. Tregoning, and M. Kleiver. 1982. "Ghanaian National Policy towards Indigenous Healers." *Social Science and Medicine* 16 (21): 1873–81.

Wilk, C. M., and P. Bolton. 2002. "Local Perceptions of the Mental Health Effects of the Uganda Acquired Immunodeficiency Syndrome Epidemic." *Journal of Nervous and Mental Disease* 190 (6): 394–97.

World Health Organization. 2005. *Mental Health Atlas.* Geneva: World Health Organization.

Wylie, D. 2001. *Starving on a Full Stomach: Hunger and the Triumph of Cultural Racism in Modern South Africa.* Charlottesville: University Press of Virginia.

Yoder, P. S., ed. 1982. *African Health and Healing Systems.* Los Angeles: Crossroads.

Young, A. 1997. *The Harmony of Illusions: Inventing Post-Traumatic Stress Disorder.* Princeton, NJ: Princeton University Press.

2 COMMON MENTAL DISORDERS IN SUB-SAHARAN AFRICA

The Triad of Depression, Anxiety, and Somatization

VIKRAM PATEL AND DAN J. STEIN

ANY UNDERSTANDING OF depression and anxiety in sub-Saharan Africa—indeed, in all developing countries, and in all probability in developed countries too—must highlight the fact that depression and anxiety more commonly occur together than separately, at least in community and primary health care settings. For example, the World Health Organization's multinational study on general health care found that the comorbidity of depression and anxiety exceeded 50 percent (Goldberg and Lecrubier 1995), confirming previous observations made in primary care. Even if there are valid differences between depression and anxiety in terms of phenomenology, risk factors, and treatment, from a clinical and public health point of view there is significant utility in emphasizing the overlap between these two states of emotional distress. This overlap has prompted some psychiatrists to propose a return to the older concept of neuroses, albeit using new names such as "cothymia" (Tyrer 2001). In this chapter, we use the term "common mental disorders" (CMDs), first coined in 1992 (Goldberg and Huxley 1992). CMDs are a group of mental disorders that, according to the World Health Organization's classification of mental disorders (World Health Organization, 1992), include depressive disorders, anxiety disorders, and disorders characterized by the clinical presentation of physical complaints where no obvious physical cause can be determined (labeled as "somatoform" or "somatic symptom" disorders). Evidently, this rubric is similar to the old category of neuroses. Although we do not discuss substance use disorders in this chapter, that omission is not intended to underplay the high prevalence and morbidity of these disorders, as well as that of a number of other psychiatric disorders.

The recent World Mental Health Surveys that have been conducted in many countries (Demyttenaere et al. 2004) around the world have shown that although the prevalence of these disorders varies widely across study populations, they are relatively common in all populations. A range of twelve-month prevalence of 5–20 percent may be considered to be a reasonable estimate in most populations. In Nigeria, the estimated prevalence of CMDs (including substance use disorders) was around 5 percent, while in South Africa it was approximately 16 percent. These disorders are of great global health significance, not only because they are extremely common but also because of their impact on the health of populations. CMDs are a leading cause of disease burden in the world. For example, depressive disorder is one of the top five causes of disease burden (estimated using the disability-adjusted life-year indicator) today (Lopez et al. 2006), and is projected to become the second leading cause of disability (after HIV/AIDS) by 2030 (Mathers and Loncar 2006). Apart from their impact on disability, CMDs are also associated with mortality. For example, they are known to increase the risk of mortality due to other health problems such as heart disease (Penninx et al. 2001), and they are a major risk factor for suicide. Suicide, in turn, is now the leading cause of death in young people in many developing countries (Aaron et al. 2004; Phillips et al. 2002). CMDs are strongly associated with the targets of the Millennium Development Goals (Miranda and Patel 2005), in particular poverty, gender equity, maternal and child health, and HIV/AIDS. Some of these linkages are discussed in more detail below. Evidence from developing countries shows that CMDs are among the commonest health problems in people who consult their family doctors or primary health care providers. On average, between a quarter and a third of all adults receiving primary care suffer from a CMD (Goldberg and Lecrubier 1995). Although these disorders are associated with the seeking of health care, the vast majority of patients receive inappropriate or inadequate treatments for their mental disorder (Wang, Aguilar-Gaxiola et al. 2007).

THE EVIDENCE BASE FOR CMDS IN SUB-SAHARAN AFRICA

This chapter is based in good part on work carried out in Harare, the capital of Zimbabwe, by researchers affiliated with the University of Zimbabwe Medical School. A major component of the evidence presented here comes from the Primary Mental Health Care Project (see the textbox "The Primary Mental Health Care Project") (Patel 1998). Some of the data came from studies sponsored by the Medical Research Council Unit on Anxiety Disorders in Cape Town. Other material came from a systematic review of the explanatory models of mental illness in sub-Saharan Africa (Patel 1995a). Recent reviews of the epidemiological literature and evidence base for treatments for CMDs in developing countries (Patel et al. 2007; Prince et al. 2007) was also considered. This chapter, however, is not based on a systematic review of the literature, and potentially relevant research

TEXTBOX 2.1. THE PRIMARY MENTAL HEALTH CARE PROJECT

This was a three-year project in primary care in Harare, Zimbabwe, aimed at describing the epidemiology of common mental disorders (CMDs), in primary health care centers and among the patients of traditional medical practitioners in the city of Harare. Before embarking on the study, the researchers conducted extensive networking and held consultations with key health providers, policy makers, academics, and representatives of nongovernmental organizations to explore local concepts of CMDs. The most common condition was *kufungisisa* (which literally means thinking too much or worrying excessively), and most subjects with this complaint appeared to suffer from anxiety or depression. The next step in the research was to elicit the common symptoms, explanatory models, and disease idioms of primary care patients with conspicuous CMDs (Patel, Gwanzura, et al. 1995; Patel, Musara, et al. 1995; Patel, Simunyu, and Gwanzura 1995).

These idioms were incorporated into a preliminary fourteen-item questionnaire, the Shona Symptom Questionnaire, which was evaluated and found to be a locally valid measure of CMD (Patel, Simunyu, et al. 1997). For example, the first question uses the notion of kufungisisa with the question "Did you have times (in the last week) in which you were thinking deep or thinking too much?" This questionnaire was then used in a case-control investigation of the risk factors for CMD among people who were consulting primary care doctors and among another group of people who were consulting traditional medical practitioners (a mixed group of spirit mediums, diviners, herbalists, and apostolic Christian leaders) (Patel, Todd, et al. 1997). The cohorts of cases and controls were reviewed after a twelve-month period to provide information on the outcome and incidence of CMDs (Patel, Todd, et al. 1998; Todd et al. 1999).

that may have been published in journals that are not indexed, particularly those from Africa, was not reviewed. This is an important omission that must be acknowledged at the outset.

Colleagues in the Department of Psychiatry of the University of Zimbabwe have also carried out a series of research studies since the 1980s that described various aspects of CMDs in Zimbabwe. A summary of the major findings were published some years ago (Patel et al. 2001). Notable investigations included a series of studies on depression in women and its association with life events (Abas

and Broadhead 1997; Broadhead and Abas 1998; Broadhead et al. 2001), studies of depression in mothers (Nhiwatiwa, Patel, and Acuda 1998), and CMDs in
refugees from and survivors of conflict in the region (Reeler 1994). In summary,
three major lessons were learned, around which this chapter is structured. First,
although the symptoms characteristically associated with the psychiatric condition of CMD are largely universal, they are expressed and experienced in unique
ways in different settings. Second, depression is more common among marginalized populations than in other groups, and a knowledge of both the miseries
of everyday life and of the nature of psychiatric diagnoses is needed to fully understand these health conditions. Third, irrespective of how one may explain or
conceptualize the human experience of CMDs, they have a profound impact on
the life of the patient.

SYMPTOMS AND CATEGORIES

The prominent finding of studies in Africa, as in almost all developing countries,
is that the core symptoms of CMD can be detected in a similar presentation in most
cultures. Although this conclusion may change as globalization continues, the
commonest presenting complaints associated with CMD have been somatic—in
particular, tiredness, weakness, multiple aches and pains, dizziness, palpitations,
and sleep disturbances. However, this does not mean that emotional and cognitive symptoms are not experienced also—they are simply not volunteered as readily to the treating health care providers. But when asked, most patients will report
psychological symptoms that are considered the hallmark of these disorders in
biomedical classifications, such as loss of interest in daily or social activities, suicidal thoughts, poor concentration, and anxiety or worry. Indeed, these psychological symptoms may have greater validity than the somatic complaints in distinguishing mental disorders from physical ones (Okulate, Olayinka, and Jones
2004), because many of the somatic complaints can occur in both types of disorders. Furthermore, when multiple somatic complaints affecting several organ
systems occur together, then there is a strong likelihood they are associated with a
CMD. For example, an analysis of the World Mental Health Surveys on the association between pain and CMDs showed that in all cultures the prevalence of specific
mood and anxiety disorders followed a linear pattern, with the lowest rates found
among people reporting no pain, intermediate rates among those with one pain,
and the highest rates among those with multisite pain. The authors concluded that
the "consistent pattern of associations suggests that diffuse pain and psychiatric
disorders are generally associated, rather than diffuse pain representing an idiom
for expressing distress that is specific to particular cultural settings or diffuse pain
solely representing a form of masked depression" (Gureje et al. 2008, 84).

Earlier theories had suggested that, in developing countries, somatic symptoms were the cultural equivalent of depression and that somatization—the process by which psychological distress was converted to somatic symptoms—was typical. This hypothesis has now been shown to be wrong in two respects. First, somatic symptoms are also the commonest presenting features of depression in developed societies (Bhatt, Tomenson, and Benjamin 1989; Gureje et al. 2008; Katon and Walker 1998). And second, the classic psychological symptoms of CMD can also usually be elicited in developing countries (Araya et al. 1994; Patel, Gwanzura, et al. 1995). Acute cases of CMDs are more likely to be somatic, consistent with an emphasis on such symptoms in concepts of illness; when the condition becomes chronic, the patient reevaluates the illness experience and is more likely to become aware of psychological symptoms (Weich et al. 1995). Although many psychiatric patients in the developed world may have somatic symptoms, may employ religious constructs to explain their life course, and may use herbs and complementary treatments, there seem to be some differences between them and patients in Africa: many people in the former group prefer psychological explanations, while many people in the latter group prefer supernatural explanations. Still, patients throughout the world use multiple explanatory models, and people with chronic diseases may be particularly likely to employ a range of—often contradictory—constructs. On balance, then, the key message is that somatic symptoms are classic presenting symptoms of CMDs in Africa, but psychological symptoms are often elicited on inquiry.

Why do CMD patients present with somatic complaints? There is a growing appreciation that the language we use to describe mental states is metaphorical, stemming from more concrete bodily experiences. Throughout the world, for example, psychological anger is described in terms of bodily or internal heat (Lakoff 1987). Recent work has emphasized the connection between psychological loss and body pain (Panksepp 2003). Ultimately such concrete bodily experiences may depend on physiological facts, such as sympathetic arousal during anger and various alterations during separation. Still, there is great variation in the nature of metaphors used by patients. P. O. Ebigbo, N. Janakiramaiah, and N. Kumaraswamy (1989) report on the phenomenology of patients treated in a Nigerian psychiatric hospital and given biomedical diagnoses. Sixty-five somatic and other symptoms relating to the head and body were included in a rating scale that effectively distinguished psychiatric patients from people without mental disorders. Although many of the symptoms bear close similarity to phenomena described in biomedical classifications—such as insomnia, loss of appetite, headache, fearful thoughts, palpitations, dizziness, suicidal wishes, aggressiveness, excessive talkativeness, hypersomnia, restlessness, and bodily pains—there were several symptoms that appear to be unique, including heat and a crawling sensation in the head, feeling as if the tongue was trembling, a turning sensation in the head, and a feeling that the heart wanted to fly out of the body (Ebigbo 1982). Feelings such as guilt were much less emphasized in Ebigbo's patients, giving credence to the traditional belief that depression represents an attack from the outside, such as through witchcraft or aggression by a spirit. In studies in Zimbabwe, phenomena such as thinking too much, feelings of pressure or heat in the head, the sensation of something moving under the skin, dizziness, body aches, and palpitations have been reported by people with CMDs. L. J. Kirmayer, T. H. T. Dao, and A. Smith (1998) suggest that many patients in developing countries present with a confluence of somatic, affective, and anxiety disorders, which are then experienced and expressed in terms of culture-specific idioms of distress.

Although somatic presentations and the occurrence of cognitive and emotional phenomena appear to be universal, the content of these phenomena may vary across cultures. *Kufungisisa* is one such example of a cognitive experience that has been widely described in both African and other developing countries. It bears some phenomenological similarity to worrying but also shares some features of obsessional thinking. It is clear that one cannot accurately translate *kufungisisa* simply as worry or some other biomedically defined experience—it is a unique term that captures a particular important cognitive experience with cultural validity. At the same time, it may be clinically useful to determine whether or not a specific psychiatric diagnosis has explanatory power in a particular individual. For example, although the term *amafufunyane* is commonly used in the South African context, some patients with this condition may be diagnosed with depression, while others are diagnosed with schizophrenia.

Another example is the feeling that ants or other insects are crawling under one's skin. From one perspective, this might appear to be a tactile hallucination, analogous to formication. However, if one were to explore the actual meaning and experience of this complaint, one would discover a close relationship with the tingling numbness characteristically associated with hyperventilation in people who are very anxious. Again, a simple translation of the phenomena of tingling numbness is unlikely to lead one to the idiom of ants or insects crawling under the skin. Conversely, perceptual disturbances are not restricted to psychoses; the literature in both the West and Africa emphasizes the high prevalence of hallucinations in people without a psychiatric diagnosis (Johns et al. 2002) and of phenomena such as flashbacks in patients with anxiety and related disorders such as post-traumatic stress disorder. In sub-Saharan Africa, it is important to be aware that hallucinations may occur in the context of CMD; for example, a person who wakes in the middle of the night (due to anxiety or depression) and who is in a state of heightened worry about some problem may think she sees an owl or some other medium associated with witchcraft by her window. This conforms, as Ebgibo pointed out, to a view of the emotional condition as possibly associated with an external agency, typically an evil one related to supernatural forces (Patel 1995b). More neurobiological explanations of symptom variations across groups may also be relevant. For example, it has been suggested that sleep paralysis is particularly common in African-Americans (Friedman 1997).

So we can infer that symptoms are mostly universal, though their content does vary, and a bottom-up approach to eliciting phenomena is more likely to achieve a culturally appropriate illness description for a CMD. The development of the Shona Symptom Questionnaire provides one example of such an approach that led to a screening tool for the detection of CMDs in primary care settings in Zimbabwe (Patel, Simunyu, et al. 1997). A relatively more complex issue, however, is whether the diagnostic labels employed in biomedical psychiatry—notably, depression and anxiety disorders—are valid in African cultures. This is not simply a semantic issue: if labels that organize symptoms into diagnostic categories are not valid, then the latter will not be acknowledged and appropriately addressed in health care—an all-too-common observation in primary care (Abas et al. 2003).

The first problem is where CMDs should be classified, particularly whether they should be considered a mental disorder. Although CMDs clearly have social origins, overemphasizing this point may contribute to most patients and primary health care providers understanding CMD entirely from a social context, often attributing causation to external agencies. Thus, the experiences of feeling sad, not sleeping well, suffering from headaches, and so on can be attributed to social difficulties or supernatural forces, not to a disorder—let alone a mental one (Patel 1995a; Patel, Gwanzura, et al. 1995). Two major implications of this understanding of the experience of CMDs—the stigma associated with mental disorders (Gureje et al. 2005; Stein and Gureje 2004) and the commonly held view that mental disorders are equivalent to the biomedical category of psychoses—mean that CMDs may not be considered as mental disorder. This is a crucial consideration when designing programs intended to integrate the detection and management of CMDs in community and primary heath care settings.

Second is the concern about how CMDs should be labeled. Arguments against the validity of labels often cite the fact that labels such as depression and phobias have no conceptually equivalent term in many non-European languages (Patel 1996). These terms, derived from European cultures, have made the leap from the everyday language of emotional experience to medical disorders and, in the process, acquired biomedical significance. The use of the feeling of sadness as the label by which the condition of depression is identified may in fact lead to a significant degree of underreporting, because sadness does not feature prominently in the clinical presentation of the mood disorder (Bebbington 1993). Terms such as CMDs, though offering some advantages over depression because they do not imply a specific mood state, can be criticized because of their vagueness. Furthermore, the notion of mental disorders rarely extends beyond the severe psychoses to encompass what many might wrongly perceive as the natural consequence of the difficulties of daily life (Patel 1995a, 1996). Clearly, educating the public about the nature of these conditions and their available treatments is a public health challenge. We often use terms that are culturally appropriate (such as "nerves" or "chemical imbalance" in the West) but that bear little relationship to core psychosocial and neurobiological mechanisms. In addition, the use of a language of illness rather than a language of resilience may inappropriately encourage patients to seek health services (Stein et al. 2007). Nevertheless, in view of advances in the efficacy and cost-efficiency in the treatment of CMDs, culturally appropriate education is critical for the successful integration of CMD care in routine health care settings in Africa.

KEY MESSAGES: SYMPTOMS AND CATEGORIES

- Many symptoms of CMDs are universal. For example, the somatic presentations of tiredness, aches, pains, and sleep problems are common in developed and developing countries.
- With sympathetic inquiry, emotional and cognitive symptoms are commonly elicited from patients.
- Perceptual abnormalities may be seen in patients with depression and anxiety disorders.
- Local idioms—for example, *kufungisisa* ("thinking too much," in Shona)— are commonly used to express complex conditions.
- Some typical symptoms, such as loss of appetite, are not specific to particular conditions due to the high prevalence of somatic disorders.
- Multiple explanatory models (both natural and supernatural) are used in both the developed world and in Africa. In less modernized groups, a prominent explanatory model is that of the supernatural.

MARGINALIZATION AND MISERY

Two major multinational studies have described the prevalence of CMDs: the World Health Organization's study of mental illness in primary care (World Health Organization 1995) and the World Mental Health Surveys in community settings (Demyttenaere et al. 2004). Both these impressive exercises in descriptive epidemiology have included centers in sub-Saharan Africa. Below we will consider some of the major findings on the burden of CMDs, but here it is pertinent to note a remarkable result of both studies: the enormous variation—up to eightfold—in the prevalence of CMDs across sites. Because of their design, cross-sectional studies can shed only some light on the reasons for such variations (other than those due to the unpredictable influence of methodological variations—such as the varying content and significance of symptoms used to diagnose CMDs, as discussed above; selection bias; and response bias). Indeed, much more work is needed to further our understanding of variations in risk and protective factors across cultures. Importantly, there is discordance between individual-level and ecological-level rates of CMDs. For example, individual-level data often show that marginalization and disadvantage are risk factors for CMDs, while ecological comparisons often show lower overall rates in countries with higher levels of such disadvantage. Ecological comparisons, of course, are likely to be heavily confounded, but they remain important alternative data for the confirmation of etiological hypotheses. One example of how ecological data may be used to investigate the determinants of CMDs is the work of Kate Pickett, Oliver James, and Richard Wilkinson (2006). Using the World Mental Health Survey data, they concluded that higher national levels of income inequality are linked to a higher prevalence of mental illness.

There are four major sources of marginalization that increase the risk for CMDs: poverty; female gender; trauma and displacement; and suffering from a physical disease, including stigmatized disorders such as HIV/AIDS. In an international meta-analysis of data from twenty-five countries, Vincent Lorant and coauthors (2003) found compelling evidence for an association between socioeconomic inequality and depression. People of low socioeconomic status (SES) had higher odds of being depressed than other people (odds ratio: 1.81), but their odds of a new episode (1.24) were lower than their odds of persisting depression (2.06). Furthermore, greater levels of inequality in a country may play a role in explaining the higher risk for people of lower SES. The evidence base from Africa is generally—but not always (Gureje et al. 2006; Stein et al. 2008)—consistent with this finding. Five recent cross-sectional surveys of people seeking treatment and community samples from four developing countries—including Zimbabwe—were collated to examine the economic risk factors for depression. In all five studies, there was a consistent and significant relationship between low income and risk of CMDs (Patel et al. 1999). There was also a relationship between proxy indicators of impoverishment and CMDs. For example, people who had experienced food insecurity recently and those who were in debt were more likely to suffer from CMDs. C. Todd and coauthors (1999) found that subjects in Zimbabwe who reported difficulty getting enough money to buy food were four times more likely to suffer from a CMD in the following twelve months. In the same study, economic difficulties at baseline predicted the persistence of CMDs twelve months later (Patel, Todd, et al. 1998). Thus, although 31 percent of those with a CMD at baseline but whose economic problems had been solved during the year showed a persistence of their mental health problem, more than half of those who experienced new problems showed persistent symptoms. The causal pathways between poverty and CMDs have been described elsewhere (Patel and Kleinman 2003).

Both community-based studies and studies of treatment seekers indicate that women are disproportionately affected by CMDs (World Health Organization 2000). The World Health Organization's study of mental illness in primary care found an overall sex ratio of 1.89 (based on the 25,000 subjects who were screened), indicating that female rates of CMDs are almost double the male rates. However, there was considerable variation across centers where the study was conducted, suggesting a cultural basis for some of this variation. In Ibadan, Nigeria, an *International Statistical Classification of Diseases and Related Health Problems,* tenth edition, diagnosis of current CMD was more common among men (5.3 percent) than among women (3.8 percent) with a sex ratio of 0.70. Although the reversed sex ratio found in this center—with men being more likely than women to be suffering from a CMD—may be a chance finding or the result of differential access to primary care for men and women with CMDs, the huge cross-cultural variability in the sex ratio for CMD does call into question any simplistic biological or hormonal explanations for the increased vulnerability experienced by women. Although some other studies have replicated the lack of sex difference for the risk of CMDs (Gureje et al. 2006), most other studies from Africa and developing countries elsewhere in the world report consistently elevated rates for women (for example, this was the case in the World Mental Health Surveys). Sociocultural explanations for women's increased vulnerability to CMDs in developing countries may include the pervasive influence of gender disadvantage, which is manifested at various levels of society—from women's lack of political participation to their reduced opportunities for education and health care, lack of access to the better occupations, and increased risk of violence at the hands of a spouse or other sexual partner. It may be more acceptable for males to express psychopathology primarily in terms of externalizing symptoms, such as substance abuse. The reproductive roles of women in developing countries—including the expected provision of sexual services and bearing children—and the severe adverse consequences of infertility have been linked to rape, partner violence, and CMDs. A study of life events and depression in women in Zimbabwe is illustrative of the impact of gendered life difficulties on the risk for CMDs in women (see the textbox "Life Difficulties and Depression in Women in Zimbabwe").

The third major factor associated with CMDs is the consequence of trauma and conflict, tragically a common occurrence in sub-Saharan Africa. It is not

TEXTBOX 2.2. LIFE DIFFICULTIES AND
DEPRESSION IN WOMEN IN ZIMBABWE

The research of Jeremy Broadhead and Melanie Abas (1998) on the social
origins of depression in women in townships of Harare, Zimbabwe, is an
important contribution to our understanding of the universal role of life
difficulties in the etiology of depression. The authors screened 172 women
with the Present State Examination and the Bedford Life Events and Difficulties Scale (LEDS) (Brown and Harris 1978) and found that nearly 31
percent were experiencing an episode of depression or anxiety. About 18
percent were suffering from a depression. This was in contrast, to 9 percent
of the women in Camberwell, a deprived inner district of London thought
to have a relatively high rate of depression. The researchers investigated
potential reasons for the high rates of depression found in Harare using the
LEDS. More women in Harare had suffered a severe life event (54 percent)
than those in Camberwell (31 percent) in the preceding twelve months.
Rates for both severe events and major difficulties, a combination known
to predispose to depression, were as high as 55 percent in Harare, compared with only 28 percent in Camberwell. It appeared that the doubling
of the rate of depression in Harare could be largely explained by the increased rates of severe life events and major difficulties experienced by the
women. Most of the events that were rated severe in Harare but nonsevere
in Camberwell were accounted for by widespread beliefs in witchcraft and
the power of the spirit world among the women in Harare. For example,
certain events such as lightning striking one's house would be rated as
severe, with high levels of danger. A notable finding in Harare was the
high proportion of events involving humiliation and entrapment related to
marital crises, such as being deserted by one's husband and being left with
several children; premature death; illness in family members; and severe
financial difficulties occurring in the absence of an adequate welfare safety
net. The study confirmed that severe life events and long-term difficulties
were universally important as correlates of depression. The higher rates of
depression among the African women than among those in Camberwell
could largely be accounted for by the greater number of severe life experiences of the women in Harare.

difficult to understand why people exposed to conflict—with its attendant risks of displacement, bereavement, injury, and horrific abuses—may be associated with an increased risk of CMDs. During conflicts, women are particularly vulnerable to displacement, rape and other sexual violence, and witnessing atrocities committed against family members. A number of studies from war-affected countries in Africa bear testimony to the enormous mental health consequences, mostly CMDs, for survivors of conflict (Reeler 1994; de Jong, Komproe, and Ommeren 2003; Bolton, Neugebauer, and Ndogoni 2002). For example, a survey that sought to estimate the prevalence of major depressive disorder among Rwandans five years after the genocidal civil war in 1994, and that used a combination of symptoms and functional impairment criteria for the diagnosis of depression, reported a prevalence of 15.5 percent for current depression. Depressive symptoms were strongly associated with functional impairment in major roles for men and women (Bolton, Neugebauer, and Ndogoni 2002). Subjects exposed to trauma, including human rights violations in South Africa, have a high prevalence of CMDs (Kaminer et al. 2001).

In the African setting, the association of CMDs with HIV/AIDS has important public health implications (Freeman 2004; Stein et al. 2005). Some of this association may be explained on the basis of psychological factors: HIV and AIDS are stigmatizing conditions, with a poor prognosis in countries that do not provide antiretroviral treatment. At the same time, some of this association is certainly neurobiological: the HIV virus has quite specific detrimental effects on neuronal function. Irrespective of etiology, the HIV/AIDS epidemic in Africa has led to a significant strain on mental health services. Thus, a systematic review of the evidence base identified thirteen studies of mental disorder in HIV-positive people, with a considerable heterogeneity in reported prevalence (Collins et al. 2006). The largest and best-designed of these studies (which compared HIV-positive recipients of health care services and matched controls in Bangkok, Kinshasa, Nairobi, and Sao Paulo) reported a higher prevalence of depression and more symptoms of depression among symptomatic HIV-positive people than among people who were not symptomatic or who were HIV-negative (Maj et al. 1994). One study, from Uganda, used a diagnostic assessment for depression and found no association between depression and adherence to antiretroviral therapy (Byakika-Tusiime et al. 2005), but another study, from Ethiopia, reported that depression was associated with less than 95 percent self-reported adherence in the week prior to being interviewed by the researchers (Tadios and Davey 2006).

Here we are faced with an old conundrum. If CMDs are more common in people who face social disadvantages, as described above, how does one distinguish between an understandable misery and a disorder with epidemiological characteristics and public health implications? Part of the answer lies in the analysis of the impact of CMDs, as described in the next section—thus, irrespective of whether we call it misery or disorder, this human condition is associated with health outcomes that include increased disability, mortality, and health care–seeking behavior. But another critical observation is that only a minority of individuals faced with these social disadvantages actually develop the symptoms that, when clustered together in a diagnostic algorithm, signify CMDs. In our experience, it is truly remarkable how free of CMDs so many African people are, in spite of their harsh daily lives. Thus, CMDs are not the natural consequence of disadvantage, but a consequence that is seen in some individuals who experience disadvantage. Why they develop CMDs when others do not remains a mystery, but clearly gene-environment interactions and the role of protective factors must all be considered as potential influences (Yehuda and McFarlane 1995; Patel and Goodman 2007).

KEY MESSAGES: MARGINALIZATION AND MISERY

- Marginalization and disadvantage are risk factors for CMDs. In Africa, this particularly applies to women, the poor, and those exposed to trauma and conflict or to infectious diseases such as HIV/AIDS.
- CMDs are not the natural consequence of misery and marginalization— most people faced with such adversities remain in good mental health

THE IMPACT OF DEPRESSION

We can assess the burden of CMDs by examining the impact of the condition on functioning (indicated by levels of disability), mortality, and help-seeking behavior. A recent review of the impact of mental disorders has systematically documented the evidence on these indicators (Prince et al. 2007). Here, we focus on the evidence base from Africa.

The high prevalence of CMDs, the great burden posed by these disorders on daily functioning, the inadequate health care received by most people, and the often chronic nature of these conditions are the primary reasons why they are the leading mental health cause of disability around the world. Depression is now one of the five leading causes of the burden of disease in all regions of the world apart from sub-Saharan Africa, where the condition accounts for about 1 percent of the total burden of disease, estimated by disability-adjusted life-years (Lopez et al. 2006). It is probable that depression figures much lower in the list for that region largely as a result of HIV/AIDS—which, although not appearing in the leading ten causes of burden of disease for any other region in the world, is the leading cause in sub-Saharan Africa, accounting for an incredible 16 percent of the total burden of disease. Indeed, when neuropsychiatric disorders as a whole are analyzed, these account for the second largest proportion of disease burden in South Africa (Bradshaw 2003). The three leading causes of global burden of disease in 2030 are projected to include HIV/AIDS, unipolar depressive disorders, and ischemic heart disease (Mathers and Loncar 2006).

The disability associated with depression is greater than that experienced as a consequence of other chronic diseases such as diabetes and hypertension. The findings of the recent World Health Surveys of adults eighteen and older, which studied health outcomes related to chronic disease, are instructive (Moussavi et al. 2007). Observations were available for 245,404 participants from sixty countries, in all regions of the world; fifteen were in Africa. Overall, one-year prevalence of an episode defined as depressive using the *International Statistical Classification of Diseases and Related Health Problems,* tenth edition, was 3.27 percent. An average of 5.9–13.1 percent of participants with at least one chronic physical disease (angina, arthritis, asthma, or diabetes) had comorbid depression. This was significantly higher than the likelihood of having depression in the absence of a chronic physical disease. After the researchers adjusted for socioeconomic factors and health conditions, depression had the largest effect on worsening mean health scores—indicating disability—compared to the other chronic conditions alone. Consistently across countries and different demographic characteristics, respondents with depression that was comorbid with one or more chronic diseases had the worst health scores of all. Thus, depression produces a greater decrement in health than the chronic diseases of angina, arthritis, asthma, and diabetes. The comorbid state of depression worsens health more than depression alone, any of the chronic diseases alone, and any combination of chronic diseases without depression. The reasons are likely both psychological and biological, but for public health the implications are clear: an integrated treatment service is needed.

There is much less information on the impact of CMDs on mortality. A population-based longitudinal study from Ethiopia, which followed for up to five years three hundred participants with current major depression and another three hundred who had no lifetime history of depression, reported a mortality ratio for people with depression—standardized for age and gender—of 3.55 (the 95 percent confidence interval was 1.97 to 6.39) (Mogga et al. 2006). Suicide, which for some individuals is strongly associated with CMDs, is not reliably counted in most developing countries and is therefore not currently a very useful indicator of mortality. As alluded to above, CMDs may also contribute to mortality via their association with infectious disease; subjects with particular kinds of disorders may be particularly likely to contract sexually transmitted diseases, and, once acquired, CMDs may be associated with poorer adherence to treatment, faster progression of disease, and worse prognosis (Collins et al. 2006).

In South Asia associations between perinatal CMD and infant undernutrition at six months have been consistently demonstrated in a number of studies (Patel et al. 2004). However, results from African studies are inconsistent. One of the first studies, from a South African informal settlement, reported no association between maternal depression and infant growth—although there was a trend toward an association at eighteen months postpartum, and the study was small and relatively underpowered (Tomlinson et al. 2006). In a multicountry study, in which maternal CMD and child growth were assessed contemporaneously at six to eighteen months postpartum, there was no cross-sectional association between maternal CMD and child undernutrition in Ethiopia (Harpham et al. 2005). However, more recent studies have not consistently replicated this finding (Medhin et al. 2010). Clearly, given the high prevalence of CMDs during motherhood (Nhiwatiwa, Patel, and Acuda 1998; Cooper et al. 1999; Adewuya et al. 2008), this is a subject that deserves further investigation.

Finally, we consider health care seeking in patients with CMDs. The different pathways by which patients sought care in eleven different countries were first systematically examined in the Pathways to Care Study (Gater et al. 1991), which included seven developing countries in Asia, Africa, and Latin America. However, this study focused on patients seeking psychiatric care, which would be expected to reflect a small, and unrepresentative, fraction of the population suffering from CMDs. By far the commonest route of referral was the general medical practitioner based in a family practice or a hospital outpatient clinic. A study from Harare, Zimbabwe, described the pathways to primary care for patients with conspicuous CMDs attending primary care clinics and traditional medical clinics (Patel, Simunyu, et al. 1997). Except for people with an acute illness, patients usually consulted more than one care provider; three-quarters of those with a history of prior consultations had consulted both traditional and biomedical care providers. The first care provider consulted for the illness was most often a biomedical provider. This finding is consonant with multiple concepts of illness: the illness at its onset is considered to be a normal illness, and the patient goes to a biomedical provider. If this treatment fails, or if the patient's expectations are not fulfilled, he or she then consults a traditional provider (Patel 1995a). CMDs were rarely considered to be mental disorders, and thus mental health professionals were perceived to have a limited role in their management (Patel 1996). Thus, attitudes and beliefs about illness causation, which are considerably influenced by culture, determine the pathways to care (Okello and Neema 2007).

The World Mental Health Surveys provide new data on help seeking for mental disorders for over 84,848 community-living adult respondents in sixteen countries, including two in sub-Saharan Africa (Wang, Aguilar-Gaxiola, et al. 2007). Only a fifth of the respondents in Nigeria and a quarter in South Africa with severe CMDs had accessed any form of health care for their mental health problem in the previous twelve months. Almost all of the treatment seekers in Nigeria sought help in the nonspecialist sector, as did about two-thirds of those in South Africa. Only 10 percent of those with any mental disorder in Nigeria who had sought help received minimally adequate treatment (these data were not available for South Africa). Gender, education, and income did not influence help seeking in these two countries. In another analysis of these data, the median duration of delay in seeking treatment in Nigeria was about six years, in contrast to one or two years for respondents in European countries (Wang, Angermeyer, et al. 2007). Even when patients seek treatment at primary care settings in developing countries, there may be unacceptable underdiagnosis and undertreatment (Carey, Stein, and Zungu-Dirwayi 2003). Unsurprisingly, then, there are high levels of persistence of CMDs in community and primary care settings. For example, in an Ethiopian study, a quarter of the subjects with depression reviewed up to five years later were still suffering from depression (Mogga et al. 2006), and in a Zimbabwean primary care sample, over 40 percent of patients with CMDs showed significant morbidity twelve months later (Patel, Todd, et al. 1998).

KEY MESSAGES: THE IMPACT OF DEPRESSION

- CMDs are associated with high levels of disability and increased mortality.
- There is a close interrelationship between CMDs and other health outcomes of public health importance in sub-Saharan Africa, such as chronic diseases and HIV/AIDS.
- Unmet needs for mental health treatment are pervasive; and in addition to low levels of access to health care services, even for those with severe disorders, most patients who do access care receive inadequate diagnosis and treatment.
- High levels of chronicity are reported in community and primary care samples.

IMPLICATIONS FOR PUBLIC HEALTH

The findings of this relatively rich evidence base on CMDs in Africa have a number of implications. First, CMDs—in the form of a mixture of depressive, anxiety, and somatic experiences that impair daily life—do exist and are not an artifact of a culturally insensitive biomedical psychiatric classification. They can be identified not only through culturally sensitive epidemiological studies, but also by the thousands of mental health professionals who work in Africa. To surrender to the criticisms of universalist approaches to psychiatry and dismiss the notion of CMDs as a genuine cause of human suffering is to do great disservice to the people who suffer from these disorders and the health systems that are struggling to address them.

Second, levels of mental health literacy are low and levels of stigmatization are high in Africa—indeed, across the developing world (Stein et al. 2001). The concept of the CMD may not be well known, either among the public or among primary care providers. Those taking a purely social-construction approach might argue that making people aware of disorders such as depression and anxiety would lead to medicalization of experiences that are best approached from other perspectives. Our own view is that, although public health responses to trauma certainly need to emphasize resilience rather than employ a disease model alone (Stein et al. 2007), in general more engagement with the public and consumer groups in the developing world to increase mental health literacy would be desirable (Stein et al. 1997). Developing pragmatic classifications for public health and using locally defined illness categories, such as those generated in studies in Zimbabwe and Uganda (Bolton et al. 2003; Patel, Simunyu, and Gwanzura 1995) may reduce the gap between psychiatric and nonpsychiatric perceptions of CMDs.

Third, people facing social and economic disadvantages are at greater risk of CMDs, and by disabling them, CMDs rob them even further of the necessary human competencies needed to address these disadvantages. CMDs are, however, not the natural consequence of disadvantage—most people who are poor or disadvantaged do not become so depressed or anxious that their daily life is impaired to a significant extent. There are undoubtedly blurred lines between the miseries of life and clinically significant CMDs. Indeed, the two are best considered not as alternative explanations for the human experience, but as points on a continuum. Nevertheless, despite some of its important limitations, a medicalization of suffering has a useful and valid role (Stein and Gureje 2004).

Fourth, CMDs are associated with profound adverse impacts and low levels of adequate treatment. This is despite the fact that there is new evidence from developing countries (Patel et al. 2007), including some in Africa, that CMDs cannot be treated effectively using low-cost interventions—for example, group therapy delivered by villagers (Bolton et al. 2003). An immediate imperative is to increase the coverage of effective treatments for all mental disorders in African countries. The recent call for action by the Lancet Global Mental Health Group (2007) provides the necessary evidence and strategies to guide such a scaling up. New evidence on the reduction of the risk factors for depression means that, for example, improving economic security and reducing gender-based violence through microfinance (Pronyk et al. 2006) should be scaled up alongside improved treatment services. Mental health must be integrated into existing health and development activities targeted to the marginalized. The recent efforts by the Millennium Villages Project to address depression as part of an integrated strategy for development in Africa is a welcome step in this direction. Unfortunately, integration has often been taken to mean that existing and hard-pressed primary care practitioners are expected to provide both general physical and mental health care. In underresourced areas this invariably leads to the neglect of mental health treatment. We would advocate a model in which, at the primary care level, specific additional investments in human resources are made that focus on lower-cost health workers who are trained and supported by specialists, where possible, and, where there are seamless pathways, allowing input from secondary and tertiary levels of health care services as needed.

NOTE

Vikram Patel is supported by a Wellcome Trust Senior Clinical Research Fellowship in Tropical Medicine. Dan Stein is supported by the Medical Research Council of South Africa. The authors acknowledge the help of Eugene Kinyanda in identifying some references for this essay.

REFERENCES

Aaron, R., A. Joseph, S. Abraham, J. Muliyil, K. George, J. Prasad, S. Minz, V. J. Abraham, and A. Bose. 2004. "Suicides in Young People in Rural Southern India." *Lancet* 363 (9415): 1117–8.

Abas, M., F. Baingana, J. Broadhead, E. Iacoponi, and J. Vanderpyl. 2003. "Common Mental Disorders and Primary Health Care: Current Practice in Low-Income Countries." *Harvard Review of Psychiatry* 11 (3): 166–73.

Abas, M., and J. Broadhead. 1997. "Depression and Anxiety among Women in an Urban Setting in Zimbabwe." *Psychological Medicine* 27 (1): 59–71.

Adewuya, A. O., B. O. Ola, O. O. Aloba, B. M. Mapayi, and J. A. Okeniyi. 2008. "Impact of Postnatal Depression on Infants' Growth in Nigeria." *Journal of Affective Disorders* 108 (1–2): 191–93.

Araya, R., R. Wynn, R. Leonard, and G. Lewis. 1994. "Psychiatric Morbidity in Primary Health Care in Santiago, Chile: Preliminary Findings." *British Journal of Psychiatry* 165 (4): 530–33.

Bebbington, P. 1993. "Transcultural Aspects of Affective Disorders." *International Review of Psychiatry* 5 (2–3): 145–56.

Bhatt, A., B. Tomenson, and S. Benjamin. 1989. "Transcultural Patterns of Somatization in Primary Care: A Preliminary Report." *Journal of Psychosomatic Research* 33 (6): 671–80.

Bolton, P., J. Bass, R. Neugebauer, H. Verdeli, K. F. Clougherty, P. Wickramaratne, L. Speelman, L. Ndogoni, and M. Weissman. 2003. "Group Interpersonal Psychotherapy for Depression in Rural Uganda: A Randomized Controlled Trial." *Journal of the American Medical Association* 289 (23): 3117–24.

Bolton, P., R. Neugebauer, and L. Ndogoni. 2002. "Prevalence of Depression in Rural Rwanda Based on Symptom and Functional Criteria." *Journal of Nervous and Mental Disease* 190 (9): 631–37.

Bradshaw, D. 2003. *Initial Burden of Disease Estimates for South Africa, 2000.* Cape Town: South African Medical Research Council.

Broadhead, J., and M. Abas. 1998. "Life Events and Difficulties and the Onset of Depression among Women in a Low-Income Urban Setting in Zimbabwe." *Psychological Medicine* 28 (1): 29–38.

Broadhead, J., M. Abas, G. Khumalo-Sakatukwa, M. Chigwanda, and E. Garura. 2001. "Social Support and Life Events as Risk Factors for Depression among Women in an Urban Setting in Zimbabwe." *Social Psychiatry and Psychiatric Epidemiology* 36 (3): 115–22.

Brown, E., and T. Harris. 1978. *Social Origins of Depression.* London: Tavistock.

Byakika-Tusiime, J., J. H. Oyugi, W. A. Tumwikirize, E. T. Katabira, P. N. Mugyenyi, and D. R. Bangsberg. 2005. "Adherence to HIV Antiretroviral Therapy in HIV+ Ugandan Patients Purchasing Therapy." *International Journal of Sexually Transmitted Disease and AIDS* 16 (1): 38–41.

Carey, P. D., D. J. Stein, and N. Zungu-Dirwayi. 2003. "Trauma and Posttraumatic Stress Disorder in an Urban Xhosa Primary Care Population: Prevalence, Co-Morbidity and Service Use Patterns." *Journal of Nervous and Mental Disease* 191 (4): 230–36.

Collins, P. Y., A. R. Holman, M. C. Freeman, and V. Patel. 2006. "What Is the Relevance of Mental Health to HIV/AIDS Care and Treatment Programs in Developing Countries? A Systematic Review." *AIDS* 20 (12): 1571–82.

Cooper, P., M. Tomlinson, L. Swartz, M. Woolgar, L. Murray, and C. Molteno. 1999. "Post-Partum Depression and the Mother-Infant Relationship in a South African Peri-Urban Settlement." *British Journal of Psychiatry* 175 (6): 554–58.

de Jong, J. T. V. M., I. H. Komproe, and M. V. Ommeren. 2003. "Common Mental Disorders in Postconflict Settings." *Lancet* 361 (9375): 2128–30.

Demyttenaere, K., R. Bruffaerts, J. Posada-Villa, I., Gasquet, V. Kovess, J. P. Lepine, et al. 2004. "Prevalence, Severity, and Unmet Need for Treatment of Mental Disorders in the World Health Organization World Mental Health Surveys," *Journal of the American Medical Association* 291 (21): 2581–90.

Ebigbo, P. O. 1982. "Development of a CultureSpecific (Nigeria) Screening Scale of Somatic Complaints Indicating Psychiatric Disturbance." *Culture, Medicine and Psychiatry* 6 (1): 29–43.

Ebigbo, P. O., N. Janakiramaiah, and N. Kumaraswamy. 1989. "Somatization in Cross-Cultural Perspective." In *Clinical Psychology in Africa,* edited by K. Peltzer and P. O. Ebigbo, 233–50. Enugu, Nigeria: Chuka.

Freeman, M. 2004. "HIV/AIDS in Developing Countries: Heading towards a Mental Health and Consequent Social Disaster?" *South African Journal of Psychology* 34 (1): 139–59.

Friedman, S. 1997. *Cultural Issues in the Treatment of Anxiety.* New York: Guilford.

Gater, R., De B. Almeida E. Sousa, G. Barrientos, J. Caraveo, C. R. Chandrashekhar, M. Dhadphale, et al. 1991. "The Pathways to Psychiatric Care: A Cross-Cultural Study." *Psychological Medicine* 21 (3): 761–74.

Goldberg, D., and P. Huxley. 1992. *Common Mental Disorders: A Biosocial Model.* London: Tavistock/Routledge.

Goldberg, D., and Y. Lecrubier. 1995. "Form and Frequency of Mental Disorders across Cultures." In *Mental Illness in General Health Care: An International Study,* edited by T. B. Ustun and N. Sartorius, 323–334. Chichester, UK: John Wiley and Sons.

Gureje, O., V. O. Lasebikan, O. Ephraim-Oluwanuga, B. O. Olley, and L. Kola. 2005. "Community Study of Knowledge of and Attitude to Mental Illness in Nigeria." *British Journal of Psychiatry* 186 (5): 436–41.

Gureje, O., V. O. Lasebikan, L. Kola, and V. A. Makanjuola. 2006. "Lifetime and 12-Month Prevalence of Mental Disorders in the Nigerian Survey of Mental Health and Well-Being." *British Journal of Psychiatry* 188 (5): 465–71.

Gureje, O., M. Von Korff, L. Kola, K. Demyttenaere, Y. He, J. Posada-Villa, et al. 2008. "The Relation between Multiple Pains and Mental Disorders: Results from the World Mental Health Surveys." *Pain* 135 (1–2): 83–91.

Harpham, T., S. Huttly, M. J. De Silva,. and T. Abramsky. 2005. "Maternal Mental Health and Child Nutritional Status in Four Developing Countries." *Journal of Epidemiology and Community Health* 59 (12): 1060–64.

Johns, L., J. Y. Nazroo, P. Bebbington, and L. Kuipers. 2002. "Occurrence of Hallucinatory Experiences in a Community Sample and Ethnic Variations." *British Journal of Psychiatry* 180 (2): 174–78.

Kaminer, D., D. J. Stein, I. Mbanga, and N. Zungu-Dirwayi. 2001. "The Truth and Reconciliation Commission in South Africa: Relation to Psychiatric Status and Forgiveness among Survivors of Human Rights Abuses." *British Journal of Psychiatry* 178 (4): 373–77.

Katon, W., and E. A. Walker. 1998. "Medically Unexplained Symptoms in Primary Care." *Journal of Clinical Psychiatry* 59 (suppl. 20): 15–21.

Kirmayer, L. J., T. H. T. Dao, and A. Smith. 1998. "Somatization and Psychologization: Understanding Cultural Idioms of Distress." In *Clinical Methods in Transcultural Psychiatry,* edited by S. O. Okpaku, 233–65. Washington: American Psychiatric Association.

Lakoff, G. 1987. *Women, Fire, and Dangerous Things: What Categories Reveal about the Mind.* Chicago: University of Chicago Press.

Lancet Global Mental Health Group. 2007. "Scaling Up Services for Mental Disorders: A Call for Action." *Lancet* 370 (9590): 1241–52.

Lopez, A., C. Mathers, M. Ezzati, D. Jamison, and C. Murray. 2006. *Global Burden of Disease and Risk Factors.* Oxford: Oxford University Press.

Lorant, V., D. Deliege, W. Eaton, A. Robert, P. Philippot, and M. Ansseau. 2003. "Socio-Economic Inequalities in Depression: A Meta-Analysis." *American Journal of Epidemiology* 157 (2): 98–112.

Maj, M., R. Janssen, F. Starace, M. Zaudig, P. Satz, B. Sughondhabirom, et al. 1994. "WHO Neuropsychiatric AIDS Study, Cross-Sectional Phase I: Study Design and Psychiatric Findings." *Archives of General Psychiatry* 51 (1): 39–49.

Mathers, C. D., and D. Loncar. 2006. "Projections of Global Mortality and Burden of Disease from 2002 to 2030." *PLoS Medicine* 3 (11): e442.

Medhin, G., C. Hanlon, M. Dewey, A. Alem, F. Tesfaye, Z. Lakew, et al. 2010. "The Effect of Maternal Common Mental Disorders on Infant Undernutrition in Butajira, Ethiopia: The P-MaMiE Study." *BMC Psychiatry,* 10 (32): 1–13.

Miranda, J. J., and V. Patel. 2005. "Achieving the Millennium Development Goals: Does Mental Health Play a Role?" *PLoS Medicine* 2 (10): e291.

Mogga, S., M. Prince, A. Alem, D. Kebede, R. Stewart, N. Glozier, and M. Hotopf. 2006. "Outcome of Major Depression in Ethiopia: Population-Based Study." *British Journal of Psychiatry* 189 (3): 241–46.

Moussavi, S., S. Chatterji, E. Verdes, A. Tandon, V. Patel, and B. Ustun. 2007. "Depression, Chronic Disease and Decrements in Health: Evidence from the World Health Surveys." *Lancet* 370 (9590): 851–58.

Nhiwatiwa, S., V. Patel, and S. W. Acuda. 1998. "Predicting Postnatal Mental Disorder with a Screening Questionnaire: A Prospective Cohort Study from a Developing Country." *Journal of Epidemiology and Community Health* 52 (4): 262–66.

Okello, E. S., and S. Neema. 2007. "Explanatory Models and Help-Seeking Behavior: Pathways to Psychiatric Care among Patients Admitted for Depression in Mulago Hospital, Kampala, Uganda." *Qualitative Health Research* 17 (1): 14–25.

Okulate, G. T., M. O. Olayinka, and O. B. Jones. 2004. "Somatic Symptoms in Depression: Evaluation of Their Diagnostic Weight in an African Setting." *British Journal of Psychiatry* 184 (5): 422–27.

Panksepp, J. 2003. "Feeling the Pain of Social Loss." *Science* 302 (5643): 237–39.

Patel, V. 1995a. "Explanatory Models of Mental Illness in Sub-Saharan Africa" *Social Science and Medicine* 40 (9): 1291–98.

———. 1995b. "Spiritual Distress: An Indigenous Concept of Non-Psychotic Mental Disorder in Harare." *Acta Psychiatrica Scandinavica* 92 (2): 103–7.

———. 1996. "Recognizing Common Mental Disorders in Primary Care in African Countries: Should 'Mental' Be Dropped?" *Lancet* 347 (9002): 742–44.

———. 1998. *Culture and Common Mental Disorders in Sub-Saharan Africa: Studies in Primary Care in Zimbabwe.* Hove, UK: Psychology.

Patel, V., M. Abas, J. Broadhead, C. Todd, and A. P. Reeler. 2001. "Depression in Developing Countries: Lessons from Zimbabwe." *British Medical Journal* 322 (7284): 482–84.

Patel, V., R. Araya, S. Chatterjee, D. Chisholm, A. Cohen, M. De Silva, C. Hosman, H. McGuire, G. Rojas, and M. van Ommeren. 2007. "Treatment and Prevention of Mental Disorders in Low-Income and Middle-Income Countries." *Lancet* 370 (9591): 991–1005.

Patel, V., R. Araya, M. S. Lima, A. Ludermir, and C. Todd. 1999. "Women, Poverty and Common Mental Disorders in Four Restructuring Societies." *Social Science and Medicine* 49 (11): 1461–71.

Patel, V., and A. Goodman. 2007. "Researching Protective and Promotive Factors in Mental Health." *International Journal of Epidemiology* 36 (4): 703–707.

Patel, V., F. Gwanzura, E. Simunyu, K. Lloyd, and A. Mann. 1995. "The Explanatory Models and Phenomenology of Common Mental Disorder in Harare, Zimbabwe." *Psychological Medicine* 25 (6): 1191–99.

Patel, V., and A. Kleinman. 2003. "Poverty and Common Mental Disorders in Developing Countries," *Bulletin of the World Health Organization* 81 (8): 609–15.

Patel, V., T. Musara, P. Maramba, and T. Butau. 1995. "Concepts of Mental Illness and Medical Pluralism in Harare." *Psychological Medicine* 25 (3): 485–93.

Patel, V., M. Rahman, K. Jacob, and M. Hughes 2004. "Effect of Maternal Mental Health on Infant Growth in Low Income Countries: New Evidence from South Asia." *British Medical Journal* 188 (3): 284–85.

Patel, V., E. Simunyu, and F. Gwanzura. 1995. "Kufungisisa (Thinking Too Much): A Shona Idiom for Non-Psychotic Mental Illness." *Central African Journal of Medicine* 41 (7): 209–15.

Patel, V., E. Simunyu, F. Gwanzura, G. Lewis, and A. Mann. 1997. "The Shona Symptom Questionnaire: The Development of an Indigenous Measure of Non-Psychotic Mental Disorder in Harare." *Acta Psychiatrica Scandinavica* 95 (6): 469–75.

———. 1998. "The Outcome of Common Mental Disorders in Harare, Zimbabwe." *British Journal of Psychiatry* 172 (1): 53–57.

Patel, V., C. Todd, M. Winston, F. Gwanzura, E. Simunyu, W. Acuda, and A. Mann. 1997. "Common Mental Disorders in Primary Care in Harare, Zimbabwe: Associations and Risk Factors." *British Journal of Psychiatry* 171: 60–64.

Patel, V., C. Todd, M. Winston, F. Gwanzura, E. Simunyu, W. Acuda, and A. Mann. 1998. "Outcome of Common Mental Disorders in Harare, Zimbabwe." *British Journal of Psychiatry* 172: 53–57.

Penninx, B. W. J. H., A. T. Beekman, A. Honig, D. J. Deeg, R. A. Schoevers, J. T. van Eijk, and W. van Tilburg. 2001. "Depression and Cardiac Mortality: Results from a Community-Based Longitudinal Study." *Archives of General Psychiatry* 58 (3): 227.

Phillips, M. R., X. Li, and Y. Zhang. 2002. "Suicide Rates in China, 1995–99." *Lancet* 359 (9309): 835–40.

Pickett, K. E., O. W. James, and R. G. Wilkinson. 2006. "Income Inequality and the Prevalence of Mental Illness: A Preliminary International Analysis." *Journal of Epidemiology and Community Health* 60 (7): 646–47.

Prince, M., V. Patel, S. Saxena, M. Maj, J. Maselko, M. Phillips, and A. Rahman. 2007. "No Health without Mental Health—a Slogan with Substance." *Lancet* 370 (9590): 859–77.

Pronyk, P. M., J. R. Hargreaves, J. C., Kim, L. A. Morison, G. Phetla, C. Watts, J. Busza, and J. D. H. Porter. 2006. "Effect of a Structural Intervention for the Prevention of Intimate-Partner Violence and HIV in Rural South Africa: A Cluster Randomised Trial." *Lancet* 368 (9551), 1973–83.

Reeler, A. P. 1994. "A Preliminary Investigation into Psychological Disorders among Mozambican Refugees: Prevalence and Clinical Features." *Central African Journal of Medicine* 40 (11): 309–15.

Stein, D. J., and O. Gureje. 2004. "Depression and Anxiety in the Developing World: Is It Time to Medicalise the Suffering?" *Lancet* 364 (9430): 233–34.

Stein, D. J., S. Seedat, R. A. Emsley, and B. O. Olley. 2005. "HIV/AIDS in Africa—a Role for the Mental Health Practitioner?" *South African Medical Journal* 95 (3): 167–68.

Stein, D. J., S. Seedat, A. Herman, H. Moomal, S. G. Heeringa, R. C. Kessler, et al. 2008. "Lifetime Prevalence of Psychiatric Disorders in South Africa." *British Journal of Psychiatry* 192 (2): 112–17.

Stein, D. J., S. Seedat, A. Iversen, and S. Wessely. 2007. "Post-Traumatic Stress Disorder: Medicine and Politics." *Lancet* 369 (9566): 139–44.

Stein, D. J., C. Wessels, J. van Kradenberg, and R. A. Emsley. 1997. "The Mental Health Information Centre of South Africa: A Report of the First 500 Calls." *Central African Journal of Medicine* 43 (9): 244–46.

Stein, D. J., C. Wessels, N. Zungu-Dirwayi, M. Berk, and Z. Wilson. 2001. "Value and Effectiveness of Consumer Advocacy Groups: A Survey of the Anxiety Disorders Support Group in South Africa." *Depression and Anxiety* 13 (2): 105–107.

Tadios, Y., and G. Davey. 2006. "Antiretroviral Treatment Adherence and Its Correlates in Addis Ababa, Ethiopia," *Ethiopian Medical Journal* 44 (3): 237–44.

Todd, C., V. Patel, E. Simunyu, F. Gwanzura, W. Acuda, M. Winston, and A. Mann. 1999. "The Onset of Common Mental Disorders in Primary Care Attenders in Harare, Zimbabwe." *Psychological Medicine* 29 (1): 97–104.

Tomlinson, M., P. J. Cooper, A. Stein, L. Swartz, and C. Molteno. 2006. "Post-Partum Depression and Infant Growth in a South African Peri-Urban Settlement." *Child Care and Health Development* 32 (1): 81–86.

Tyrer, P. 2001. "The Case for Cothymia: Mixed Anxiety and Depression as a Single Diagnosis." *British Journal of Psychiatry* 179 (3): 191–93.

Wang, P. S., A. Aguilar-Gaxiola, J. Alonso, M. C. Angermeyer, G. Borges, E. J. Bromet, et al. 2007. "Use of Mental Health Services for Anxiety, Mood, and Substance Disorders in 17 Countries in the WHO World Mental Health Surveys." *Lancet* 370 (9599): 841–50.

Wang, P. S., M. Angermeyer, G. Borges, R. Bruffaets, W. Chiu Tat, G. D. E. Girolamo, et al. 2007. "Delay and Failure in Treatment Seeking after First Onset of Mental Disorders in the World Health Organization's World Mental Health Survey Initiative." *World Psychiatry* 6 (3): 177–85.

Weich, S., G. Lewis, R. Donmall, and A. Mann. 1995. "Somatic Presentation of Psychiatric Morbidity in General Practice." *British Journal of General Practice* 45 (392): 143–47.

World Health Organization. 1992. *The ICD-10 Classification of Mental and Behavioural Disorders*. Geneva: World Health Organization.

———. 1995. *Mental Illness in General Health Care: An International Study*. Chichester, UK: John Wiley and Sons.

———. 2000. *Women's Mental Health: An Evidence Based Review*. Geneva: World Health Organization.

Yehuda, R., and A. C. McFarlane. 1995. "Conflict between Current Knowledge about Posttraumatic Stress Disorder and Its Original Conceptual Basis." *American Journal of Psychiatry* 152 (12): 1705–13.

3 SCHIZOPHRENIA AND PSYCHOSIS IN WEST AFRICA

URSULA M. READ, VICTOR C. K. DOKU,

AND AMA DE-GRAFT AIKINS

IN PSYCHIATRY, THE term "schizophrenia" refers to a group of major mental disorders whose etiology is still unknown and that involves a complex set of disturbances of thinking, perception, affect, and social behavior (Barbato 1998). It is characterized by psychotic symptoms, known as "positive symptoms," such as auditory hallucinations (hearing voices) and delusions, as well as by "negative symptoms" such as social withdrawal, blunted affect, and self-neglect. Schizophrenia has been viewed as the prototypical manifestation of madness. It can have a devastating effect on the person's sense of self and ability to conform to social norms and to engage successfully in personal relationships. In diagnosing schizophrenia, the clinician distinguishes between the real and the hallucinatory, between subjective experience and a presumed objective reality. Thus, the diagnosis of schizophrenia is intimately involved with judgments concerning what it means to be a functioning member of society and what is considered to be within the normal range of behavior and belief. Such judgments are undoubtedly linked to cultural norms and expectations.

Any account of schizophrenia—not only in Africa, but globally—must consider the historical and cultural origins of schizophrenia as a disease category within psychiatric practice. Psychiatric diagnoses, perhaps more than those in any other biomedical field, have undergone significant changes over time and raised considerable debate, both about their status as discrete categories of biomedical pathology and about their validity across cultures. This debate has generally been polarized between the biological or medical model of psychiatry and the psychosocial model. Transcultural psychiatry, under the influence of anthropology, has tended to take the latter perspective, emphasizing context and meaning rather than signs and symptoms (Littlewood 1990).

Schizophrenia may be the most controversial of the psychiatric diagnoses. The precise characteristics of the disorder, now one of the major diagnoses in psychiatry, have been subject to some dispute both inside and outside psychiatry since the term was first coined by Swiss psychiatrist Eugen Bleuler in 1908. Bleuler's term replaced the earlier term "dementia praecox," or premature dementia, used by German psychiatrist Emil Kraepelin in his 1893 textbook of psychiatry to describe a psychotic condition with onset in adolescence and poor outcome. Kraepelin first made the distinction between disorders of mood (affective disorders) and psychosis, and he is considered the father of the system of disease classification in psychiatry (Shorter 1997). This separation of psychotic from affective disorders represents a particular cultural and historical turn in the history of madness in Europe, with Kraepelin's identification of dementia praecox marking a move toward a scientific and biological psychiatry and away from earlier social and religious approaches to mental illness. However, the seeds of uncertainty regarding the diagnosis were sown by Kraepelin himself, when in 1904 he suggested a cross-cultural epidemiology to throw light on the etiology of mental disorder (Jablensky 1997; Jilek 1995).

Schizophrenia remains a contested diagnosis among both mental health practitioners and their patients, not least because of its status as a severe mental illness with potentially serious implications for long-term prognosis. The ongoing nature of such debates in the psychiatric community is reflected in discussions regarding the status of schizophrenia in the fifth edition of the *Diagnostic and Statistical Manual of Mental Disorders* (*DSM*) of the American Psychiatric Association. To reflect the wide variation in symptomology, course, and outcome of psychotic illness, some have argued for a descriptive dimensional approach, in which groups of correlated symptoms rather than conceptually discrete diagnostic categories are identified (Allardyce et al. 2007; Dutta et al. 2007).

In concert with the debates about schizophrenia and changes in psychiatric theory and practice, the trajectory of schizophrenia as a disease category in psychiatry in West Africa has evolved as it was subjected to influences both in the continent and worldwide. In this essay we investigate the introduction of the concept of schizophrenia in West Africa through the practice of psychiatry and the ongoing difficulties in applying a diagnosis with origins in European biomedical science to West African patients, many of whom might be subject to conflicting views of their disorder held by themselves, their families, and professional and religious specialists. We consider the usefulness of schizophrenia as a diagnosis in the West African context, and we ask how the treatment of the severely mentally ill in West Africa might benefit from a closer consideration of the specific presentation of psychosis in the region. Finally, to suggest ways forward for mental health care in West Africa, we review the resources available to people with severe mental illness in countries where psychiatric professionals are few and the burden of care remains largely on families and the community, to suggest ways forward for mental health care in West Africa.

This essay draws mainly on the English-language literature and hence is biased toward the Anglophone countries of West Africa, particularly Ghana and Nigeria. This is partly a result of the constraints in accessing the Francophone literature from the United Kingdom and Ghana, where the authors are based, as well as the dominance of English in research publications. In addition, many countries of West Africa have no significant provision of psychiatric services (Jacob et al. 2007) and thus are largely absent from the research record. The majority of research on schizophrenia and other psychotic disorders in West Africa has been conducted in Nigeria, one of the sites for early cross-national studies of schizophrenia. Nonetheless, the close cultural affinities among the countries of West Africa, as well as similarities in the development of psychiatry in the various parts of the region, permit some generalizations to be made.

THE HISTORY OF PSYCHIATRY IN WEST AFRICA

Prior to the establishment of asylums in the early years of the twentieth century, the treatment of the mad or mentally ill in West Africa was the province of what are now called traditional healers (Odejide, Oyewunmi, and Ohaeri 1989). Traditional healers in West Africa represent a great diversity of practices. However, many operate shrines devoted to particular gods, where supplicants seek healing through confession, offerings, and herbal medicines. Margaret Field, a psychiatrist and anthropologist who studied mental illness at shrines in rural Ghana in the 1950s, noted that those whom she identified as "chronic schizophrenics" were beyond the help of traditional healers and so remained in the care of the family or became vagrants (1960, 445). Indeed, it was largely such chronic schizophrenics who dominated the populations of the colonial asylums (McCulloch 1995, 30). With growing urbanization, the mad had become increasingly visible in the cities and towns of West African colonies, leading to the introduction of legislation to allow for their removal and confinement, first in prisons and later in lunatic asylums. The construction of asylums in West Africa was at first solely a British enterprise. Despite the formulation of plans as early as 1912 for the development of psychiatric services in the French West African colonies, psychiatric hospitals were not constructed there until the close of the colonial epoch. Troublesome *aliénés indigènes* (indigenous aliens—the term applied to those with mental illness in colonial times [Littlewood and Lipsedge 1997]) were shipped to asylums in France, although some rooms in the general hospitals in Senegal were allocated for psychiatric cases (Collomb 1975). In British West Africa, the first colonial hospital for the mentally ill, the Kissy Lunatic Asylum, was established in Sierra Leone in 1844, followed in 1888 by the conversion of the High Court at Victoriaborg in Accra, Ghana, into an asylum (Forster 1962). These functioned largely as custodial institutions, offering little in the way of treatment and being squalid and overcrowded. Indeed, some of the early asylums in Nigeria, for example, formed part of the prison system and had no trained clinical staff (McCulloch 1995; Sadowsky 1999). Leland Bell describes the Kissy Lunatic Asylum as "a place for the demented and dangerous, people who were burdens and created trouble for family and society" (1991, 16). Along with mental patients, the institution housed various "undifferentiated dependents" —paupers, beggars, criminals, the physically disabled, and the mentally retarded. Whatever the original intentions of their founding authorities, the asylums in Accra and Lagos followed a similar trajectory, used by families to dispose of troublesome relatives and by city authorities to rid the streets of unsightly undesirables.

It was only toward the end of the colonial era that asylums began to take on more of a medical and scientific role (Bell 1991; Forster 1962; McCulloch 1995). The appointment of psychiatrists, including African psychiatrists trained in Europe, and the recognition by the colonial authorities that Africans were capable of self-government led to the asylums being viewed as places for treatment rather than merely confinement. The same period also saw major advances in the treatment of serious and chronic mental disorders, such as schizophrenia, in Europe and North America—in particular the introduction of physical therapies, such as insulin coma and electroconvulsive therapy in the 1930s and the advent of antipsychotics in the 1950s (Shorter 1997). These therapies were introduced into the practice of psychiatry in Africa, although somewhat belatedly. Field, for example, reported that in 1957 there was no insulin therapy in Ghana, at a time when this was one of the major methods of treatment for chronic schizophrenia in Europe and North America (1960, 454). Thus, she concluded that there was little that the psychiatric hospitals could offer people with chronic schizophrenia that could not be provided at home.

Distinguishing between the criminal and the insane, or later deciding on the most appropriate means of treatment, required clarity in diagnosis, which stimulated a debate among those working in psychiatry in Africa about whether psychiatric disorders such as schizophrenia could be mapped onto the symptoms demonstrated by African patients. The 1940s and 1950s saw the growth of what came to be known as ethnopsychiatry, as European and North American psychiatrists working in the colonies began to compare what they encountered among patients in Africa with their experience of psychiatry in the West (Keller 2001; McCulloch 1995). Mindful of the influence of culture on the presentation of symptoms, both psychiatrists and anthropologists provided descriptive data on the presentation of madness among West Africans.[1] In the 1950s colonial psychiatrists were joined by African psychiatrists trained in Europe, such as Emmanuel Forster in Ghana and Thomas Lambo in Nigeria, who were conversant both with the terminology of psychiatry and, at least to some degree, with West African concepts of madness and its causes (German and Raman 1976). Psychiatrists conducting research on mental illness among West Africans generally began with psychiatric diagnoses and searched for evidence of these disorders in the group being studied (Field 1960; Fortes and Mayer 1966; Harding 1973; Leighton et al. 1963). However, others began with an indigenous concept such as a broad category of madness (Tooth 1950) or a more specialized concept such as "illnesses of the spirit" (Beiser et al. 1973) and attempted to draw parallels between the symptoms described and the diagnostic categories of psychiatry. Some psychiatrists claimed to have identified "culture-bound syndromes" (Lin 1962, 158) that were not captured by the usual Western diagnostic categories, such as what was termed "brain fag" (Prince 1960a).[2] Though Margaret Field concluded that "if the stranger asks to be shown a madman he will probably be led to a florid schizophrenic" (1960, 315), most studies in Africa more easily drew comparisons between African manifestations of madness and the broader psychiatric symptoms termed psychosis, than between madness and the more restricted diagnostic features required for a diagnosis of schizophrenia.

The consistency of reports arising from these studies of what typified madness in West African cultures is notable. Common signs of madness included nakedness, talking incoherently, dirty habits, wandering aimlessly, and aggressiveness (Field 1960; Fortes and Mayer 1966). Anthropologists and psychiatrists alike drew parallels between such symptoms and psychosis, giving rise to a "pathoplastic" view of mental illness, in which the presumed organic form remained consistent but the manifestation or content of psychopathology differed (Lambo 1955, 250). The overwhelming conclusion reached by both European and European-trained African researchers was that, despite certain cultural or environmental influences on the presentation of mental illnesses, the same diagnoses could be applied to West African patients and to European ones (Forster 1962; Leighton et al. 1963; Tooth 1950). Geoffrey Tooth, a British psychiatrist commissioned by the colonial authorities to conduct a two-year survey into the "forms of psychosis and neurosis among West Africans" (1950, 24) in what was then the Gold Coast, sums up this perspective: "While it is likely that the clinical picture of schizophrenic reactions may also be modified by the environmental and cultural background of the patient, all the varieties of schizophrenia commonly seen in Europeans may also be seen in Africans" (1950, 48). Such a conclusion may also have been influenced by a change in colonial ideology from a view of the African as biologically and psychologically inferior—as reflected in the work of colonial psychiatrists such as John Carothers and his theory of the "African mind" (1953)—to what Henri Collomb calls the "dogme égalitaire" (1975, 100) that swept aside cultural and psychological differences.

The growing confidence of psychiatrists in their ability to diagnose schizophrenia among West Africans is reflected in the clinical records of psychiatric hospitals. These reveal that in the late colonial period schizophrenia became the most common diagnosis among patients admitted. Bell (1991) reports that after the 1940s schizophrenia was increasingly used as a diagnosis at the Kissy Lunatic Asylum and by the 1960s it was the most common diagnosis among inpatients. A report of an inspection of the asylum at Accra in 1935 records that schizophrenia was diagnosed for 27.6 percent of inpatients, with another 19.2 percent diagnosed with chronic delusional insanity, a diagnosis that is now obsolete and that might now be replaced with schizophrenia in some cases (Cunyngham-Brown 1937). Forster (1962) records that diagnoses of schizophrenia at the same hospital rose from 280 out of 1,189 admissions in 1955 to 446 out of 1,010 admissions in 1960.

However, uncertainties in diagnosis remained: the high numbers of schizophrenia diagnoses were sometimes matched or exceeded by the numbers of cases "not yet diagnosed," a phenomenon which persists to the present day.[3] Forster (1958) reports that although 469 outpatients at the Accra Psychiatric Hospital in 1956 were diagnosed with schizophrenia, another 332 were uncategorized. Twenty-six years later the picture had hardly changed (Adomako 1972). Between 1909 and 1959 the majority of cases at Kissy received no psychiatric designation at all, due to the custodial role of the institution and the lack of clinical personnel qualified to make a diagnosis. However, the numbers of undiagnosed cases persisted after independence, despite the arrival of psychiatrists and the implementation of a more medical model of care. Although some patients were designated as "transient psychoses," many were admitted following incidents of violent behavior that may have raised questions about whether their behavior was pathological or criminal (Bell 1991, 109).

SCHIZOPHRENIA AS A DISORDER OF CIVILIZATION

The search for the presence or absence of schizophrenia among Africans also drew on contemporary theories of the psycho- or socio-genesis of schizophrenia.[4] In the first half of the twentieth century there were many epidemiological studies of schizophrenia and psychoses, as researchers sought to shed light on their nature and cause (Jablensky 1997). Thus, the psychiatrists and anthropologists who conducted comparative studies of schizophrenia in African countries were concerned not only with the mental health of the Africans but also with the question of the disease's origins. If schizophrenia could be shown to be absent among "primitives," as had long been argued (Demerath 1942; Faris 1934; Seligman 1932), that would help confirm the presumed etiology of schizophrenia as a disorder arising from the stresses of civilization, industrialization, and urbanization. This was explicitly stated by the authors of the Aro-Cornell project, which compared psychiatric disorders in Nigeria with those found in North America: "To study these qualitatively and quantitatively in a West African group and to compare the findings with what has been learned in epidemiological investigations in North America would, we thought, advance ideas of cause" (Leighton et al. 1963, 521).

The impact of contact by another culture was the most prominent among the environmental factors that colonial psychiatrists believed might influence the nature of psychopathology among Africans. Thus, although psychiatrists claimed to recognize the symptoms of schizophrenia among West Africans, they also suggested that it occurred largely among those in closest contact with European civilization. These theories echoed what has been called the "primitivist" theme in cross-cultural psychiatry, in which those from traditional cultures were either seen as degenerate and prone to psychotic outbursts or as free from the strains of civilization and its attendant psychopathology, protected by traditional communal values (Lucas and Barrett 1995). The concern with the effects of contact between Africa and the West often drew on an evolutionary paradigm that formed a popular theoretical justification for the colonial venture (explicitly stated in the French colonial notion of the *evolué*), as well as on fears of the potentially destabilizing impact of acculturation on the colonized. The dangers that detribalization and acculturation posed for Africans' mental health were a frequent theme in the psychiatric literature of the late colonial and early postcolonial period. The theme was discussed both by colonial psychiatrists such as Tooth (1950) and Field (1960) and by members of the new generation of African psychiatrists such as Lambo (1981) and Forster (1962).[5] Such writers commonly argued that the rapid social changes brought about by colonialism and industrialization, with the concomitant breakdown of traditional tribal life, might present particular stresses for Africans, possibly leading to a steep increase in cases of mental illness—in particular, schizophrenia and other psychoses. Field, for example, found that literacy rates were higher than average among those she diagnosed with schizophrenia and predicted a "startling outburst of acute schizophrenia" in the newly independent Ghana, arising from the stresses and ambitions fostered by programs for universal literacy and industrialization (1958, 1048). Forster, the first African psychiatrist working in Ghana, predicted that social change such as urbanization and the disruption of tribal community life" (1962, 22) would lead to an increase in "psychotic reactions" (1962, 13) and claimed that schizophrenia was most common among members of the educated classes in southern Ghana, who were torn between native and imported Western cultures (Forster 1962 and

1958). Forster held a clearly evolutionary view, portraying Africans as falling into three classes with their associated psychiatric problems—the educated "Westernized African . . . elegant and superior to his brothers," who is susceptible to anxiety and hysteria; the "illiterate African," prone to "cyclothymic reactions"; and the "very primitive people [who] present less schizophrenic and cyclothymic disorders, and more hysterical and criminal tendencies" (1962, 9).

These psychiatrists were among those who suggested that schizophrenia, as classically defined, was absent in rural areas, whose populations displayed their own distinct forms of psychopathology. Forster claimed that the experience of migration from the countryside to the city "became a source of confusion for the simple minds of the migrant labor force, most of whom came from the less evolved regions," and that such migration led to "certain atypical and catastrophic schizophreniform reactions," in particular "primary delusional patterns with persecutory tendencies leading to acts of violence in which the attacker was allegedly protecting himself" (1962, 12). Both Tooth and Forster argued that the farther north one traveled, away from Western influences, the more atypical the forms of schizophrenia became. Indeed, Tooth claimed that although among the urban literate section of the population, schizophrenia took nearly the same form as in Europeans, a typical clinical picture of schizophrenia was rare among "bush" peoples, who presented instead with what he termed "an amorphous endogenous psychosis" (1950, 49).

SCHIZOPHRENIA OR PSYCHOSIS?

Psychiatrists in West Africa thus concluded not only that those closest to the influence of European society were most at risk from schizophrenia and other disorders of European civilization, but also that the standardized categories of psychiatry might not apply to people living in rural areas relatively untouched by Western influence. Tooth claimed that "broadly speaking, it is relatively easy to recognize the standard psychoses when they occur in Africans who have been in contact with Western civilization, but among the 'bush' peoples, with a few exceptions, diagnosis is less certain" (1950, 41). Although Tooth acknowledged that the "cultural gap" between the examiner and the patient might partly explain this difficulty, he concluded that "there are real differences in the quality of the psychotic reactions of individuals with different racial and cultural backgrounds, differences which make it impossible to fit them into the accepted nosological framework" (ibid.). Tooth was not alone in wondering if psychosis among West Africans could be squeezed into the standardized syndrome required for a diagnosis of schizophrenia. In Nigeria, Lambo (1955) challenged the Kraepelinian distinction between neurotic and psychotic disorders that had been so influential in the development of psychiatric classification. Lambo hypothesized that paranoid psychosis among the Yoruba resembled a disorder midway between the psychotic and psychoneurotic illnesses of Euro-American cultures.

This bringing together of affective and psychotic symptoms was linked to the debates in psychiatry in Africa about how Africans responded to stresses and life events that in Europe and North America were considered potential etiological factors in affective disorders such as depression. The primitivist view of the mental health of Africans was reflected in the assumption of many colonial psychiatrists that depression was rare among Africans (Forster 1962, 35, Tooth 1950, 38).[6] A complementary hypothesis was that whereas Europeans under stress tended to develop symptoms of depression, such as withdrawal and feelings of guilt and sadness, Africans reacted to stress with chaotic symptoms that were suggestive of a psychotic reaction (Sow 1990). Several writers argued for the recognition of transient reactive psychoses distinct from schizophrenia among Africans. These have been labeled variously "fear psychoses" (Field 1960, 201–74), "hysterical psychosis" (Langness 1967), and "*bouffées délirantes*" (Collomb 1965) and are characterized by a short-lived acute and intense disturbance of perception, mood, and behavior that often occurs in response to a stressful event and that usually has a spontaneous resolution. This characterization of the African response to stress carries traces of the view held by colonial psychiatrists such as Carothers (1947) of Africans as psychologically unsophisticated and overly emotional. In a review of psychiatry in Africa, Allen German described such brief psychoses as "an acute reaction pattern to psychic trauma expressed in an exotic form due to other factors such as cultural expectations and traditional beliefs" (1972, 466). This definition clearly contrasts a psychotic reaction to stress—described as atypical and "exotic"—with a depressive reaction.

Although the notion of such reactive psychoses points to the potential relationship of sociocultural factors and stressful or traumatic life events to the onset of psychosis, it has also been recognized that biological factors such as malnutrition or febrile illnesses may play a role in the etiology of psychosis in countries with high levels of poverty and tropical diseases. German speculated that "acute transient psychoses appear to be characteristic of people living in poverty who are illiterate, undernourished and diseased," and he suggested that with improved nutrition and health, such conditions might be expected to decrease (1972, 467). Undoubtedly some acute psychoses can be attributed to an organic cause such as viral infections or fever, which are common in African countries. However, one of the few studies to examine the role of biological as well as psychosocial factors in the etiology of acute brief psychoses within two developing countries (India and Nigeria) found evidence for the presence of both fever and significant life events prior to the onset of psychosis, albeit it within a small sample (Collins et al. 1996). A more thorough study of the occurrence of significant life events in the six months prior to the onset of schizophrenia, again among a Nigerian sample, did not find more life events among those diagnosed with schizophrenia than among controls (Gureje and Adewunmi 1988). However, these researchers did not measure the subjective appraisal of such events nor the level of social support, which could mitigate their impact.

The debates about whether African patients were suffering from schizophrenia or from acute transient psychoses also reflect the inconsistencies in the classification of schizophrenia in the American Psychiatric Association's DSM and the World Health Organization's *International Statistical Classification of Diseases and Related Health Problems* (ICD). Duration of symptoms is one of the key diagnostic markers employed by both classification systems. Although the most recent revision of DSM, DSM-V, has sought to eliminate its differences from the ICD in the definition of schizophrenia, the difference in regard to minimum duration of symptoms has been retained, with DSM requiring a six-month duration of symptoms versus one month's duration in the ICD (Tandon et al. 2013). As Sunny Ilechukwu (1991) points out, some psychiatrists in Africa, such as Lambo, included brief psychoses under the schizophrenia rubric, but others, such as Forster, excluded them.

What is striking in these discussions is that despite the best efforts of psychiatrists to identify schizophrenia among West African patients, there remained a significant number of cases—perhaps the majority—that failed to conform to the typical schizophrenic syndrome. German concludes his review of psychiatry in Africa by stating that "confused amorphous psychoses with schizophrenic features are so common in Africa that they could hardly be termed atypical. Probably they are best separated conceptually from schizophrenia and regarded as part of the group of acute transient psychoses" (1972, 468). The question is, therefore, can schizophrenia be clinically distinguished from such brief or "amorphous" psychoses? German argued in the affirmative: "In conclusion, . . . one is impressed by the essential similarity of schizophrenia as it occurs in disparate cultures, a phenomenon which argues the formidable role of constitutional factors in etiology and suggests that environmental aspects may have been overemphasized. These environmental aspects, apart from determining a variety of transient psychoses which may be confused with schizophrenia, also add pathoplastic color to the clinical picture and appear to soften the impact of chronicity and deterioration. They do not, however, seem to alter the structure and form of schizophrenia" (ibid, 469). This argument, however, seems to point two ways—both toward a form of psychosis resulting from biological determinism (schizophrenia) and toward a form of psychosis resulting from environmental stress but sharing enough characteristics with schizophrenia to be mistaken for it.

CHRONICITY OR RECOVERY?

These debates revolved around the possible influence of etiology and nosological status on the outcome of psychotic illness, but others focused on the possible influence on recovery of supportive factors in the sociocultural environment. In contrast with the characterization of schizophrenia as a chronic, recurring disorder, many researchers observed that Africans seemed to make a rapid recovery from psychotic breakdowns. Some, such as Lambo (1962) in Nigeria, related this to the support available to the mentally ill in African villages. Alfa Sow, a Guinean doctor and social scientist who took an anthropological approach, argued that "chronicity is generally less pronounced in Africa than it is in the West. This difference seems to be due mainly to great tolerance on the part of the community, which facilitates rapid reintegration into the family group, as well as to the quality of human relationships" (1990, 30). This argument was lent support by studies suggesting that people who broke down in urban areas, where traditional support structures such as the extended family were not available, seemed to fare much worse than those who broke down in rural areas and often required detention in hospital (Ojesina 1979). Some researchers argued that the mentally ill faced less stigma in traditional West African societies (Cunyngham-Brown 1937; Fortes and Mayer 1966; Lambo 1962). In Ghana, for example, it was claimed that in the rural north, the mentally ill were more easily accepted by the community than in the urban areas in the south. Tooth writes: "There appears to be little social stigma attached to madness, lunatics are well treated in their homes and even when shackled to a log in the traditional manner, the madman is seldom alone for long, is well fed and enjoys the company of his children and friends" (1950, 30).

Indeed, chronicity in mental illness was felt to be largely a Western phenomenon—a result of urbanization, a paucity of family support, the pressures of modernity, and the routine detention of the mentally ill in long-stay psychiatric hospitals. In his report, Tooth includes a number of accounts of atypical psychoses that he calls "delusional states," (1950, 46) using a diagnostic category that by then was already obsolete, and suggests that many of the harmless vagrant psychotics might fall into this category. Most of these cases came from the north of Ghana or from small villages in the south, and he reports that these patients were reassimilated into community life once the acute phase of their illness had passed. He suggests that "these endogenous psychotics left to fend for themselves outside the family, would have developed into the dilapidated eccentrics of the market place, but if transported into an alien and restricted environment would have produced the symptomatology of one of the familiar varieties of Schizophrenia. In short, the form of psychosis has been determined by the treatment" (1950, 48).

However, more recent studies have challenged such notions of rural African life as a protective utopia from the dangers of mental breakdown. The poverty experienced by many rural Africans undermines the notion of village life as free of stress. Indeed, researchers have demonstrated strong correlations between poverty and schizophrenia (Saraceno, Levav and Kohn 2005). In addition, a number of studies in Nigeria have also revealed widespread stigma and discrimination against those with mental illness (Adewuya and Makanjuola 2005; Gureje et al. 2005; Kabir et al. 2004; Ohaeri and Fido 2001). Stigma, along with the stresses and costs of caring for a mentally ill relative, can strain even the most supportive family network, particularly in cases of chronic or severe psychotic illness (Gureje and Bamidele 1999; Martyns-Yellowe 1992; Ohaeri 1998; Ohaeri 2000; Ohaeri and Fido 2001; Ukpong 2006). Indeed, despite the presence of large family networks that can serve as potential sources of support, measurements of family burden in Nigeria have been shown to be greater than in the United Kingdom. This may be due in part to the absence in Nigeria of state avenues of support such as social welfare and facilities for rehabilitation (Ohaeri 2001). The numbers of patients abandoned in psychiatric hospitals ("The Mantle of Mental Health Recovery" 2005; Jegede, Williams, and Sijuwola 1985) and healing facilities such as prayer camps in Ghana[7] testify to the absence or breakdown of family support for many.

A final challenge to the enduring view that the chance of recovery from schizophrenia and other psychotic disorders is better in lower-income countries has come through a reappraisal of schizophrenia as a chronic disorder. Outcome studies in both high- and low-income countries suggest a heterogeneous course, ranging from a single episode with complete remission to a chronic and deteriorating condition (Davidson and McGlashan 1997). A World Health Organization–sponsored study of the fifteen- and twenty-five-year course of schizophrenia found that over 50 percent of subjects from both "industrialised" and "non-industrialised" countries were rated as "recovered." The authors concluded that "schizophrenia and related psychoses are best seen developmentally as episodic disorders with a rather favorable outcome for a significant proportion of patients" (Harrison et al. 2001, 515). Such a conclusion suggests that in some cases "brief psychotic disorders" could be rather instances of recovery from schizophrenia (Edgerton 1980, 172–73).

CHALLENGES IN THE EPIDEMIOLOGY OF SCHIZOPHRENIA IN WEST AFRICA

Today the extent of psychotic illness in West Africa remains largely unknown. In Africa as a whole there is little funding for research, particularly in mental health, and limited research expertise. Official statistics from health facilities are often unreliable (Gureje and Alem 2000). The few international epidemiological studies that included Africa illustrate the enduring difficulties in applying diagnostic concepts whose roots are in Europe and North America to African populations, as well as the continuing dominance of European and North American diagnostic standards in international psychiatric research. In the 1960s the developers of the ICD and the DSM attempted to establish an internationally recognized nosology of psychiatric diagnoses. However, the coexistence of these two major classificatory systems points to the ongoing difficulties in delineating watertight diagnostic categories in psychiatry. Accusations of ethnocentric bias have accompanied the development of the DSM and the ICD since their creation.[8] Despite this, assessment instruments derived from these diagnostic manuals have been adopted as the gold standard for accurate diagnosis of schizophrenia and other mental disorders in international research.

These instruments have their origins in countries not nearly so culturally diverse as those of Europe and Africa, but they come from the differing diagnostic traditions of the United Kingdom and the United States. This led to the development of a standardized assessment instrument in an attempt to produce reliable diagnoses of schizophrenia on both sides of the Atlantic. The result of this endeavor was the Present State Examination, which received its first major cross-cultural exposure through its use in the first international study of schizophrenia, the World Health Organization's International Pilot Study of Schizophrenia, which was launched in 1967. This study set out to establish whether schizophrenia could be reliably identified cross-culturally, using the Present State Examination to find cases that conformed to the standardized diagnostic criteria. The study was conducted in nine countries, and it purported to show a similar incidence of schizophrenia across all nine. Two- and ten-year follow-up studies suggested that patients with a diagnosis of schizophrenia in what were termed "developing" countries had better outcomes than patients in other countries (Jablensky et al. 1992).[9]

However, the World Health Organization studies have since been widely criticized, both for their methodology—they used diagnostic categories and instruments derived from studies in North American and European populations— and for the essentializing distinctions made between developing and developed countries (Edgerton and Cohen 1994; Cohen 1992; Fernando 1991; Williams 2003). Furthermore, the patients in developing countries who were included in the study were selected from those who had presented to Western-style psychiatric facilities, thus effectively screening out a large number of people who may have presented with similar symptoms but had been treated by traditional healers or who had not sought help at all. Importantly for the study of schizophrenia in Africa, only one African country, Nigeria, was included in the International

Pilot Study of Schizophrenia. In fifteen-year follow-up studies, no African country was included (Harrison et al. 2001). As for the supposed evidence of a better outcome for schizophrenia in the developing world, this echoed many earlier primitivist arguments and has been questioned by several researchers. Alex Cohen and coauthors (2008), who reviewed studies of schizophrenia outcomes in twenty-three countries, found a much greater variation. They cautioned that the outcome measures employed in the World Health Organization studies provided insufficient detail, for example in relation to cultural specificities surrounding family relationships, marriage, and employment. In respect to measures of outcome in West Africa, the crude distinction between "unemployed" and "employed" failed to capture much of the informal work that many people in these societies perform (Edgerton and Cohen 1994, 228). Similarly, using the categories of married, divorced, or single might also fail to reflect either the significance of marital status in West African societies or the variety of relationships covered by the term "marriage" in a region where conjugal relationships have been viewed as "a bundle of interactional possibilities with associated political, economic, legal or other implications" (Burnham 1987, 50).

Despite these criticisms, policy makers, practitioners, and researchers in the field of mental health in West Africa have since drawn heavily on the results of the International Pilot Study of Schizophrenia and epidemiological studies conducted predominantly in the countries of Europe and North America to estimate prevalence and incidence rates of mental illnesses. This is largely due to the paucity of population-based studies that have been conducted in West African countries. Those that do exist have continued to use instruments based on ICD and DSM diagnostic syndromes, with the most recent in Nigeria using the Yoruba translation of the Composite International Diagnostic Interview (Gureje et al. 2006). However, such instruments—written in English and designed largely for use in the EuroAmerican context—continue to present difficulties because they do not reflect the specificity of symptoms in diverse settings and they must be translated into the large number of vernacular languages in West Africa. In a population-based epidemiological study of schizophrenia in Ghana that used the Schedules for Clinical Assessment in Neuropsychiatry, which succeeded the Present State Examination, Victor Doku identified a number of terms in the instrument that had no equivalents in Twi, the language of translation. Furthermore, the study identified more cases that fit the category of unspecified psychosis in the tenth edition of the ICD (F28), than that of schizophrenia (Doku 2005). In West Africa somatic symptoms such as crawling peppery and burning sensations have been recorded in both psychotic and mood disorders (Ilechukwu 1991; Ohaeri and Adeyemi 1990). However, these are not captured using internationally standardized instruments, and in the interests of international equivalence, few local instruments are developed. Peter Ebigbo (1982) in Nigeria did develop a scale to measure such somatic symptoms, and it has been suggested that this could be used alongside standardized instruments to capture some of the expressions of mental distress that might be missed by the use of international instruments alone (Ilecukwu 1991, 183).

Nonetheless, the danger with such epidemiological studies of mental disorder is that researchers will encounter only the symptoms that match the stringent requirements of the diagnosis (Kleinman 1977).[10] Those aspects of psychotic illnesses that fall outside the narrow category of schizophrenia and that are most influenced by culture are the ones most likely to be missed. Assen Jablensky acknowledges that sampling a population with a "checklist" of psychopathic criteria, such as those of the ICD and the DSM, is likely to exclude "less severe, transient or atypical cases" (1997, 116). German (1987) has suggested that research by black African clinicians may overcome some of the problems of ethnocentric bias, since the "emic" perspective of African clinicians should enable them to make more reliable judgments about what is normal and what is deviant behavior. However, African psychiatrists have been trained in the use of psychiatric theory and practice that may blind them to aspects of their patients' experience that do not fit into the language and concepts of psychiatric categories. The use of French and English in both clinical practice and international research results in the translating of vernacular vocabularies and concepts of madness and distress into language that concords with psychiatric terminology, leading inevitably to distortion of the illness experience.[11] Laurence Kirmayer and Harry Minas argue: "The emphasis on large-scale epidemiology to resolve issues of fact will inevitably suppress the voices of small groups and contribute to the homogenization and standardization of world cultures and traditions of healing. What we gain in methodological rigor we lose in diversity" (2000, 444). In order to address some of these issues, Joop de Jong and Mark Van Ommeren have suggested a combination of qualitative and quantitative methods in order to conduct a "culture-informed epidemiology," including focus groups to explore contextual issues; in-depth interviews to gather illness narratives of people with mental illness; and careful translation, back translation, and piloting of instruments (2002). Illness taxonomies such as that described by Helga Fink (1989) in Ghana may also help elucidate local categories and concepts of mental illness, which can be used to supplement standard epidemiological data.

In addition to such diagnostic dilemmas, many epidemiological studies in West Africa draw on hospital-based samples, since this remains the most feasible means of accessing a cohort of people with mental illness, given the absence of reliable census data, the inaccessibility of many rural areas, and the limited numbers of clinicians able to conduct research (Ilechukwu 1991).[12] However, there are methodological problems with conducting epidemiological research solely in hospitals. Such samples are inevitably biased toward those who have already interpreted their symptoms in such a way as to lead them to seek help from biomedical facility. Hospital-based samples may also distort perceptions of the presentation of mental illness in African societies, since the people who are brought to psychiatric hospitals are likely to be those who are most disturbed and aggressive and, therefore, most likely to prompt the family to seek external help. As German argues, the tendency to select violent patients for hospital admission may mean that researchers fail to adequately describe "the occurrence and nature of psychoneurotic disorders, or of the 'quieter' psychoses such as psychotic states of depression" (1972, 465). Furthermore, in view of a number of factors—including the scarcity of psychiatric facilities and personnel, poor road transportation, inadequate funds to travel to treatment centers and pay for treatment, and commonly held views of mental illness as a spiritual condition—only a minority of people with mental illness may seek help from psychiatric services.[13] There are also a significant number of vagrants in many West African countries with possible symptoms of mental illness who are excluded from most studies because of the difficulties in successfully engaging and following up such people. Finally, hospitals may admit only those patients who conform most nearly to standardized psychiatric diagnoses. As Sow argues, "Are not 'hospitalizable' (or hospitalized) patients precisely the persons who happen to correspond, at least in part, to the nosographic categories characteristic of Western hospitals?" (1990, 13).

CULTURAL AND SOCIOPOLITICAL INFLUENCES ON PSYCHOPATHOLOGY

Debates about the status of schizophrenia in West Africa have focused largely on causative factors and outcomes, and few studies have examined the content as well as the form of psychotic symptoms that West Africans experience. The limited research available appears to show that the content of symptoms such as delusions and hallucinations reflects the patient's cultural and social milieu. Forster, for example, argued that contact with "the Western style of life" in the south of Ghana influenced the content of patients' psychopathology: "Thus, in this region, delusions may appear concerning political parties and government, operations by means of electricity, wireless and telephone agencies" (Forster 1958, 39). This pathoplastic view of schizophrenic symptoms continues in more contemporary studies. A study of the auditory hallucinations of ninety-nine psychotic patients in the psychiatric unit of the Military Hospital in Yaba, a part of Lagos, found that "life circumstances of cultural significance" (Okulate and Jones 2003, 539) were manifested in the content of hallucinations. The authors concluded that "culture-based differences" may occur in the phenomenology of auditory hallucinations (2003, 540). Case studies from Nigeria and Ghana illustrate the ongoing influence of magical or supernatural effects such as witchcraft or curses on the content of psychopathology such as hallucinations and delusions (Okulate and Jones 2003; Read 2012; Farmer and Falkowski 1985).

However, in viewing the peculiarities of African pathology as merely cultural manifestations of a universal disorder, psychiatrists may overlook the extent to which the experience of mental illness may also reflect the inequities and racial politics of colonial and post-colonial societies.[14] Psychiatrists working in Africa frequently asserted that the chief pathology of the African was persecutory delusions, which were often related to fears of witchcraft (Carothers 1947; Forster 1962; Sow 1990). None of these psychiatrists addressed the fact that in the context of the periods in which they were studying African psychopathology, such feelings may have had some basis in the colonial regime and contemporary racial politics. In a study of West African students admitted to psychiatric hospitals in the United Kingdom between 1955 and 1965, a period when there was considerable overt racism directed against black immigrants, John Copeland noted the extremely high incidence of persecutory symptoms among the cohort studied (57 out of 60 students, and 104 out of 116 admissions) (1968). This included people diagnosed with depression as well as those diagnosed with schizophrenia, whose version of reality may have been more open to question. Copeland observed that those diagnosed with schizophrenia "tended to make accusations against non-coloured people" (ibid., 11). However, despite his earlier noting of the "social difficulties" confronting West African students living in Britain, including "colour," (ibid., 8) this did not prompt Copeland to consider that such persecutory delusions could have been caused by racism. Instead, he saw them as the result of "cross-cultural influences" (ibid., 11) resulting from contact with Western culture. Indeed, he concluded that it is only such persecutory ideas about "non-coloured people" that can safely be taken as indications of pathology, since persecutory ideas about fellow Africans are commonplace: "It seems therefore, that as long as paranoid persecutory ideas remain consistent with the original cultural setting, and are attributed to the activities of other Africans and centre around magic, poisoning and hypnotism (when this is regarded as supernatural), they are of no diagnostic specificity" (ibid.).

In such cases, vaguely defined notions of cultural influences on psychopathology may become a catchall that obscures the sociopolitical realities confronted by those experiencing mental illness. Jonathan Sadowsky (1999 and 2004) conducted a historical study of the content of Nigerian psychiatric patients' delusions and hallucinations that had been preserved in archival sources of the colonial period. This work differs from many clinically oriented studies in demonstrating how the content of delusions reflected the political events of the time. Sadowsky shows how the writings of psychiatric patients address with "splintered eloquence" (2004, 243) the themes of Nigeria's imminent independence and anxieties about ethnic conflicts, anxieties that were only too tragically fulfilled in the Biafran war. The hyperbole of patients' letters when framed as grandiosity may have allowed them to say what they could not have said had they been judged to be sane: "To the extent that these inmates were mad, their madness allowed sentiments to flourish that might otherwise have been concealed" (ibid., 247). Sadowsky concludes that "the mad can have an unsettling degree of insight into social inequities and existential dilemmas—even as they may not, from a clinician's point of view, show comparable insight into the nature of their illness" (ibid.). This approach recognizes the specific content of psychopathology as both personally, culturally, and historically meaningful, rather than as simply an aid to diagnosis. If incorporated into the assessment and treatment of mental illness, such an approach has potential for grounding problem identification and intervention in the experience of the patient, moving the influence of culture on the manifestation of mental illness beyond broad pathoplastic generalizations.

DIAGNOSING SCHIZOPHRENIA IN CLINICAL PRACTICE

The realities of clinical practice in West Africa contrast sharply to the more reified and better-funded sphere of international mental health research, yet West African practice reflects the ongoing dominance of biomedical models of mental illness in practice. Most data derived from psychiatric services in West African countries indicate that schizophrenia is the most common diagnosis (Ikwuagwu et al. 1994; Turkson 1998; Bell 1991; Gesler and Nahim 1984). However, in contemporary psychiatric practice in West Africa, the lack of trained psychiatrists and psychiatric nurses raises questions as to the reliability of current diagnostic statistics gained from hospital populations. Because of the number of patients relative to the number of clinicians available to assess them, clinical interviews are often very brief. Furthermore, there are possibilities for misunderstanding and misdiagnosis arising from the linguistic complexity of West African societies. In psychiatry, language is the major method through which patients convey their symptoms (Westermeyer and Janca 1997). As mentioned above, the language of psychiatry in West Africa remains English or French, and clinical notes, textbooks, notices, and medical charts are all written in these European languages. Yet these languages are not spoken fluently by the majority of people living in West Africa, particularly those who have received limited education and may thus be among the poorest and most disenfranchised. Most West African countries use several language groups; therefore, the potential for diagnostic confusion is heightened, as the clinician and the patient may not use the same language. Trained interpreters are not used, which leads to a complex chain of translation and retranslation. For example, the patient or his relatives may translate his complaints from a local language into a West African lingua franca such as Yoruba, Hausa, or Twi. Concepts used in these languages to express madness, emotional states, or mental distress must then be translated into equivalents in English or French in order to fit into psychiatric syndromes. It is inevitable in this process that meaning is lost or distorted, thus adding to the difficulty in reaching an accurate diagnosis, particularly when time is limited.

Given these difficulties, it is likely that schizophrenia may be overdiagnosed or, conversely, missed—particularly when the patient presents with negative symptoms, such as social withdrawal, rather than the typical positive symptoms of hallucinations and delusions. Furthermore, it may be difficult in practice to distinguish between schizophrenia and other psychoses. The treatment and prognosis for the two would differ, with long-term prophylaxis with antipsychotic medication being considered an important step for patients with schizophrenia as a way to prevent relapse and significant implications for the person's everyday functioning. Indeed, some have argued that the "negative syndrome" may be of more diagnostic and prognostic value in schizophrenia than positive symptoms (Gureje, Aderibigbe, and Obikoya 1995, 715). This emphasizes the value of assessing the impact of illness on function—for example, through instruments such as the World Health Organization's Disability Assessment Schedule (World Health Organization 2000)—rather than focusing solely on psychopathology.

The legacy of the so-called Kraepelinian dichotomy between affective and psychotic disorders may also result in a tendency among clinicians to overlook depressive symptoms in those with psychosis. Diagnoses such as schizoaffective disorder, and bipolar affective disorder point to the fact that psychotic and affective symptoms are not mutually exclusive. The prevalence of brief and acute psychoses suggested by research from West Africa could prompt clinicians to investigate the potential affective and reactive components in the presentation of psychosis, which may suggest psychosocial methods of treatment in addition to medication.

There is a danger that schizophrenia may come to be associated with violent behavior by staff in psychiatric services since, as noted above, cases with such behavior are most likely to precipitate a crisis in families that may lead the family to bring the patient to the psychiatric hospital. Quieter manifestations of schizophrenia and negative symptoms, such as social withdrawal and self-neglect, may not be so readily associated with madness and thus not lead to the same help-seeking behavior. Mental illness has also become strongly associated with cannabis use in popular discourse and professional practice in

West Africa, leading to a frequent diagnosis of cannabis psychosis in hospital-ized patients, particularly young men. Cannabis use has proliferated in West Africa since World War II (Lambo 1965, see also Akyeampong, this volume). Hospital-based studies in West Africa confirm the frequency of cannabis use among young male patients with psychotic symptoms (Rolfe et al. 1993; Sijuwola 1986). A study in the Gambia found that psychotic patients were 4.4 times more likely to have a positive cannabinoid result than nonpsychotic controls. The au-thors concluded that "cannabis is a major factor in the etiology of psychosis" (Rolfe et al. 1993, 800). However, although cannabis psychosis as a diagnosis may be popularly employed in psychiatric practice, some have argued that it is indistinguishable from schizophrenia (Imade and Ebie 1991; Sijuwola 1986). A review of the case notes on 272 individuals with psychotic illness in Nigeria was unable to discover "any consistency of symptoms among the cannabis psychosis that could lead to its classification as an independent diagnostic category dif-ferent from schizophrenia" (Imade and Ebie 1991, 136). Furthermore, once can-nabis use is identified as a cause of psychosis, clinicians may overlook other potential precipitating factors of which cannabis use may itself be symptomatic. For example, Lambo (1965) linked cannabis use to socioeconomic causes such as unemployment and migration from a rural area to an urban one. Forty years later, unemployment and underemployment remain a major problem for young males in West Africa in both urban and rural areas (United Nations Office for West Africa 2006), which is likely to have psychological effects in some cases. Cannabis use may also mask prodromal or actual symptoms of psychosis, which may have led to its use. For example, a person might use cannabis to cope with difficulties managing social interactions or to block out distressing auditory hallucinations.

TREATMENT FOR SCHIZOPHRENIA AND PSYCHOSIS

Treatment for schizophrenia and other psychotic illnesses in West Africa has inevitably followed a different trajectory from that in higher-income countries. Despite the optimism of postcolonial psychiatrists and ambitious plans in some countries for the expansion of mental health care in the early years of indepen-dence (Forster 1962), the political chaos and economic decline experienced in several West African countries in the 1970s and 1980s meant that many of these plans failed to come to fruition. Health institutions collapsed, and there was an exodus of health professionals, including psychiatrists and psychiatric nurses, to Europe and North America.[15] In countries such as Sierra Leone and Guinea Bissau, which have experienced civil war, psychiatric services are only now very slowly being rebuilt, often with the support of international agencies.

The difficult economic and political situation of many West African countries has had a deleterious effect on psychiatric care in the region. The lack of trained professionals, the paucity of opportunities for professional development, and the neglect of mental health care in the budgets of many governments mean that individuals with schizophrenia and their families receive very limited support from the state and are frequently unable to access a high standard of psychiatric care. The number of psychiatrists and other professionals working in mental health care is insufficient to meet the mental health needs of the population in West Africa, as is the case in many other low-income countries (Jacob et al. 2007). In Ghana, many professionals working in psychiatry are approaching retirement, including most psychiatrists and many community psychiatric nurses, and others have returned to work from retirement to help fill the gap in human resources.

In the early postcolonial period, African psychiatrists were active in drawing on resources in the local environment in caring for those with serious mental illnesses such as schizophrenia, with Lambo's "village psychiatry" being the most famous example (Asuni 1979).[16] Another innovation in Senegal was the use of an *accompagnant*, a family member who remains with the patient during his or her hospital stay (Diop and Dores 1976; Franklin et al. 1996). However, there now appears to be a tendency towards what Jean-Francois Bayart (2000) calls "extraversion," in which the impetus for the majority of initiatives in mental health care does not come from other countries in the subregion or even in Africa, but from external international agencies—in particular, the World Health Organization, aid agencies, and nongovernmental organizations. These agencies tend to import models of psychiatric treatment and care that originated in Europe or North America and that may have little relevance or feasibility in the West African context. Yet because these agencies have access to significant funding and resources for research and service development, they may become indispensable in the context of scarcity.

Mental health care is frequently a low priority in countries with limited resources. The vision of a decentralized mental health service, with psychiatry provided within primary care, that Forster (1962) outlined has barely begun to be implemented in West Africa. Despite evidence of the value of community mental health care to support patients with chronic psychiatric conditions such as schizophrenia in low- and middle-income countries (Alem 2002, Wiley-Exley 2007), most service provision remains concentrated in inpatient services (Saxena et al. 2007). In West Africa the provision of community mental health care is hampered by the scarcity of personnel and resources. In Ghana, for example, there are only 115 community psychiatric nurses for a population of twenty-one million, and many of them struggle to reach the more distant communities due to poor roads, scarce public transportation, and the lack of funds to reimburse them for transportation costs. Many West African countries have no psychiatric nurses at all. This means that there is no follow-up care available in the community for many people who are diagnosed and treated for schizophrenia and psychosis in psychiatric hospitals. They may have difficulties obtaining regular supplies of medication following discharge, which in turn has implications for their possible relapse and outcome. Those most in need of psychiatric services may be the least able to access them, as those with the most serious symptoms are likely to also be those for whom the economic consequences of the illness are most severe. Those most disabled by mental illness will be unable to work and hence may be unable to meet the costs of transportation and treatment (Ojesina 1979).

Little research has been conducted in West Africa to suggest what treatment might be most effective for people in the region with diagnoses of schizophrenia and psychosis. However, several studies of patients treated with antipsychotic medication in psychiatric hospitals in Nigeria suggest that improved outcomes reduced family burden (Ohaeri 1998; Ohaeri 2001). As noted above, pharmaceutical treatment for schizophrenia and psychosis appears to have arrived later in West Africa than in Europe and North America, but it is now well established in psychiatric practice. However, the revolution in antipsychotic prescription that has taken place with the arrival of so-called atypical antipsychotics in high-income countries has not occurred in most of West Africa. The range of drugs available is far less than that available elsewhere. Chlorpromazine and haloperidol are available in most African countries (Kohn et al. 2004), but atypicals such as risperidone and olanzapine are much scarcer. Thus, medication at government health institutions is largely restricted to the older antipsychotics, which have potentially serious and debilitating side effects such as prolonged drowsiness and movement disorders. As elsewhere, such side effects are often a factor in many patients' stopping antipsychotic medication. In addition, as noted above, psychotropic medication and follow-up care in the community may not be locally available. This can lead to frequent relapses and hospital readmissions. Depot antipsychotics that are administered by injection and release the drug slowly over time are frequently used in high-income countries for the control of psychotic symptoms, particularly for patients unwilling or unable to take oral medication. A trial of a depot antipsychotic (haloperidol decanoate) in Guinea Bissau demonstrated that this form of medication had a favorable effect on outcomes for patients with schizophrenia, significantly reducing their need for hospital admissions (de Jong and Komproe 2006). However, depot medication is rarely available in West Africa, and, again, there are often no community-based psychiatric nurses to administer the drug and monitor its effects.

Given the evidence for the equal efficacy of older and atypical antipsychotics, some people have argued that replacing lower-cost antipsychotics, such as chlorpromazine, with expensive atypicals in low-income countries may not warrant the additional cost (Patel et al. 2007, Saxena et al. 2007). Atypicals also have serious side effects that are unpleasant for patients, and research in the United States indicates that attrition from atypical antipsychotics is nearly as high as that for the older drugs (Dolder et al. 2002). With limited resources for mental health care, West African health care planners must decide whether atypical antipsychotics are a worthwhile investment. In the meantime, ensuring reliable access to medication remains a challenge for many countries. In Ghana, for example, although major antipsychotics such as chlorpromazine and haloperidol are included in the essential medicines list, there are frequently problems of supply, which have led to hospitals being without sufficient quantities of the drugs. When that happens, patients or their families must purchase medication from pharmacies at their own expense. For some the expense is unsustainable, and the problem may lead people not to use psychiatric hospitals.

Psychological interventions are so rare as to be unavailable for the vast majority of patients in West African countries. Though occupational therapy and group therapy were implemented in some psychiatric hospitals in the 1960s and 1970s—for example, Aro, in Nigeria (Asuni 1979)—talking therapies, psychosocial treatments, and rehabilitation are now rarely available. The lack of psychologists, social workers, and occupational therapists means that care in psychiatric hospitals is largely focused on the management of aggressive and agitated patients, and psychotic disorders are treated predominantly through psychotropic medication. Thus, the psychosocial care of those with serious mental illness is largely the domain of the patient's family, religious practitioners, and traditional healers.

It is notable that the vast majority of studies on schizophrenia in West Africa have been written by psychiatrists, and that by far the largest share of these studies come from Nigeria. Very limited research has been published by other mental health professionals such as nurses, psychologists, or social workers, or by social scientists such as anthropologists and sociologists. This is perhaps inevitable given the very limited numbers of mental health professionals working in most West African countries. However, it does mean that research is largely quantitative rather than qualitative, and focused on biomedical rather than psychosocial or anthropological approaches. There is also a tendency to use standardized scales that may mask the specific cultural factors pertinent to the study of schizophrenia in West Africa. Even scales that are used to measure psychosocial factors such as life events tend to have been developed in Europe or America. They may not reflect the specific meaning of life events in the context of West African societies and may omit some altogether (Jadhav 2004). Significantly, in contrast to the proliferation of firsthand accounts of schizophrenia in Europe and North America—including autobiographical works, academic publications, and items in the media—the voices of the mentally ill in West Africa have largely been unheard in the international research literature. Yet the lived experiences of those with mental illness and their families could provide many insights into the meaning and impact of mental illness in West African societies. Such experiences could elucidate the needs of those with mental illness and their families and could inform the development of interventions grounded in local experience and resources. Very recently Ghana has witnessed the gradual emergence of a rights-based movement, which draws its inspiration from the psychiatric service user movement in Europe. In addition, a mental health nongovernmental organization, BasicNeeds, has collected a number of firsthand accounts of mental illness from those affected, which it publishes in its monthly magazine and uses for research and advocacy. However, the serious stigma attached to mental illness in West African societies may prevent many people with mental illness from speaking out. Many are hidden away at home or in prayer camps or shrines; many become vagrants (Asuni 1980, see also de-Graft Aikins, this volume). These are the invisible mentally ill, who may never enter the statistics of epidemiological studies nor receive psychiatric treatment.

LAY CONCEPTIONS OF SCHIZOPHRENIA

As a consequence of such silences, the question of what schizophrenia means to those diagnosed with it, their families, and the communities in which they live is largely unexplored. Outside of the specialized realm of psychiatry, the concept of schizophrenia remains largely unknown among the general population in West African countries, and even many patients may not be aware that they have been diagnosed with such a disorder. The paucity of information on mental health is compounded by lack of education and high levels of illiteracy. Terms used to describe madness in vernacular languages cannot be said to be exact equivalents of syndromes such as schizophrenia. However, behaviors which are identified as "mad" (*dam* in Twi and *were* in Yoruba, for example) seem to be those that bear a strong resemblance to the schizophrenic or psychotic syndrome as Field (1960) observed. A survey of general knowledge of mental disorders among 120 adults in Nigeria, found that "the symptoms most commonly recognized, and described as indicative of mental disorder, may be classified under psychotic reactions" (Ugorji and Ofem 1976, 297). These included incoherent speech, shouting, dancing or singing inappropriately, public nakedness, and aggressive behavior. Other studies in Nigeria and Cape Verde similarly report that mental illness is typically identified with violence, nudity, talking nonsense, uncleanliness, wandering, and eccentric behavior (Gureje et al. 2005; Kabir et al. 2004; Mateus, dos Santos, and de Jesus Mari 2005). There are also reported distinctions between different kinds of madness in popular knowledge, such as madness with elements of danger and madness as odd or antisocial behavior (Weinberg 1965).

If schizophrenia becomes equated with madness in West Africa, patients and families may resist the diagnosis due to the attendant stigma (Mateus, dos Santos, and de Jesus Mari 2005). Ultimately, diagnostic labels may be of more importance to researchers and clinicians than they are to patients, particularly since—as noted above—the language of psychiatry in the region is English or French, while the people treated mostly speak African languages. As Sow observes, "what is of greatest interest to the African patient from the very beginning and above everything else is the cause or, more importantly, meaning of his illness, since it is felt to be a misfortune—indeed, much more interesting than the syndromic, even significant, pattern of some objective morbid structure that would be extraneous to him" (1990, 51). Psychiatric care may be the most "culturally unfamiliar" treatment option for many families in West Africa (Franklin et al. 1996, 326), with the asylum being only one treatment choice among a range of therapeutic options. It has long been observed in several West African countries that most families consult traditional or religious healers for the treatment of mental illness either before or after their first hospital consultation (Osei 2001; Jahoda 1979; Mullings 1984; Lamptey 1977; Appiah-Poku et al. 2004; Franklin et al. 1996). Although the use of traditional and religious healers has often been attributed to beliefs regarding the spiritual etiology of mental illness (Franklin et al. 1996; Jahoda 1979; Lamptey 1977), the inaccessibility of biomedical treatment may also play a role. Where it is available, the often free treatment provided by psychiatric hospitals can appeal to families struggling to care for a relative with psychotic illness. Megan Vaughan suggests that with the introduction of asylums in the colonial period, "the idea that insanity was a condition sometimes calling for confinement in a distant institution at no cost to the insane or their relatives, held some attractions" (1991, 106).

Throughout West Africa it is also common for people to approach different healing resources as they search for the cure of an illness (Read 2012a; de-Graft Aikins 2005; Franklin et al. 1996). The simultaneous use of spiritual and biomedical treatment also reflects a desire on the part of many Africans to address the perceived spiritual and physical aspects of mental illness (Fink 1989; Read 2012b). Traditional healers' views of madness are diverse and represent a panoply of approaches, from those of the *marabouts* of Senegal (Franklin et al. 1996) to those of the *bosomfo* of Ghana (Yeboah 1994); a thorough exploration is beyond the scope of this chapter. However, in the traditional view madness may result from the breaking of taboos, sorcery or witchcraft, or the actions of ancestral spirits or genies (Franklin et al. 1996; Appiah-Kubi 1981; Mullings 1984). Robert Franklin and coauthors write that in Senegal for example: "Psychiatric patients often suspect the cause of their illness to be magic spells initiated by rivals in conflicts involving love, money, or professional activities" (1996, 325). Nigerian films, which are popular throughout Anglophone West Africa, frequently include a story line in which an individual develops a psychosis through the actions of sorcery, witchcraft, or curses (Aina 2004). Treatment by traditional healers usually combines herbal treatment (Prince 1960b) and a ritual, such as the sacrifice of animals (Yeboah 1994). Recently the Pentecostal and charismatic churches in West African countries with large Christian populations have become a popular resource for the treatment of mental illness (Appiah-Poku et al. 2004; Ohaeri and Fido 2001). They have developed their own models of mental illness, which often combine the belief systems of traditional religion and Christianity, and sometimes biomedicine. Psychotic symptoms such as hallucinations and delusions may be seen as evidence of demonic possession. For patients and their families, biomedical and spiritual approaches may not be mutually exclusive, despite their differing epistemologies. A study of the caregivers of patients with diagnoses of schizophrenia in Nigeria found that psychoses were most often attributed to the work of Satan, even though the families had sought hospital care (Ohaeri and Fido 2001). Dag Heward-Mills (2005), a prominent healing evangelist and medical doctor in Ghana, explicitly links schizophrenia with demonic possession in one of his publications.

EXPERIENCES OF SCHIZOPHRENIA

The impact of schizophrenia and psychosis on the individual West African affected and on his or her family can be considerable. The personal and social effects of mental illness are influenced by culture, which shapes the response to madness of the patient, the family, and the local community. Functional impairment and disability arising from the illness may lead to significant loss of income, exacerbating existing conditions of poverty for many people in West Africa. A survey of fifty-five patients diagnosed with schizophrenia in Nigeria found that for two-thirds of them social and leisure activities were restricted, and the majority had their domestic routines and trading disrupted. Many of their marriages broke down, and thirty-one of the fifty-five were unemployed. Although those from rural areas found it "relatively easy to get back to their farming or petty trading," those in cities found it much harder to find work, which led to a worsening of their condition (Ojesina 1979, 100). Another Nigerian longitudinal study of fifty people with schizophrenia found that at a ten-year follow-up, twenty-two were unemployed and twenty had no income at all (Suleiman et al. 1997).

In the absence of state avenues of support, families are a vital resource for the care of people with serious mental illness (Jegede, Williams, and Sijuwola 1985). Studies in Nigeria emphasize the importance of the extended family in improved outcomes for patients with schizophrenia (Ohaeri 1998; Ohaeri 2001; Ohaeri and Fido 2001). A study of patients with schizophrenia and psychotic disorders found that the patients generally gave high ratings to their quality of life and attributed this to the level of family support and tolerance (Olusina and Ohaeri 2003). However, the patients in these studies had been treated and discharged from the hospital, and the majority of them were comparatively free of symptoms. Caregiver burden was shown to be higher among families caring for family members with active psychotic symptoms. In addition, in one study of 123 patients with schizophrenia diagnoses, the duration of illness was significantly negatively correlated with receipt of material, social, and emotional support and the regularity of social interaction. Jude Ohaeri suggests that there is "a cycle in the care of chronic mentally ill patients whereby effective treatment begets further social support and vice versa, leading to the possibility that relatives as caregivers could experience 'burn out' in poor outcome cases" (1998, 1471).

There was a significant financial impact on all families caring for those with serious mental illness, including schizophrenia, and psychological distress on the part of caregivers (Ohaeri 2001; Ohaeri and Fido 2001). Considerable time may be devoted by family members to caring for the patient, often impairing their own ability to work and resulting in loss of income (Ojesina 1979; Suleiman et al. 1997; Read forthcoming). Qualitative research with families in Ghana has revealed the high emotional and financial impact of mental illness, including prolonged dependence on family care; managing agitated, antisocial, or aggressive behavior; costs of treatment; and loss of earnings of both carers and the person affected (Read forthcoming; Quinn 2007). Some family members may spend many months at prayer camps or shrines with the sick person, leading to further loss of income (Read forthcoming). The costs of treatment and of travel to treatment centers may also be considerable.

In addition to the impact of disability, including its financial burden, patients and their families may experience stigma and social exclusion. The person affected by mental illness may be unable to fulfill expected social roles and responsibilities, such as marriage and parenthood. In many societies mental illness is viewed as contagious and hereditary. Many people would be unwilling to marry someone who has experienced mental illness, particularly if they are unable to earn enough to support children (Fink 1989; Gureje et al. 2005). In West African societies marriage and bearing children is often highly valued, and someone who is unable to fulfill these social roles may not be seen as a responsible adult member of society (Appiah-Kubi 1981). Other social relationships with family, friends, and peers may well be impaired, leading to isolation. Some of those with mental illness in West Africa become vagrants (Asuni 1980; Gureje and Alem 2000; Jegede, Williams, and Sijuwola 1985). Some mentally ill vagrants may have withdrawn from society because they are unable to meet the norms of social life or maintain a livelihood, or they may be abandoned by their families. Maltreatment, such as keeping a person in chains, is common both at shrines and Christian healing centers, as well as at home (Ndetei and Mbwayo 2010; Read, Adiibokah, and Nyame 2009). Often it is a last resort by family members who must deal with symptoms of aggression, agitation, or wandering.

CONCLUSION

It is to such worlds of suffering and social exclusion that psychiatry in West Africa addresses itself, yet its impact remains barely felt in many countries, and the standard of care is sometimes little better than that provided by nonmedical healers. Whether schizophrenia exists or not in West Africa could perhaps be said to be of little import to those most affected. More important is to improve the quality of life of some of the most neglected and stigmatized members of society. To discover how to accomplish this remains the task for researchers and clinicians in the region, together with those families affected by mental illness and international collaborators who are willing to consider an African solution to what in its everyday experience is an African problem, whatever its global status. Adewunmi Olusina and Jude Ohaeri argue that "adequate and effective medical treatment is the first step towards reducing the burden of illness and improving satisfaction and the subjective quality of life (QOL) of community-living psychiatric patients, though effective treatment may also help to reduce stigma through improving the individual's level of functioning and social participation. The significant role of the family in improving outcomes for those with schizophrenia and psychoses also suggests that, where possible, mental health services should work to strengthen family support" (2003, 713).

Since its introduction into West Africa through colonial psychiatry, the diagnosis of schizophrenia has become one of the most common in the region's rare psychiatric services. However, there remain uncertainties about the validity of the diagnosis and schizophrenia's status as a chronic deteriorating condition, both internationally and locally. We suggest that an uncritical application of diagnoses derived from Euro-American psychiatric practice risks excluding or distorting the particularities of the West African experience of mental breakdown. Questions remain as to the universal usefulness of schizophrenia as a diagnosis, and it is possible that a more fluid and inclusive concept of psychosis has greater potential to reflect the experience of severe mental illness in the West African context. In addition, although taking an ethnographic approach to clinical assessment as advocated in cultural formulation may hinder the quest for objectivity in diagnosis, it may more clearly reflect the specific manifestation of psychotic illness within West African societies and thus open the way for a better understanding of sociocultural and environmental influences and implications for treatment and support.

Whatever the nosological uncertainties, it is clear that those who suffer from psychosis in West Africa face difficulties in reaching psychiatric services. Although family support and traditional and faith healers go some way toward treating psychotic illness, and there may be some spontaneous remission, many patients suffer from neglect, stigmatization, and a high level of subsequent disability. The strengthening of the mental health care systems in West African countries through initiatives such as the training of psychiatrists and psychiatric nurses, and the provision of mental health care at the community level may be the ideal, but it is evident that there are insufficient resources for comprehensive mental health care systems along the lines of those in Europe and North America. Nor is it clear that this is the most appropriate model in the West African context. Innovative approaches need to be found that draw on resources in the local environment. This may include greater engagement with traditional or religious healers and practical and educational support for families who are providing care for a mentally ill relative. There remains a need for anthropologically informed studies to examine the lived experiences of people with serious mental illness and their family members in the varying contexts of West African societies. Such studies might help elucidate the meaning of mental illness for those most nearly affected—the patient and his or her family and community. This in turn could inform the development of services that draw on local social, cultural, and material resources to respond to people's expressed needs and preferences rather than reproducing the limitations and uncertainties of European and North American practice.

NOTES

1. In Ghana this included Margaret Field, who trained first in anthropology and then in psychiatry; and Doris Mayer, who joined her husband, the anthropologist Meyer Fortes, to collect data on psychosis among the Tallensi. In Nigeria Jane Murphy conducted fieldwork with the Yoruba, in which she set out to identify local definitions of madness. She found that the Yoruba term *were* was used to identify those who in English would be termed "crazy" or "insane," and that persons thus labelled were distinguished from those who underwent spiritual experiences that may also have involved periods of deviant behavior. Based on her findings, Murphy argued that "relativism has been exaggerated" and that "in widely different cultural and environmental situations

sanity appears to be distinguishable from insanity by cues that are very similar to those used in the Western world" (1976, 1019).

2. The concept of culture-bound syndromes, one of the favorite themes of early cross-cultural psychiatry, led to some of these, including brain fag, being listed in the third edition of the DSM and the *International Statistical Classification of Diseases and Related Health Problems* (ICD), tenth edition, although not classified as standardized diagnoses. However, the concept has been heavily criticized. Some have claimed that all illnesses, including the standard psychiatric diagnoses such as schizophrenia, should be seen as culture-bound and that the notion of culture-bound syndromes serves only to exoticize psychiatric symptoms in non-Western societies. Others have argued for the inclusion of Western syndromes, such as anorexia nervosa, among the categories of culture-bound syndromes. See Tseng (2006) for an overview of these debates.

3. For example, at Accra Psychiatric Hospital in 2005 there were 511 recorded cases of schizophrenia and other psychotic disorders—the most frequently recorded diagnoses—and 639 cases recorded as "other," representing 18 percent of inpatients.

4. From the 1940s to the 1960s, a period when psychoanalysis was dominant in psychiatry, several theories were proposed to suggest that the causes of schizophrenia were intrapsychic and/or environmental. Famous among these were the "schizophrenogenic mother" and the "double bind." Such theories have largely been discredited in current psychiatric orthodoxy (see Shorter 1997, 177).

5. See also Sow (1990); Fortes and Mayer (1966). A different perspective is taken by the Ghanaian writer Ayi Kwei Armah in his novel *Fragments* (1974). He describes the disillusionment and subsequent mental breakdown of the protagonist, Baako, whose dreams of contributing to the creative development of the newly independent Ghana are frustrated by the materialistic aspirations of his relatives and fellow countrymen.

6. This view was later challenged by Field (1960), who claimed that women who confessed to witchcraft in Ghana were in fact displaying symptoms of self-reproach equivalent to depression. Raymond Prince provides a review of the literature concerning the discrepancy between writings from the colonial period, which reported a virtual absence of depression among Africans, and those of the postcolonial era, which contradicted these earlier writers. He suggests that rather than an actual increase in depression, the greater number of reported cases in the later period may result from a greater tendency among clinicians to recognize and diagnose depression. In addition, most colonial studies had used hospital-based population samples. However, it was known that those with depression were unlikely to present to psychiatric hospitals, and thus later studies that included people presenting to outpatient clinics and traditional healers had revealed more cases of depression. Prince also hypothesises that "as patients become more Westernised, so their illness patterns conform more with those of Western patients" (Prince 1967, 190).

7. Prayer camps, many established by Pentecostal churches, have proliferated in Ghana since the early 1990s. The camps usually center on a charismatic prophet or pastor who is perceived to have special healing powers and who treats a variety of illnesses, including mental ones. As in the shrines, patients may stay for many months, praying, fasting, and seeking deliverance from evil spirits (Gifford 2004; van Dijk 1997; Tetteh 1999; Meyer 1998; Larbi 2001). However, the prayer camps have been the source of some controversy, as there are reports of the use of physical restraints, beatings, neglect, and financial exploitation of patients there, who are often chained, denied shelter, and forced to fast (Commonwealth Human Rights Initiative 2008).

8. The development of the cultural formulation in the fourth edition of the DSM (DSM-IV) represented an attempt to address issues of cultural bias in the diagnosis of mental illness. However, this has not allayed concerns about the cross-cultural validity of the DSM. Indeed, members of the National Task Force on Culture and Psychiatric Diagnosis, who served as consultants in the development of DSM-IV, later heavily criticized the American Psychiatric Association for overriding many of their recommendations (Good 1996; Lewis-Fernandez 1996).

9. The "developing country" category included Columbia and India as well as Nigeria. "Developed countries" included the Soviet Union, United States, and United Kingdom.

10. Arthur Kleinman has criticized the methodology of many studies conducted under the rubric of cross-cultural psychiatry, arguing that the application of Western diagnostic categories to symptoms seen in people in non-Western societies constitutes a "category fallacy." He points out that such methodology imposes artificially stringent boundaries on what constitutes a diagnosis and thereby specifically excludes constellations of symptoms that are most influenced by culture. He suggests that "the 'ideal' cross-cultural study of schizophrenia or depression . . . would begin with detailed local phenomenological descriptions" (Kleinman 1977, 4), a point recently reiterated by Sushrut Jadhav (2004).

11. Jadhav provides an example from India that also applies to West Africa. Psychiatric professionals use textbooks written in high-income countries, and "culture blind" language in order to reduce rich local idioms—for example, of bodily experience—into standard English psychiatric terminology such as "somatisation." Thus, "local worlds, their core moral and cultural values, and the rich (non-English) vocabulary associated with bodily problems . . . are often glossed over or pruned to fit into conventional psychiatric nosology" (2004, 7). Similarly, one of the authors of this chapter (Doku) found that his psychiatric training in Ghana equipped him with more appropriate skills to assess patients in Europe than in his homeland.

12. Methods of identifying a cohort of psychotic patients without using hospital samples were employed by Tooth (1950), who consulted local chiefs to identify people in their communities considered mad, and Field (1960), who selected her cases from those attending shrines in Ghana. A later study in Ibarapa, in western Nigeria, also identified cases of psychosis at the shrines of traditional healers, as well as interviewing vagrants (Harding 1973).

13. In Ghana, for example, there are approximately 2,500 psychiatric hospital beds for a population of twenty-one million, and over 90 percent of these beds are located in three large psychiatric hospitals in the south of the country, which could take up to two days to reach for people in the north. In comparison to many West African countries, Ghana is comparatively well resourced in terms of psychiatric services (Jacob et al. 2007).

14. A notable exception is Frantz Fanon (1986, 2001), who argued extensively for the possible origins of mental illness in the experience of racism and colonialism. However, his theories on the colonial psyche were rooted in his experiences in the Antilles and colonial Algeria. Jock McCulloch criticizes Fanon's writings for ignoring differences in the colonial experience and for glossing over the organic reality of at least some of the cases Fanon treated in his clinical work. McCulloch argues that Fanon's "clinical writings do not so much provide an intricate model of the colonial personality as suggest

the existence, under colonial conditions, of a heightened propensity towards illness and breakdown" (1983, 134–35).

15. The problem of the brain drain continues. A report from 2004 states that 2,697 medical doctors who trained in West Africa (predominantly Nigeria and Ghana) are now working in the United States (Hagopian et al. 2004).

16. Lambo began his experiment in "village psychiatry" in 1954, in an attempt to draw on the resources available in village settings in Africa. Suitable patients from the hospital in Aro, Nigeria, were sent to live with their families in village locations close to the hospital where they could also consult with traditional healers. They continued to come to the hospital for consultation and treatment such as medication. Aspects of this system were replicated in Benin city in Nigeria (Asuni 1979), Senegal (Collomb 1976), and Tanzania (Swift 1976).

REFERENCES

Adewuya, A. O., R. O. Makanjuola. 2005. "Social Distance towards People with Mental Illness amongst Nigerian University Students." *Social Psychiatry and Psychiatric Epidemiology* 40 (11): 865–68.

Adomako, C. C. 1972. "Mental Hospital Patients: A Castle Road Profile." *Ghana Medical Journal* 11 (2): 65–71.

Aina, O. F. 2004. "Mental Illness and Cultural Issues in West African Films: Implications for Orthodox Psychiatric Practice." *Medical Humanities* 30 (1): 23–26.

Alem, A. 2002. "Community-Based vs. Hospital-Based Mental Health Care: The Case of Africa." *World Psychiatry* 1 (2): 98–99.

Allardyce, J., W. Gaebel, J. Zielasek, and J.van Os. 2007. "Deconstructing Psychosis Conference February 2006: The Validity of Schizophrenia and Alternative Approaches to the Classification of Psychosis." *Schizophrenia Bulletin* 33 (4): 863–67.

Appiah-Kubi, K. 1981. *Man Cures, God Heals: Religion and Medical Practice among the Akans of Ghana*. Allanheld, NJ: Osmun.

Appiah-Poku, J., R. Laugharne, E. Mensah, Y. Osei, and T. Burns. 2004. "Previous Help Sought by Patients Presenting to Mental Health Services in Kumasi, Ghana." *Social Psychiatry and Psychiatric Epidemiology* 39 (3): 208–11.

Armah, A. K. 1974. *Fragments*. London: Heinemann.

Asuni, T. 1979. "Therapeutic Communities of the Hospital and Villages in Aro Hospital Complex in Nigeria." *African Journal of Psychiatry* 1 (2): 35–42.

———. 1980. "Vagrant Psychotics in Abeokuta." *African Journal of Psychiatry* 6 (3–4): 15–23.

Barbato, A. 1998. *Schizophrenia and Public Health*. Geneva: World Health Organization.

Bayart, J.-F. 2000. "Africa in the World: A History of Extraversion." *African Affairs* 99 (395): 217–67.

Beiser, M., W. A. Burr, J.-L. Ravel, and H. Collomb. 1973. "Illnesses of the Spirit among the Serer of Senegal." *American Journal of Psychiatry* 130 (8): 881–86.

Bell, L. V. 1991. *Mental and Social Disorder in Sub-Saharan Africa: The Case of Sierra Leone, 1787–1990*. New York: Greenwood.

Burnham, P. 1987. "Changing Themes in the Analysis of African Marriage." In *Transformations in African Marriage,* edited by D. Parkin and D. Nyamwaya, 37–54. Manchester, UK: Manchester University Press.

Carothers, J. C. 1947. "A Study of Mental Derangement in Africans, and an Attempt to Explain Its Peculiarities, More Especially in Relation to the African Attitude to Life." *Journal of Mental Science* 93: 548–97.

———. 1953. *The African Mind in Health and Disease: A Study in Ethnopsychiatry*. Geneva: World Health Organization.

Cohen, A. 1992. "Prognosis for Schizophrenia in the Third World: A Re-Evaluation of Cross-Cultural Research." *Culture, Medicine and Psychiatry* 16 (1): 53–57.

Cohen, A., V. Patel, R. Thara, and O. Gureje. 2008. "Questioning an Axiom: Better Prognosis for Schizophrenia in the Developing World?" *Schizophrenia Bulletin* 34 (2): 249–50.

Collins, P. Y, N. N. Wig, R. Day, V. K. Varma, S. Malhotra, A. K. Misra, B. Schanzer, and E. Susser. 1996. "Psychosocial and Biological Aspects of Acute Brief Psychoses in Three Developing Country Sites." *Psychiatric Quarterly* 67 (3): 177–93.

Collomb, H. 1965. "Bouffées délirantes en psychiatrie Africaine." *Psychopathologie Africaine* 1 (1): 167–239.

———. 1975. "Histoire de la psychiatrie en Afrique Noire Francophone." *African Journal of Psychiatry* 1 (2): 87–115.

———. 1976. "Le besoin et la demande pour une assistance psychiatrique." *African Journal of Psychiatry* 1: 95–102.

Commonwealth Human Rights Initiative. 2008. "Human Rights Violations in Prayer Camps and Access to Mental Health in Ghana." Accra: Commonwealth Human Rights Initiative Africa, 2008.

Copeland, J. R. M. 1968. "Aspects of Mental Illness in West African Students." *Social Psychiatry and Psychiatric Epidemiology* 3 (1): 7–13.

Cunyngham-Brown, R. 1937. *Report on Mission to the British Colonies of the West Coast of Africa on the Care and Treatment of Lunatics: The Gold Coast Colony*. London: Crown Agents.

Davidson, L., and T. H. McGlashan. 1997. "The Varied Outcomes of Schizophrenia." *Canadian Journal of Psychiatry* 42 (1): 34–43.

de Jong, J. T. V. M., and I. H. Komproe. 2006. "A 15-Year Open Study on a Cohort of West-African Out-Patients with a Chronic Psychosis." *Social Psychiatry and Psychiatric Epidemiology* 41 (11): 897–903.

de Jong, J. T. V. M., and M. Van Ommeren. 2002. "Toward a Culture-Informed Epidemiology: Combining Qualitative and Quantitative Research in Transcultural Contexts." *Transcultural Psychiatry* 39 (4): 422–33.

de-Graft Aikins, A. 2005. "Healer-Shopping in Africa: New Evidence from a Rural-Urban Qualitative Study of Ghanaian Diabetes Experiences." *British Medical Journal* 331 (7519): 737–43.

Demerath, N. J. 1942. "Schizophrenia among Primitives: The Present Status of Sociological Research." *American Journal of Psychiatry* 98 (5): 703–707.

Diop, D., and M. Dores. 1976. "L'admission d'un acccompagnant du malade a l'hôpital psychiatrique." *African Journal of Psychiatry* 2 (1): 119–30.

Doku, V. 2005. "Risk Factors for Schizophrenia in Rural Ghana." Unpublished manuscript.

Dolder, C. R., J. P. Lacro, L. B. Dunn, and D. V. Jeste. 2002. "Antipsychotic Medication Adherence: Is There a Difference between Typical and Atypical Agents?" *American Journal of Psychiatry* 159 (1): 103–108.

Dutta, R., T. Greene, J. Addington, K. McKenzie, M. Phillips, and R. M Murray. 2007. "Biological, Life Course, and Cross-Cultural Studies All Point toward the Value of Dimensional and Developmental Ratings in the Classification of Psychosis." *Schizophrenia Bulletin* 33 (4): 868–76.

Ebigbo, P. 1982. "Development of a Culture Specific (Nigeria) Screening Scale of Somatic Complaints Indicating Psychiatric Disturbance." *Culture, Medicine and Psychiatry* 6 (1): 29–43.

Edgerton, R. B. 1980. "Traditional Treatment for Mental Illness in Africa: A Review." *Culture, Medicine and Psychiatry* 4 (2): 167–89.

Edgerton, R. B., and A. Cohen. 1994. "Culture and Schizophrenia: The DOSMD Challenge." *British Journal of Psychiatry* 164 (23): 222–31.

Fanon, F. 1986. *Black Skin, White Masks*. Translated by Charles Lam Markmann. London: Pluto.

———. 2001. *The Wretched of the Earth*. Translated by Constance Farrington. London: Penguin.

Faris, R. E. L. 1934. "Some Observations on the Incidence of Schizophrenia in Primitive Societies." *Journal of Abnormal and Social Psychology* 29 (1): 30–31.

Farmer, A. E., and W. F. Falkowski. 1985. "Maggot in the Salt, the Snake Factor and the Treatment of Atypical Psychosis in West African Women." *British Journal of Psychiatry* 146 (4): 446–48.

Fernando, S. 1991. *Mental Health, Race and Culture*. London: Macmillan.

Field, M. J. 1958. "Mental Disorder in Rural Ghana." *Journal of Mental Science* 104 (437): 1043–51.

———. 1960. *Search for Security: An Ethno-Psychiatric Study of Rural Ghana*. London: Faber and Faber.

———. 1968. "Chronic Psychosis in Rural Ghana." *British Journal of Psychiatry* 114 (506): 31–33.

Fink, H. E. 1989. *Religion, Disease and Healing in Ghana: A Case Study of Traditional Dormaa Medicine*. Munich, Germany: Trickster Wissenschaft.

Forster, E. B. 1958. "A Short Psychiatric Review from Ghana." In *Health, Mental Disorders and Mental Health in Africa South of the Sahara CCTA/CSA-WFMH-WHO Meeting of Specialists on Mental Health*, 37–41. Bukavu, Democratic Republic of Congo: Commission for Technical Co-Operation South of the Sahara.

———. 1962. "The Theory and Practice of Psychiatry in Ghana." *American Journal of Psychotherapy* 16 (1): 7–51.

Fortes, M., and D. Y. Mayer. 1966. "Psychosis and Social Change among the Tallensi of Northern Ghana." *Cahier D'Etudes Africaines* 6 (21): 5–40.

Franklin, R. R., D. Sarr, M. Gueye, O. Sylla, and R. Collignon. 1996. "Cultural Response to Mental Illness in Senegal: Reflection through Patient Companions—Part 1. Methods and Descriptive Data." *Social Science and Medicine* 42 (3): 325–38.

German, G. A. 1972. "Aspects of Clinical Psychiatry in Sub-Saharan Africa." *British Journal of Psychiatry* 121 (564): 461–79.

———. 1987. "Mental Health in Africa." *British Journal of Psychiatry* 151 (4): 435–46.

German, G. A., and A. C. Raman. 1976. "From Birth to Maturity: Historical Aspects of the Association of Psychiatrists in Africa." *African Journal of Psychiatry* 2:255–65.

Gesler, W. M., and E. A. Nahim. 1984. "Client Characteristics at Kissy Mental Hospital, Freetown, Sierra Leone." *Social Science and Medicine* 18 (10): 819–25.

Gifford, P. 2004. *Ghana's New Christianity: Pentecostalism in a Globalising African Economy*. London: Hurst.

Good, B. J. 1996. "Culture and DSM-IV: Diagnosis, Knowledge and Power." *Culture, Medicine and Psychiatry* 20: 127–32.

Gureje, O., Y. A. Aderibigbe, and O. Obikoya. 1995. "Three Syndromes in Schizophrenia: Validity in Young Patients with Recent Onset of Illness." *Psychological Medicine* 25 (4): 715–25.

Gureje, O., and A. Adewunmi. 1988. "Life Events and Schizophrenia in Nigerians: A Controlled Investigation." *British Journal of Psychiatry* 153 (3): 376–75.

Gureje, O., and A. Alem. 2000. "Mental Health Policy Development in Africa." *Bulletin of the World Health Organization* 78 (4): 475–82.

Gureje, O., and R. Bamidele. 1999. "Thirteen-Year Outcome among Nigerian Outpatients with Schizophrenia." *Social Psychiatry and Psychiatric Epidemiology* 34 (3): 147–51.

Gureje, O., V. O. Lasebikan, O. Ephraim-Oluwanuga, B. O. Olley, and L. Kola. 2005. "Community Knowledge of and Attitude to Mental Illness in Nigeria." *British Journal of Psychiatry* 186 (5): 436–41.

Gureje, O., V. O. Lasebikan, L. Kola, and V. A. Makanjuola. 2006. "Lifetime and 12-Month Prevalence of Mental Disorders in the Nigerian Survey of Mental Health and Well-Being." *British Journal of Psychiatry* 188 (5): 465–71.

Hagopian, A., M. J. Thompson, M. Fordyce, K. E. Johnson, and L. G. Hart. 2004. "The Migration of Physicians from Sub-Saharan Africa to the United States of America." *Human Resources for Health* 2(1): 17.

Harding, T. W. 1973. "Psychosis in a Rural West African Community." *Social Psychiatry* 8 (4): 198–203.

Harrison, G., K. Hopper, T. Craig, E. Laska, C. Siegel, J. Wanderling, K. C. Dube, and K. Ganev. 2001. "Recovery from Psychotic Illness: A 15- and 25-Year International Follow-Up Study." *British Journal of Psychiatry* 178 (6): 506–17.

Heward-Mills, Dag. *Demons and How to Deal with Them*. Accra: Parchment House, 2005.

Ikwuagwu, P. U., J. C. Nafziger, U. H. Iheuze, and J. U. Ohaeri. 1994. "A Study of the Social and Clinical Characteristics of In-Patients at a Psychiatric Unit in Northern Nigeria." *West African Journal of Medicine* 13 (4): 191–95.

Ilechukwu, S. T. C. 1991. "Psychiatry in Africa: Special Problems and Unique Features." *Transcultural Psychiatric Research Review* 28 (3): 169–308.

Imade, A. G. T., and J. C. Ebie. 1991. "A Retrospective Study of Symptom Patterns of Cannabis-Induced Psychosis." *Acta Psychiatrica Scandinavia* 83 (2): 134–36.

Jablensky, A. 1997. "The 100-Year Epidemiology of Schizophrenia." *Schizophrenia Research* 28 (2): 111–25.

Jablensky, A., N. Sartorius, G. Ernberg, M. Anker, A. Korten, J. E. Cooper, R. Day, A. Bertelsen. 1992. "Schizophrenia: Manifestations, Incidence and Course in Different Cultures, A World Health Organization Ten-Country Study," *Psychological Medicine Monograph Supplement* 20 (1): 1–97.

Jacob, K. S., P. Sharan, I. Mirza, M. Garrido-Cumbrera, S. Seedat, J. J. Mari, V. Sreenivas, and Shekhar Saxena. 2007. "Mental Health Systems in Countries: Where Are We Now?" *Lancet* 370 (9592): 1061–77.

Jadhav, S. 2004. "How 'Culture-Bound' Is 'Cultural Psychiatry'?" *International Psychiatry* 4 (April): 6–7.

Jahoda, G. 1979. "Traditional Healers and Other Institutions Concerned with Mental Illness in Ghana." In *African Therapeutic Systems,* edited by Z. Ademuwagun, J.A. Ayoade, I. E. Harrison, and D. M. Warren, 98–109. Waltham, MA: African Studies Association.

Jegede, R.O., A. O. Williams, and A. O. Sijuwola. 1985. "Recent Developments in the Care, Treatment, and Tehabilitation of the Chronically Mentally Ill in Nigeria." *Hospital and Community Psychiatry* 36 (6): 658–61.

Jilek, W. G. 1995. "Emil Kraepelin and Comparative Sociocultural Psychiatry." *European Archives of Psychiatry and Clinical Neuroscience* 245 (4–5): 231–38.

Kabir, M., Z. Iliyasu, I. Abubakar, and M. Aliyu. 2004. "Perception and Beliefs about Mental Illness among Adults in Karfi Village, Northern Nigeria." *BMC International Health and Human Rights* 4 (1): 3.

Keller, R. 2001. "Madness and Colonization: Psychiatry in the British and French Empires, 1800–1962." *Journal of Social History* 35 (2): 295–326.

Kirmayer, L. J., and H. Minas. 2000. "The Future of Cultural Psychiatry: An International Perspective." *Canadian Journal of Psychiatry* 45 (5): 438–46.

Kleinman, A. 1977. "Depression, Somatization and the 'New Cross-Cultural Psychiatry.'" *Social Science and Medicine* 11 (1): 3–10.

Kohn, R., S. Saxena, I. Levav, and B. Saraceno. 2004. "The Treatment Gap in Mental Health Care." *Bulletin of the World Health Organization* 82 (11): 858–66.

Lambo, T. A. 1955. "The Role of Cultural Factors in Paranoid Psychosis among the Yoruba Tribe." *Journal of Nervous and Mental Disease* 101 (423): 239–66.

———. 1962. *African Traditional Beliefs, Concepts of Health and Medical Practice.* Ibadan, Nigeria: Philosophical Society, University of Ibadan.

———. 1965. "Medical and Social Problems of Drug Addiction in West Africa (with Special Emphasis on Psychiatric Aspects)." *United Nations Bulletin on Narcotics* 17 (1): 3–13.

———. 1981. "Mental Health of Man in Africa." *African Affairs* 80 (319): 277–88.

Lamptey, J. J. 1977. "Patterns of Psychiatric Consultations at the Accra Psychiatric Hospital in Ghana." *African Journal of Psychiatry* 3: 123–27.

Langness, L. L. 1967. "Hysterical Psychosis: The Cross-Cultural Evidence." *American Journal of Psychiatry* 124 (2): 143–52.

Larbi, E. K. *Pentecostalism: The Eddies of Ghanaian Christianity.* Accra: Centre for Pentecostal and Charismatic Studies, 2001.

Leighton, A. H., T. A. Lambo, C. C. Hughes, D. C. Leighton, J. M. Murphy, and D. B. Macklin. 1963. "Psychiatric Disorder in West Africa." *American Journal of Psychiatry* 120 (6): 521–27.

Lewis-Fernandez, R. 1996. "Cultural Formulation of Psychiatric Diagnosis." *Culture, Medicine and Psychiatry* 20: 133–44.

Lin, T. 1962. "The Role of Epidemiology in Transcultural Psychiatry." *Acta Psychiatrica Scandinavica* 38 (3): 158–63.

Littlewood, R. 1990. "From Categories to Contexts: A Decade of the 'New Cross-Cultural Psychiatry.'" *British Journal of Psychiatry* 156 (3): 308–27.

Littlewood, R., and M. Lipsedge. 1997. *Aliens and Alienists: Ethnic Minoirities and Psychiatry.* 3rd ed. Hove, UK: Brunner Routledge.

Lucas, R. H., and R. J. Barrett. 1995. "Interpreting Culture and Psychopathology: Primitivist Themes in Cross-Cultural Debate." *Culture, Medicine and Psychiatry* 19 (3): 287–326.

"The Mantle of Mental Health Recovery." 2005. *Ghanaian Chronicle,* October 27.

Martyns-Yellowe, I. 1992. "The Burden of Schizophrenia on the Family: A Study from Nigeria." *British Journal of Psychiatry* 161 (6): 779–82.

Mateus, M. D., J. Q. dos Santos, and J. de Jesus Mari. 2005. "Popular Conceptions of Schizophrenia in Cape Verde, Africa." *Revista Brasileira de Psiquiatria* 27(2): 101–107.

McCulloch, J. 1983. *Black Soul White Artifact: Fanon's Clinical Psychology and Social Theory.* Cambridge: Cambridge University Press.

———. 1995. *Colonial Psychiatry and "The African Mind."* Cambridge: Cambridge University Press.

Meyer, B. 1998. "'Make a Complete Break with the Past': Memory and Postcolonial Modernity in Ghanaian Pentecostalist Discourse." *Journal of Religion in Africa* 28 (3): 316–49.

Mullings, L. 1984. *Therapy, Ideology and Social Change: Mental Healing in Urban Ghana.* Berkeley: University of California Press.Murphy, J. M. 1976. Psychiatric labelling in cross-cultural perspective. *Science* 191 (4231): 1019–28.

Ndetei, D. M, and A. W.Mbwayo. 2010. "Another Side of African Psychiatry in the 21st Century—Chaining as Containment." *African Journal of Psychiatry* 13:3–5.

Odejide, A. O., L. K. Oyewunmi, and J. U. Ohaeri. 1989. "Psychiatry in Africa: An Overview." *American Journal of Psychiatry* 146 (6): 708–16.

Ohaeri, J. U. 1998. "Perception of the Social Support Role of the Extended Family Network by Some Nigerians with Schizophrenia and Affective Disorders." *Social Science and Medicine* 47 (10): 1463–72.

———. 2000. "Caregiver Burden and Psychotic Patients' Perception of Social Support in a Nigerian Setting." *Social Psychiatry and Psychiatric Epidemiology* 36: 86–93.

———. 2001. "Caregiver Burden and Psychotic Patients' Perception of Social Support in a Nigerian Setting." *Social Psychiatry and Psychiatric Epidemiology* 36 (2): 86–93.

Ohaeri, J. U., and J. D. Adeyemi. 1990. "The Pattern of Somatization Symptoms at the Ibadan Teaching Hospital Psychiatric Clinic." *West African Journal of Medicine* 9 (1): 26–34.

Ohaeri, J. U., and A. A. Fido. 2001. "The Opinion of Caregivers on Aspects of Schizophrenia and Major Affective Disorders in a Nigerian Setting." *Social Psychiatry and Psychiatric Epidemiology* 36 (10): 493–99.

Ojesina, J. O. 1979. "Some Social and Psychological Problems of Schizophrenics in Nigeria." *African Journal of Psychiatry* 5 (3–4): 97–101.

Okulate, G. T., and O. B. E. Jones. 2003. "Auditory Hallucinations in Schizophrenic and Affective Disorder Nigerian Patients: Phenomenological Comparison." *Transcultural Psychiatry* 40 (4): 531–41.

Olusina, A. K., and J. U. Ohaeri. 2003. "Quality of Life of Recently Discharged Nigerian Psychiatric Patients." *Social Psychiatry and Psychiatric Epidemiology* 38 (12): 707–14.

Osei, A. O. 2001. "Types of Psychiatric Illness at Traditional Healing Centres in Ghana." *Ghana Medical Journal* 35 (3): 106–10.

Patel, V., R. Araya, S. Chatterjee, D.Chisholm, A. Cohen, M. De Silva, C. Hosman, H. McGuire, G. Rojas, and M. van Ommeren. 2007. "Treatment and Prevention of Mental Disorders in Low-Income and Middle-Income Countries." *Lancet* 370 (9591): 991–1005.

Prince, R. 1960a. "The 'Brain Fag' Syndrome in Nigerian Students." *Journal of Mental Science* 106 (443): 559–70.

———. 1960b. "The Use of Rauwolfia for the Treatment of Psychoses by Nigerian Native Doctors." *American Journal of Psychiatry* 117 (2): 147–49.

———. 1967. "The Changing Picture of Depressive Syndromes in Africa: Is It Fact or Diagnostic Fashion?" *Canadian Journal of African Studies* 1 (2): 177–92.

Quinn, N. 2007. "Beliefs and Community Responses to Mental Illness in Ghana: The Experiences of Family Carers." *International Journal of Social Psychiatry* 53 (2): 175–88.

Read, U. M. 2012a. "Between Chains and Vagrancy: Living with Mental Illness in Kintampo, Ghana." Ph. D. diss., University College London.

———. 2012b. "'I Want the One That Will Heal Me Completely So It Won't Come Back Again': The Limits of Antipsychotic Medication in Rural Ghana." *Transcultural Psychiatry* 49 (3): 1–23.

———. Forthcoming. "'No Matter How The Child Is, She Is Hers': Practical Kinship in the Care of Mental Illness in Kintampo, Ghana." *Ghana Studies*.

Read, U. M., E. Adiibokah, and S. Nyame. 2009. "Local Suffering and the Global Discourse of Mental Health and Human Rights: An Ethnographic Study of Responses to Mental Illness in Rural Ghana." *Globalisation and Health* 5:13.

Rolfe, M., C. M. Tang, S. Sabally, J. E. Todd, E. B. Sam, and A. B. Hatib N'Jie. 1993. "Psychosis and Cannabis Abuse in the Gambia: A Case-Control Study." *British Journal of Psychiatry* 163 (6): 798–801.

Sadowsky, J. 1999. *Bedlam: Institutions of Colonial Madness in Southwest Nigeria.* Berkeley: University of California Press.

———. 2004. "Symptoms of Colonialism: Context and Content of Delusion in South West Nigeria, 1945–1960." In *Schizophrenia, Culture and Subjectivity: The Edge of Experience,* edited by J. H. Jenkins and R. J. Barrett, 238–52. Cambridge: Cambridge University Press.

Saraceno, B., I. Levav, and R. Kohn. 2005. "The Public Mental Health Significance of Research on Socio-Economic Factors in Schizophrenia and Major Depression." *World Psychiatry* 4 (3): 181–85.

Saxena, S., G. Thornicroft, M. Knapp, and H. Whiteford. 2007. "Resources for Mental Health: Scarcity, Inequity and Inefficiency." *Lancet* 370 (9590): 878–89.

Seligman, C. G. 1932. "Anthropological Perspective and Psychological Theory." *Journal of the Royal Anthropological Institute of Great Britain and Ireland* 62 (July–December): 193–228.

Shorter, E. 1997. *A History of Psychiatry: From the Era of the Asylum to the Age of Prozac.* New York: John Wiley and Sons.

Sijuwola, O. A. 1986. "Comparative Study of Psychosis Associated with Cannabis." *West African Journal of Medicine* 5 (4): 271–76.

Sow, A. I. 1990. *Anthropological Structures of Madness in Black Africa.* Translated by Joyce Diamanti. New York: International Universities Press.

Suleiman, T. G., J. U. Ohaeri, R. A. Lawal, A. Y. Haruna, and O. B. Orija.. 1997. "Financial Cost of Treating Out-Patients with Schizophrenia in Nigeria." *British Journal of Psychiatry* 171 (4): 364–68.

Swift, C. R. 1976. "Mental Health Programming in a Developing Country: Any Relevance Elsewhere?" *African Journal of Psychiatry* 1: 79–86.

Tandon, R., W. Gaebel, D. M. Barch, J. Bustillo, R. E. Gur, S. Heckers, D. Malaspina, et al. 2013. "Definition and Description of Schizophrenia in the DSM-5." *Schizophrenia Research* 150 (1): 3–10.

Tetteh, J N. 1999. "The Dynamics of Prayer Camps and the Management of Women's Problems: A Case Study of Three Camps in the Eastern Region of Ghana." MPhil thesis, University of Ghana.

Tooth, G. 1950. *Studies in Mental Illness in the Gold Coast.* London: Her Majesty's Stationery Office.

Tseng, W.-S. 2006. "From Peculiar Psychiatric Disorders through Culture-Bound Syndromes to Culture-Related Specific Syndromes." *Transcultural Psychiatry* 43 (4): 554–76.

Turkson, S. N. A. 1998. "Psychiatric Diagnosis among Referred Patients in Ghana." *East Africa Medical Journal* 75 (6): 336–38.

Ugorji, R. U., and O. U. E. Ofem. 1976. "The Concept of Mental Illness among the Yakkur of Nigeria." *African Journal of Psychiatry* 2: 295–98.

Ukpong, D. I. 2006. "Demographic Factors and Clinical Correlates of Burden and Distress in Relatives of Service Users Experiencing Schizophrenia: A Study from South-Western Nigeria." *International Journal of Mental Health Nursing* 15 (1): 54–59.

United Nations Office for West Africa. 2006. *Youth Unemployment and Regional Insecurity in West Africa.* Dakar, Senegal: United Nations Office for West Africa.

van Dijk, R. 1997. "From Camp to Encompassment: Discourses of Transsubjectivity in the Ghananian Pentecostal Diaspora." *Journal of Religion in Africa* 27 (2): 135–59.

Vaughan, M. 1991. *Curing Their Ills: Colonial Power and African Illness.* Oxford: Polity.

Weinberg, S. K. 1965. "Cultural Aspects of Manic-Depression in West Africa." *Journal of Health and Human Behavior* 6 (4): 247–53.

Westermeyer, J., and A. Janca. 1997. "Language, Culture and Psychopathology: Conceptual and Methodological Issues." *Transcultural Psychiatry* 34 (3): 291–311.

Wiley-Exley, E. 2007. "Evaluations of Community Mental Health Care in Low- and Middle-Income Countries: A 10-Year Review of the Literature." *Social Science and Medicine* 64 (6): 1231–41.

Williams, C. C. 2003. "Re-Reading the IPSS Research Record." *Social Science and Medicine* 56: 501–15.

World Health Organization. 2000. *Disability Assessment Schedule: WHO-DAS II.* Geneva: World Health Organization.

———. 2001. *Mental Health: New Understanding, New Hope.* Geneva: World Health Organization.

———. 2004. *World Mental Health Survey Consortium.* Geneva: World Health Organization.

Yeboah, B. Kwaku. 1994. "The Mframah Shrine and the Practice of Contemporary Social Work. *Journal of Black Studies* 24 (3): 290–307.

4 MENTAL ILLNESS AND DESTITUTION IN GHANA
A Social-Psychological Perspective

AMA DE-GRAFT AIKINS

> In several parts of the town [Accra] mentally deranged people, almost all of them men, are seen semi-clothed or naked, their hair and skin caked with dirt. This points to a need for greater institutional provisions. At present, unless such people become dangerous, they are left in the town where they sleep in the open, begging or stealing food.
>
> —Ione Acquah, *Accra Survey*

THE AFRICAN LITERATURE on mental illness and destitution has limited itself to "vagrant psychotics." A typical definition of a vagrant psychotic would be the one that guided Taha Baasher and colleagues in their work in Lesotho and Egypt in the 1980s: "A person who was without permanent accommodation, employment, money or regular sources of food and who lived a socially and geographically unsettled life. He should also manifest gross abnormality of behaviour in such a way that his general conduct, emotional reactions, or cognitive functions were such that a psychotic illness could clearly be established" (1983, 35).

In that cross-country study—and in other studies on "vagrant psychotics" elsewhere in Africa, such as Nigeria (Asuni 1971), Ghana (Acquah 1958) and Sierra Leone (Bell 1991)—evidence suggests that although all vagrants are characterized by "socially and geographically unsettled" lives, not all vagrants are psychotics. Of the sixty-seven vagrants that Baasher and colleagues interviewed in Maseru, Lesotho, in the 1980s, "approximately half of these were psychotic and appeared to subsist by begging. At least two were alcoholics and two epileptics. The remainder were beggars without an immediately apparent physical or mental handicap" (1983, 35). In Ghana's capital, Accra, a survey was conducted by the country's Department of Social Welfare in 1953 to capture profiles of "others who wander about the streets of the municipality in an apparent state of destitution"

(Acquah 1958, 81). The survey identified 170 destitute individuals and grouped them into three categories: the economically destitute, the disabled destitute, and the mentally ill destitute. The mentally ill destitute were largely "feeble minded" and "senile" (ibid.); none was psychotic.

More compelling evidence comes from official efforts in a number of African countries to rid major cities of vagrants and beggars prior to important national events. Baasher and colleagues (1983) report that in Addis Ababa in 1973, 650 beggars were cleared from the streets prior to the tenth anniversary of the founding of the Organization of African Unity, and only 5 percent of these were chronic psychotics. In Ghana over the last few decades, official efforts to clear city streets of vagrants prior to important national events, such as the fiftieth anniversary of Ghana's independence in March 2007, has resulted in a mix of former psychotic or schizophrenic patients, disabled beggars, and filthy—but quite mentally healthy—car mechanics ending up in overcrowded hospital wards.

The literature suggests, therefore, that using the term "vagrant psychotics" is limiting. The state of vagrancy may cause psychological distress and physical want, stress, and disorders,[1] but it does not necessarily always coincide with psychosis. Thus using "vagrant psychotics" as a conceptual lens excludes other categories of mentally ill groups whose members may choose a life of vagrancy or have that life imposed on them. In this chapter the term "mentally ill destitute" is adopted. The use of "mentally ill" moves empirical attention beyond psychosis and includes a wider range of mental illnesses that may result in destitution. In *The African Poor*, John Iliffe distinguishes between structural and conjunctural poverty. Structural poverty refers to "long-term poverty of individuals due to their personal or social circumstances," while conjunctural poverty refers to "temporary poverty into which ordinarily self-sufficient people may be thrown by crisis" (1987, 4). Iliffe also distinguishes between the poor and the destitute (very poor) in Africa. The African poor have struggled "continuously to preserve themselves and their dependents from physical want," but the destitute have "*permanently or temporarily* failed in that struggle and have fallen into physical want" (2; emphasis added). Iliffe describes the social reality of the destitute as one marked by extreme material deprivation (through personal misfortune or exclusion of themselves from land and labor), psychological struggles (with solitude, neglect, and chronic want), and psychological strength (resilience in the face of adversity). In this complex psychological, material, and structural formulation, "destitution" has a broader empirical reach than "vagrancy." It encompasses the classic vagrant psychotic, as well as those at risk of vagrancy and those who weave in and out of vagrancy. It also draws attention to other forms of "socially and geographically unsettled" lives that may not be as publicly visible as vagrancy, such as sequential institutionalization in pluralistic mental health systems.

RESEARCH QUESTIONS AND CONCEPTUAL FRAMEWORK

This chapter explores the context of destitution for mentally ill individuals in Ghana through a social-psychological lens. It addresses the following questions:

1. Which groups of mentally ill individuals are at risk of destitution?
2. What factors mediate the relationship between mental illness and destitution?
3. What can experiences of actual and potential mentally ill destitutes teach us about preventing destitution and/or minimizing its impact on the mentally ill?
4. What is the state of current interventions for the (potential) mentally ill destitute, and what are the future challenges?

Baasher and colleagues note that vagrancy is "dependent on the complex interaction of personal characteristics and social conditions" (1983, 30). Examining this "complex interaction" requires a systematic approach. The classical social psychology approach to everyday experiences situates its level of analysis at the interface of the individual and society (see, for example, Bartlett 1932; Doise 1986; Markova 2003). Based on the premise that there is a mutual relationship between the individual and his or her society, this approach aims to "conceptualise, simultaneously, both the power of society and the agency of individuals" (Gervais, Morant, and Penn 1999, 422). Willem Doise provides a useful typology of this approach when he identifies four interrelated levels of analyses that social psychologists must be concerned with:

1. The "intra-personal" or the intrasubjective level, which shapes the "mechanisms by which the individual organises her/his experience" (1986, 11).
2. The "inter-personal" or the intersubjective level, where "the dynamics of the relations [are] established at a given moment by given individuals in a given situation" (12).
3. The social (group) level, where "the social experiences and social positions of subjects" are determined (14).
4. The "ideological" or structural level, where societal "ideologies, systems of beliefs and representations, values and norms, which validate and maintain the established social order" play a role (15).

To understand the relationships between mental illness and destitution, it is important to keep the experience of mental illness at the forefront. In the literatures of social psychology and the sociology of illness, chronic illness causes biographical disruption. The sociologist Michael Bury (1982) defines biographical disruption as the disruption that chronic illness causes to both the physical body and the life trajectory of the sufferer. In the case of mental illness, disruption would also affect a third area: the mind or psyche. Biographical disruption draws attention to the interrelationship between self and illness, on the one hand, and that between the ill self and society, on the other hand.

In terms of the self-illness relation, the individual has to deal with the symptoms, impairments, and/or disabilities the illness brings, as well as the course and impact of treatment.[2] A mentally ill individual living with depression, for example, has to deal with the physical symptoms of depression—such as listlessness, sleeplessness, and undereating or overeating—as well as coping with medical treatment and its potential side effects. Although the relationship of self to illness is a crucial dimension of the chronic illness experience, the chronically ill "live with illness in a world of health" (Radley 1994, 136). This brings the self-society relationship to the fore. The experience of illness is not only informed by the biophysical aspect. It is also structured by shared ideas circulating within society about the body, health, illness, life, and death (Kleinman 1988; Bury 1997). The impairments and disabilities that an individual may experience do not remain private individual matters. They become focal points around which societal perceptions, responses, and relationships revolve and are reshaped. The changes can have a profound impact on shared experiences, role expectations, values, and identities. Kathy Charmaz's (1983, 1991) social-psychological study of disability introduced the notion of "loss of self." "Loss of self" constitutes four social-psychological conditions that mediate—in interconnecting ways—the relationship between self and society. First, there is the impact of living a restricted life, which comes into play particularly in cases where illness brings about disability, and the lack of mobility causes an individual to be homebound. Second, there is a sense of social isolation. Fears and anxieties may arise from feeling or being made to feel by others that one's social worth is diminished. Third, individuals experience discrediting definitions of self or negative feelings about the self. Such negative sentiments are strongly linked to the difficulties of having a handicap in one's own life and one's community.[3] They occur when others react negatively to the individual's condition, especially when the condition reshapes his or her physical identity or when the condition is stigmatized. Fourth, there is the fear of becoming a burden on family, friends, and caregivers. When their illness becomes debilitating, individuals may find themselves unable to fulfill their formerly ascribed social roles and obligations and can no longer "claim with authority the identities that are based on doing these things" (Radley 1994, 148). This creates a feeling of being useless both to one's self and to others, which may in turn have a negative impact on the capabilities of caregivers. Family relationships can become strained as a result.

Using Doise's multilevel typology of the individual-society interface and Bury's concept of biographical disruption, the mental illness and destitution relation can be conceptualized at four interrelated levels (table 4.1). This multilevel conceptualization guides the discussion in the rest of this chapter.

Table 4.1. A Multilevel Conceptualization of the Relationship
between Mental Illness and Destitution

LEVEL OF ANALYSIS	KEY DIMENSIONS
Intrasubjective	Biographical disruption caused to body, mind, and life trajectory by the illness and the individual's responses to biographical disruption
Intersubjective	Shared responses to biographical disruption by sufferers and significant others, caregivers, or health care providers
Social (group)	Community and other social ideas about, and responses to, the illness category and the ill individual
Structural	Structural context of mental illness (for example, poverty, social exclusion, and a stressful workplace); established sociocultural or sociopolitical social orders regarding responses to and caring for the mentally ill

The chapter is divided into three main parts. The first part describes the contexts of destitution for mentally ill individuals in Ghana with a range of diagnoses, including psychosis, and it draws on expert and insider accounts of this phenomenon. It examines the way that intrasubjective, intersubjective, group, and structural processes mediate destitution or destitution risk. The second part focuses on the profiles and experiences of two categories of the mentally ill destitute: vagrants and "revolving door" patients. The experiences of these groups illuminate the complex relationship between structural poverty, mental illness, and destitution and offer insights into preventing and/or minimizing the impact of destitution on the mentally ill. The third part presents and discusses three sets of past and current interventions to address destitution among the mentally ill in Ghana: village settlements, Christian outreach interventions, and humanitarian and rights-based approaches offered by mental health nongovernmental organizations (NGOs). I conclude the chapter by considering challenges for the future of the mentally ill destitute in Ghana, drawing on insights from discussions on mental health rehabilitation inside and outside Africa.

CONTEXTS OF DESTITUTION FOR THE MENTALLY ILL

Intrasubjective and Intersubjective Contexts

Some mental illnesses have symptoms that highlight the way intrasubjective processes (or the self-illness relation) might lead to destitution. Neuropsychiatric conditions such as dementia and Alzheimer's disease cause memory lapses and blurred spatial boundaries. Sufferers may often wander out of their homes or care institutions into the streets and remain there for hours, days, or weeks until they are found (Akpalu et al. 2007). The auditory hallucinations that accompany schizophrenia often present concrete experiential worlds for sufferers. Voices of known and unknown persons, often malevolent, speak to sufferers, creating an extra layer of intersubjectivity that is not accessible to observers but is real to the sufferers. In the psychiatric literature, the contents of voices heard by psychotics and schizophrenics have been grouped into several categories: those that undermine the self-worth and self-belief of sufferers, those that undermine the integrity and intentions of significant others of sufferers, those that instruct sufferers to harm themselves, and those that instruct the sufferer to harm others. Auditory hallucinations may lead to voluntary destitution. This has been reported in the Ghanaian context:

> The "mental sickness" started when she was 33 years old in this time when she was "trying to make ends meet." She experienced pains in her head and was losing weight. She stopped going out and attending to her business and seeing friends . . . she heard voices telling her to go into the sea and to go to the bush, so she left her home and went far away into the bush where she wandered for 8 months. Her family and friends tried unsuccessfully to find her. Eventually she returned home and her elder sister took her to a prayer camp run by a spiritualist church. (Read 2005, 66)

As noted above, Charmaz's (1983 and 1991) concept of "loss of self" facilitates the examination of the self-society relation with respect to chronic illness and disability. Of the four social-psychological conditions characterizing loss of self, two are strongly implicated in destitution risk in the Ghanaian context. The first is discrediting definitions of self; the second is the fear of being a burden on one's family.

Discrediting definitions of self, or negative self-sentiments, are strongly linked to the difficulties of having a handicap. As noted above, they occur when others react negatively to the individual's condition. Within the individual's life, negative self-sentiments can arise when the sufferer can no longer undertake tasks and activities with significant others that were previously taken for granted. Crucially, discrediting definitions of self can also occur when individuals expect or wrongly think that significant and generalized others will react negatively to their condition. In other words, although discrediting definitions of self usually occur as a response to an actual handicap, they can also occur as a response to misperceived handicap. "Stigma consciousness" has been defined as the expectation or anticipation of being stigmatized (quoted in Link and Phelan 2001, 374). Stigma consciousness can lead to the internalization of anticipated stigma or the projection of it onto others. There is evidence to suggest that this psychological process can undermine relationships and life chances even in the absence of actual discrimination (Deacon, Stephney, and Prosalendis 2005; de-Graft Aikins 2006; Link and Phelan 2001).

Studies on depression among elderly Ghanaian women offer concrete examples of the ways negative self-sentiments occur in the context of the self-society relation and lead to destitution risks. Margaret Field's (1960) ethnopsychiatric work among the Akan in the 1950s highlighted self-accusations of witchcraft among Akan women presenting with clinical depression at the traditional shrines. An important symptom of depression is self-stigmatization; this process is often informed by prevailing norms of credible and discredited social identities. In Ghana, women are more likely than men to be labeled and stigmatized as witches (Adinkra 2004; Akrong 2007; Dovlo 2007; Kirby 2006). The risk of labeling and stigmatization increases as a woman's age increases. In Ghana's northern region, for example, a high prevalence of witchcraft accusations and the link of that prevalence to violations of women's human rights has led to the establishment of witches' "camps" (Adinkra 2004; Akrong 2007; Kirby 2006). Some camps are transitory, but most are permanent.[4] Most women seek refuge in the camps after being stigmatized and persecuted by their families and communities. Others, in anticipation of being labeled a witch and discriminated against, seek refuge before actual stigmatization occurs. Women who seek refuge in transitory camps live there for several years until they are reintegrated into their communities. Those who seek refuge in permanent camps live there for the rest of their lives. In this cultural context we can speak of a coexistence between what might be called witchcraft consciousness and actual witchcraft-related stigma that structures the contents of discrediting definitions of the depressed self. This intersubjective process informs the choice of elderly women to live lives of isolation and destitution in shrines or at witch camps.

Fear of being a burden on one's family presents destitution risks in two ways. First, the specific intersubjective dynamics outlined by Charmaz (1983 and 1991) hold true. As noted above, individuals with debilitating illnesses can lose their old identities and feel useless. The African literature on the stigma associated with HIV/AIDS suggests that women living with chronic diseases tend to be disproportionately stigmatized compared to men because gender relations constitute key sites within which embodied discourses and power struggles around illness and morality unfold (Deacon, Stephney, and Prosalendis 2005). The woman living with debilitating illness has the additional burden of being unable to fulfill her important sociocultural role and meet her obligations as mother and wife. In Ghana—where polygamy is practiced, although not legally sanctioned—women with debilitating chronic illnesses such as diabetes and cancer face greater risks of marital conflict and breakdown compared to men for these reasons (de-Graft Aikins 2006).

Second, health care is expensive, and long-term illness is viewed as an economic and psychosocial burden by many people in Ghana. The fear of becoming a burden on family, friends, and caregivers when one is ill is rooted in well-documented material facts. Compelling evidence comes from the numbers of mentally ill individuals—both female and male, and of different ages and marital statuses—who have been abandoned in the nation's three psychiatric hospitals. It may be that since some families view psychiatric hospitals as the last resort, and since shopping for healers in traditional healing systems is very common, abandonment at psychiatric hospitals comes after lengthy engagement with different health services and the family's depletion of its material and symbolic resources. Nevertheless, the fear of being a burden on one's family is a rational emotion based on shared sociocultural expectations of the economic (cost of treatment and travel) and psychosocial (in particular, stigma) burden of mental illness. Ironically the expression of this fear, in the context of complex emotions evoked by disruption of the lives of the patient and his or her family, may create strains and conflicts within the home and other significant spaces of support. These then exacerbate risks of isolation, social exclusion, and destitution.

Group and Structural Contexts

The world of health, to which the mentally ill individual fully belonged before becoming ill, constructs shared ideas about the body, health, illness, life, and death (Kleinman 1988; Bury 1997). These shared ideas shape definitions of illnesses and the ways individuals understand distinct illnesses and respond to them. Shared ideas incorporate those that influence the handicap. Sufferers and their caregivers must negotiate these shared ideas and (the potential) handicap to maintain psychological, physical, and social security. Two concepts—differentiation and legitimation—provide insights into how shared ideas and responses, including handicaps, affect the mentally ill and shape social and structural contexts for destitution.

Psychologists use the term "differentiation" to describe how individuals, families, and communities categorize mental illness along a continuum from mild to severe. Across many cultures—in Africa, Ghana (Field 1958), Nigeria (Kabir et al. 2004), and Kenya, Uganda, and Tanzania (Edgerton 1966); in Europe, Britain (Foster 2001) and France (Jodelet 1991); and in Asia, India (Wagner et al. 1999; Wagner et al. 2000)—processes of differentiation are used to distinguish individuals exhibiting mild forms of mental illness, such as depression or behaviors deemed to be eccentric, from individuals exhibiting severe mental illnesses, such as psychoses (see table 4.2).

Legitimation is described in classical sociological discourse as "the process through which (political) authority is made credible" (Bury 1997, 456). Legitima-

Table 4.2. Differentiation between Mild and Severe
Mental Illness in Selected Countries

MILD		SEVERE
	AFRICA	
	Ghana	
Depression		Psychosis
	Kenya, Uganda, Tanzania	
Neurosis; Eccentric Behavior		Psychosis
	EUROPE	
	Great Britain	
Depression; Eccentric Behavior		Schizophrenia

tion can be viewed from the perspective of society, as described in Eliot Freidson's typology of lay legitimation, or from the perspective of the individual to whom the legitimation process is applied (1970; see also Nettleton 1995). Bury (1997) discusses self-legitimation in terms of the way the chronically ill negotiate the public and private dimensions of the experience of illness in order to minimize biographical disruption. The focus in this section of the chapter is on lay legitimation processes.

Initially developed in the context of the sick role, Freidson's typology distinguishes among three types of lay legitimation. First, "conditional legitimation" refers to the temporary rights and privileges afforded to individuals experiencing temporary periods of acute ill health. The criterion for this type of legitimation is the tacit expectation that the individuals will get well with treatment, and it is therefore likely to apply to chronically ill individuals experiencing acute phases of their illness. Thus women suffering postpartum depression may be offered conditional legitimation. Similarly, individuals with schizophrenia who have successfully managed their illnesses in the past with psychotropic medication may be offered conditional legitimation when an unexpected trauma causes relapse, for example. Second, "unconditional legitimation" refers to the process or act of granting unlimited rights and privileges to individuals living with long-term serious or severe illnesses or disabilities, who cannot take action to get well. People with neuropsychiatric disorders such as dementia and Alzheimer's among the aged may be placed in this category.[5] Finally, "illegitimation" refers to the deeming of an individual's condition and identity as illegitimate. This can occur in cases where the illness is stigmatized by society; in such cases, the rights and privileges that come with being ill are revoked. In many societies schizophrenia and psychosis are stigmatized (World Health Organization 2001). In African societies epilepsy belongs to this category (Allotey and Reidpath 2007; Jilek-Aall et al. 1997).

Table 4.3. Legitimacy Category and Hierarchy of
Destitution Risk for Selected Mental Illnesses

RISK OF DESTITUTION	LEGITIMACY CATEGORY	EXAMPLES OF ILLNESS
High	Illnesses deemed illegitimate	Schizophrenia, epilepsy
Medium	Illnesses granted conditional legitimacy	Postpartum depression, post-traumatic stress disorder
Low	Illnesses granted unconditional legitimacy	Dementia, Alzheimer's disease

How do processes of differentiation and legitimation lead to destitution for the mentally ill? The literature on differentiation suggests that in many cultures, mild and temporary forms of mental illness are often contained in the private sphere, either at home or in the community, while severe chronic forms with elements of threat and violence to the self and others result in custodial care, primarily in psychiatric institutions. In African settings severe mental illnesses that are attributed to spiritual or supernatural causes will lead to custodial care in traditional and religious institutions (Field 1960; Odejide et al. 1977; Weinberg 1965). Thus, if we were to construct a hierarchy of destitution risk, individuals living with illegitimate illnesses such as schizophrenia and epilepsy would occupy the top position (that of the highest risk), individuals living with conditions granted conditional legitimation who do not take action to get well would occupy the middle (medium risk), and individuals with conditions that receive unconditional legitimation would occupy the bottom (see table 4.3).

However, the contents of this hierarchy of destitution risk would change depending on prevailing cultural and social representations of various mental illnesses. What may be deemed a conditionally legitimate illness in one culture may be deemed illegitimate in another culture. For instance, although neuropsychiatric conditions among the elderly such as dementia may be granted unconditional legitimation in UK families, this may not be the case in Ghana, where dementia is little understood by the public and is likely to be conflated with negative afflictions of aging, such as the practice of witchcraft among elderly women.

Differentiation, Legitimation, and Destitution among the Mentally Ill

In the first few decades of formal psychiatry in Ghana, psychiatric patients were not subjected to diagnosis or sophisticated pharmacotherapy. Emmanuel Forster, the first African psychiatrist south of the Sahara and first Chair of Psychiatry for the University of Ghana Medical School, notes that the function of the first asylum, established in the late nineteenth century was "purely one of custodial segregation. No treatment was given and the main function of the staff was to supervise the feeding of patients and report on their physical health to the appropriate authority" (1962, 26). By the 1930s some treatment was offered to patients in the form of "mind suiting drugs, chiefly arsenicals"; restless or violent patients were restrained physically with handcuffs or leg irons, or through seclusion; and able-bodied patients were offered occupational therapy in the form of farming. However diagnoses were still rudimentary affairs. Thus during this period there were references in the archives to "harmless deviants" and "harmful lunatics," and wards were allocated to "criminal, general, weak and female" patients (ibid.). Even so, the majority of individuals who received custodial care in the hospital were those living with illegitimate conditions: in lay discourse, the "harmful lunatics" would be considered "mad," and the harmless deviants considered socially disruptive.

These early decades also illuminated the processes of legitimation, with families, psychiatrists, and institutions (such as the police and the judiciary) agreeing on or debating what illnesses could be granted illegitimate or conditional status. Emmanuel Akyeampong (2006, 3–5) describes the case of Yaw Kyei, a goldsmith from Akwamu who was "declared insane by the colonial court" in 1931. In this case the legitimation process was straightforward: both the family and the traditional and colonial legal and psychiatric institutions agreed on the status of the illness. From the perspective of the medical officer, Yaw Kyei's symptoms—which included "shouting," "talking nonsense," and not wearing clothes—confirmed the presence of mental illness. From the family's perspective, Yaw Kyei's symptoms confirmed the presence of madness: he set his hut on fire, disappeared into the bush for days, physically attacked his family, and went naked. Crucially, Akyeampong notes two culturally driven delegitimation processes that converged with psychiatric processes. Yaw Kyei's disappearance into the bush, in Akan culture, showed "a loss of distinction between bush and settlement, between nature and culture"; in psychiatric terms, voluntary vagrancy was a symptom of severe mental illness. Second, "in Akan culture irrefutable evidence of madness came when a sick person took off his or her clothes and went stark naked"; in the psychiatric literature, nudity was increasingly seen as a manifestation of African psychosis (see Read, Doku, and de-Graft Aikins, this volume). Similar straightforward legitimation processes are described in the West African context. Writing about psychiatric experiences in colonial Nigeria, Jonathan Sadowsky notes that although asylum inmates were "not even representative of the mad generally," they "were understood as mad by their kin and neighbors and not only by the colonial state" (1999, vii).

However, the legitimation process is not always so straightforward. Often, lay and professional processes come into conflict. During the same period that Yaw Kyei's case was reported, another case focused on a situation in which family members sought to have a relative hospitalized, while the policeman documenting the request refused to endorse such a course of action because he did not agree that the illness presented—most likely what psychiatrists would characterize as harmless deviance—was illegitimate. Psychiatric reports prepared by the British alienist (nineteenth and early twentieth century forerunners of psychiatrists) Dr. F. MacLagan dated May 12, 1930, also suggested that conflicts between institutions and families about recovery, reintegration into society, and rehabilitation were common (Public Records and Archives Administration Department, Accra, CSO 11/8/02). Generally, individuals admitted to the psychiatric hospital tended to be abandoned by their family, to become institutionalized, or to become destitute after their discharge (see the second part of the chapter).

As mainstream psychiatric practices (Forster 1958) were adopted in the mid- to late 1950s, diagnoses of both outpatient and inpatient cases became important. Categories shifted from broad distinctions between "harmless deviants" and "harmful lunatics" to nuanced categories following diagnostic criteria developed in the West (see Read, Doku, and de-Graft Aikins, this volume). What became apparent was the dominance in hospital cases of severe mental illnesses within the psychotic spectrum. By 1960, for example, schizophrenia and manic depression (now called manic depressive illness or bipolar mood disorder) constituted 60 percent of admitted cases (Weinberg 1965). In contrast, milder conditions such as depression and neuroses were virtually absent in the hospital. Geoffrey Tooth conducted a survey of the Gold Coast colony in the 1940s and suggested that hospital cases constituted less than 10 percent of mental illnesses cases there. However, an absence of depressive illness was reported at the hospital (1950). Deferring to the psychiatric spirit of the times that stressed the rarity of neuroses and depression in African populations both inside and outside the continent (see, for example, Thomas and Sillen 1993; see also Read, Doku, and de-Graft Aikins, this volume), Tooth extrapolated from the lack of hospital cases to a lack of depression in Ghana. This notion soon changed.

An emerging body of community-based work and more sophisticated psychiatric observations suggested that depression and neuroses did exist in Ghana but that people suffering from them remained at home or within their community. Field (1958) suggested that families and communities could contain depression and neuroses, as well as nonviolent psychoses. Field also drew attention to community-based forms of therapy enforced by shrine priests in "shrine villages" that cared for people with mild conditions in community spaces. Individuals with severe conditions like chronic schizophrenia who could not be helped by shrine priests were returned to the care of their families or became vagrants. The social psychologist Gustav Jahoda (1961) examined the work of traditional healers, Christian religious healers, and the psychiatric hospital in Accra in the 1950s. His study demonstrated the continued popularity of traditional healers for treating mild conditions such as anxiety and depression, as well as the important healing functions of the new churches:

> Traditional healers are widely patronized by literates, and the evidence suggests the support and reassurance they provide often prevents the occurrence of serious breakdowns. A similar need is served by the healing churches for those literates who, whilst more remote from purely traditional beliefs, are still receptive to a mixture of traditional beliefs, Christian doctrine and occult notions as a means of assuaging their problems and conflicts. Were it not for this extensive preliminary screening . . . mental hospitals would be overwhelmed by a flood of cases with whom they could not possibly deal. (Jahoda 1961, 268)

In time both locally based psychiatrists and foreign psychiatric observers corroborated these community-based findings. Samuel Kirson Weinberg, an American psychiatrist who conducted a survey of diagnoses and care at the Accra Psychiatric Hospital, made this observation about Ghana and other sub-Saharan African countries (Kenya, South Africa, and Nyasaland, which is now Malawi):

> The preponderant proportion of hospitalized patients in these sub-Sahara societies were dangerous or troublesome to the community or were unable to care for themselves; the more oriented and socially manageable psychotics were not hospitalized. Many depressives were sufficiently conformist and oriented, and thus were not hospitalized; others who interpreted their behavior as witchcraft or as being bewitched, sought fetish priests or native doctors for treatment of their distress. Consequently, agitated depressives and acting-out schizoaffectives were hospitalized more readily than were immobile, less troublesome depressives. Perhaps these socially troublesome depressives were hospitalized more frequently in Ghana than in the other sub-Saharan countries. (1965, 249)

These lay processes of differentiation and legitimation have held true for hospital communities from the 1960s to present.

PROFILES AND EXPERIENCES OF THE MENTALLY ILL DESTITUTE

Vagrants and "Vagrant Patients"

In the early decades of formal psychiatry, vagrant patients were referred to as the "destitute insane." Predominantly male, the destitute insane were either "harmless deviants" or "harmful lunatics" wandering around the streets and market-

Table 4.4. Characteristics of Vagrants in Accra, 1953, and
Vagrant Patients at the Accra Psychiatric Hospital, 2006

CHARACTERISTIC	VAGRANTS, 1953	VAGRANT PATIENTS, 2006
Number	170	91
Age range	18–60[a]	11–70
Number female	—[b]	48
Number male	—[b]	43
Diagnoses	Able-bodied, physically defective (blind, crippled), or mentally defective (feeble-minded, senile)	Schizophrenia, epilepsy, hypomania
Regional distribution		
Greater Accra	17%	47%
Other	Elsewhere in southern Ghana, 11%; northern Ghana, 12%; French West Africa, 22%; Nigeria, 37%, Liberia <1%; unknown, <1%	Eastern, 16%; Volta, 9%, Central, 6%; Ashanti, 3%; Western, 3%; rest of Ghana: 13%, foreign, 3%
Occupation	Beggars (85%); unknown (15%)	Unskilled, 50%; professionals, 22%; unemployed, 9%; students, 6%; unknown, 13%

Sources: Acquah 1958, Banson et al. 2006.
[a] 109 were in the 19–40 age bracket.
[b] Data not available

places, in villages and towns and in the bush (Field 1960; Tooth 1950). The typical person in this category arrived at the hospital through legal processes—most commonly, mediation by the police and the judiciary—if and when he began to pose a physical threat to the community that had previously tolerated and supported him. Tooth's late 1940s survey suggested that many harmless vagrant psychotics came from the north or from southern villages (1950).

Between 1953 and 1956 in Ghana's capital Accra, the colonial Department of Social Welfare conducted a survey to capture profiles of "others who wander about the streets of the municipality in an apparent state of destitution" (Acquah 1958, 81). The survey identified 170 destitute individuals and grouped them into three categories: the economically destitute, the disabled destitute, and the mentally ill destitute. The mentally ill destitute were largely "feeble minded" and "senile" (ibid.); none was psychotic. Almost half (40 percent) of these 170 vagrants in Accra municipality came from Accra, other parts of southern Ghana, and northern Ghana (see table 4.4). However, more than half (59 percent) were foreigners from French West Africa, Nigeria, or Liberia. This international profile of vagrants reflected the changing face of Accra in the era just after independence, when large numbers of West Africans migrated to Ghana, especially Accra, in search of work (Agyei-Mensah and de-Graft Aikins 2010; Akyeampong 2007). It may also have reflected the conscious marketing of Accra Psychiatric Hospital by Forster, the Gambian psychiatrist then in charge, as an institution catering to the West African region.

In 1970 Forster observed that although the majority of patients arrived at the hospital after shopping for healers in traditional and religious systems, "the destitute insane . . . went direct to [the] mental hospital for treatment" (quoted in Twumasi 2005, 87). It is important to note that it was difficult to ascertain what prior treatment the vagrant patient had received because he was likely to be a long-term destitute, with no accompanying caregiver or friend to provide personal details and illness history. He was likely to be diagnosed with psychosis or schizophrenia, although other conditions such as dementia and mental retardation are reported. He would fit the description of the vagrant used by Baasher and colleagues quoted above in this chapter, someone "who lived a socially and geographically unsettled life" (1983, 35). A male vagrant ward was established at the Accra Psychiatric Hospital to accommodate this group of vagrants.

In the decades since then, the gender profile of vagrant patients has changed. Now there are as many women as men.[6] The women are accommodated in a general female ward, with people who have voluntarily committed themselves and court-committed cases. The geographical origins of vagrants have also changed. Ghanaians from different parts of the country far outnumber foreigners from the subregion. However, how the vagrant patients reached the hospital, their socioeconomic status, and the diagnoses they receive have not changed. In 2006 a survey was conducted of the vagrant patients then in the hospital (Banson et al. 2006; see table 4.4). The patients had been brought to the hospital by mass sweeps for vagrants conducted jointly by the Accra Metropolitan Assembly and the police; or by social service agencies, church groups, good Samaritans, anonymous relatives, and unspecified people (Banson et al. 2006). More than half (59 percent) were unskilled or unemployed. About 90 percent of the male vagrants were diagnosed with schizophrenia. Female vagrants, like the patients in the general female ward, were diagnosed with schizophrenia, epilepsy, or hypomania. Both male and female vagrants had records of long stays in the wards, ranging from a few months to over forty years. Sixty percent of these vagrant patients preferred living on the streets and had attempted or would attempt to escape from the hospital. Some held out hope for being reintegrated into their family. Others, like the institutionalized patients Emmanuel Forster and Samuel Danquah observed in the 1970s, "were unable to give any information of their relatives and antecedents and others were unable to give their name" (1977, 109).

"Long-Stay" Patients

In Ghana a large group of mentally ill individuals, including discharged patients, remain in hospital wards for weeks or even years, ostensibly abandoned by their families; others remain at traditional shrines or Christian prayer camps for similarly extended periods awaiting absolute healing. Fundamentally, the potential or actual destitute status of these patients is less visible to the public because their lives are largely contained within institutional spaces. However, their psychosocial, physical, and material realities are similar to publicly visible vagrants.

Traditional and Christian healing centers, such as shrines and prayer camps, provide important mental health services for the mentally ill (Doku et al. 2007; Field 1960; Jahoda 1961; Read 2005). Since psychiatric services are concentrated in the south, specifically in Accra and Cape Coast, these centers are the first line of treatment for the majority of Ghanaians. The centers operate on at least two principles that ensure compliance with treatment and the family's involvement and support. Patrick Twumasi (2005) gives an account of the evolution of the structure of family support imposed by shrine priests. In the past, a family member would have to stay with the sick person at the shrine to provide daily care and support, but today family members are allowed to pay for shrine-based caregivers to carry out the traditional roles of the family member (feeding and bathing the patient, for example). Prayer camps, often modeled on these traditional religious systems, have similar treatment approaches. This institutional arrangement not only ensures initial family involvement, but it also minimizes the risk of family abandonment over the period of treatment. Second, families often seek help from traditional shrines and prayer camps because they share similar spiritual causal theories about the mental illnesses of their relatives. Conditions such as schizophrenia, epilepsy, and alcoholism are often attributed to spiritual causes (de-Graft Aikins 2004, 2006; Read 2005). However, both traditional healing practices and prayer camps present destitution risks for their clients.

First, reports on the experiences of mentally ill individuals in traditional shrines and prayer camps suggest that physical restraint, dietary restrictions, physical ill health, and unhappiness characterize these environments (Doku et al. 2007; Osabutey 2006; Read 2005; Twumasi 2005). Patients often attempt to escape. Second, families tend to start shopping for healers for their mentally ill relatives within and across both systems and psychiatric hospitals when traditional and Christian healing is slow or not absolute. Families' constant search for a cure often conflicts with the desires of their mentally ill relatives, and although outwardly not lacking support, often results in "socially and geographically unsettled lives" for the ill. The story of fifty-one-year-old Doris Appiah Danquah, who lived with manic depression between 1978 and 1989, illustrates this process clearly (Fondation d'Harcourt 2014; Human Rights Watch 2012). During her eleven years of illness, Doris's family took her to the Accra Psychiatric Hospital; the famous Akonedi shrine in Ghana's eastern region; Nana Ntia shrine at Gomoah Feteh in the central region; several churches in Accra; a spiritual home in Kumasi in the Ashanti region (there she was treated by a psychiatrist while she was in chains); a fetish shrine in the north (where she lived for three years), and finally another spiritual home at an undisclosed location. In Kumasi and the north she made several attempts to run away. Doris eventually recovered from her illness, completed a bachelor of science in nursing and psychology, got married, had a child, and is currently employed as the director of an orphanage. Although hers is a success story, Doris's experience demonstrates the way family-imposed healer shopping presents destitution risks for individuals living with mental illnesses, especially those attributed to spiritual causes.

In the hospital setting, the majority of patients are long-stay patients. At the Accra Psychiatric Hospital the majority of long-stay patients have been diagnosed with severe conditions that are stigmatized by the Ghanaian public, such as schizophrenia, psychosis, epilepsy, and alcoholism (see table 4.5). Over the last two decades, cases of substance abuse disorders (involving cannabis, cocaine, or heroin) have increased and become a major cause of admission. Boys of primary- or secondary-school age dominate in this category, and relapse rates are reported to be high, with family distancing and social exclusion common experiences for these patients.[7]

In 1966, after the coup d'état that overthrew Ghana's first president, Kwame Nkrumah, a committee was established to examine the country's health needs. The committee member assigned to mental health, Dr. Matthew Barnor, observed severe overcrowding, poor resources, and unsanitary conditions at Accra Psychiatric Hospital: "[The hospital] had a population of over one thousand mentally ill patients. The conditions were appalling. To begin with, the population was more than the hospital could efficiently and comfortably accommodate. . . . The place at night was simply uncomfortable and horrible to behold. It had patients packed like sardines. The walls, generally speaking, were supposed to be white but from the floor to the ceiling had become dirty and changed colour. Blood from bedbugs was evident" (2001, 249). These poor conditions have persisted into the present (Adomakoh 1972; Ewusi-Mensah 2001). Overcrowding has been a major problem for the hospital since it was established in 1906 (Acquah 1958, Adomakoh 1972, Forster 1962)

There are not enough mental health professionals to meet the needs of the Ghanaian population, especially at the community level (Munko 2006). There

Table 4.5. Top Eleven Psychiatric Conditions at the Accra Psychiatric Hospital, 1960, 1993, and 2006

DISEASE	1960 NO (%)	DISEASE	1993 NO (%)	DISEASE	2006 NO (%)
Schizophrenia	446 (44.2)	Schizophrenia	253 (9)	Depression	586 (12.6)
Manic depression	162 (16.0)	Depression	218 (7.8)	Acute organic psychosis	540 (11.6)
Epilepsy	53 (5.2)	Drug abuse	190 (6.8)	Schizophrenia	421 (9.1)
Confusional psychosis	44 (4.3)	Psychosis	184 (6.5)	Epilepsy	390 (8.4)
Mental deficiency	38 (3.8)	Hypomania	76 (2.7)	Substance abuse	293 (6.3)
Alcoholism	18 (1.8)	Alcoholism	55 (2)	Neurosis	249 (5.4)
Involutional depression	18 (1.8)	Epilepsy	43 (1.5)	Schizo-affective disorder	210 (4.5)
Senile dementia	14 (1.4)	Paranoia	40 (1.4)	Alcoholism	176 (3.8)
Primary dementia	12 (1.2)	Manic depression	31 (1.1)	Hypomania	160 (3.4)
Organic (e.g., syphilis)	8 (0.8)	Personality disorder	25 (0.9)	Dementia	30 (0.6)
Not yet diagnosed	197 (19.5)	All others (unspecified)	1,695 (60.3)	All others (unspecified)	1,579 (34)
Total	1,010 (100.0)	Total	2,810 (100.0)	Total	4,634 (99.7*)

Sources: Weinberg 1965, 248 (for 1960); Ghana Ministry of Health 1994 (for 1993); Thompson et al. 2008 (for 2006).

*Percentages do not sum to 100 due to rounding error

are 200 psychiatric nurses, 3 social workers, 4 psychologists, and 8 psychiatrists per 10,000,000 Ghanaians (World Health Organization 2005). Isaac Ewusi-Mensah notes that "the perennial problem of inadequate staffing" and the staff's "unrealistic work-load has serious implications for patient care and job satisfaction" (2001, 229). Funding allocated to mental health services is grossly inadequate. In 2005, 4.5 percent of Ghana's gross domestic product (about $8.9 billion) was allocated to health, and only 0.5 percent of this health budget went to mental health (World Health Organization 2005).

In the summer of 2006—the centenary anniversary of Accra Psychiatric Hospital—a series of newspaper articles authored by the hospital's acting director, Dr. Akwasi Osei, and by journalists depicted an institution in crisis. The hospital was overcrowded; it was operating with rapidly dwindling funds, staff numbers, and food stocks; staff morale was at an all-time low; and the acting director was considering closing it. A crucial product of institutional crisis over the last two decades has been poor patient care. In 2006 the majority of patients admitted to the hospital were diagnosed as schizophrenic after brief psychiatric consultations (Banson et al, 2006). The number of "not yet diagnosed" or "unspecified" cases has been relatively high over the last four decades (see table 4.5). These often exceed the number of diagnosed cases; a substantial number of patients with undiagnosed conditions are admitted and put on psychotropic medication. Improper treatment strategies, such as the excessive use of physical restraint, are reported.

These poor hospital conditions engender "socially and geographically unsettled lives" similar to the lives of patients at shrines and prayer camps. Recent surveys of patient experiences document poor response to treatment, unhappiness at hospital conditions, and the desire to escape (Adrah et al. 2006; Banson et al. 2006). One of the key routes of destitution for revolving-door patients at Accra Psychiatric Hospital and the remaining two psychiatric hospitals in Ghana, Pantang Psychiatric Hospital on the outskirts of Accra and Ankaful Psychiatric Hospital in Cape Coast, is through patients escaping: there is a high level of absconding, particularly among substance abuse patients. Another route to destitution is through family abandonment. Without a home to return to, discharged patients end up on the streets. Informal accounts by hospital staff suggest that family abandonment increases the longer patients stay at the hospital and that poor diagnostic, treatment, and care processes are implicated in lengthy hospital stays.[8] The final route to destitution is through periodic mass evictions from the hospitals. With no welfare safety nets, the collapse of social services, and the unwillingness of families to accept their mentally ill relatives back home and into their communities, these mass evictions create greater numbers of vagrants with various mental illnesses on the streets of Accra and other Ghanaian cities.

The hospital data on vagrant and long-stay patients suggest a complex relationship between structural poverty, mental illness, and destitution. On the one hand, poverty is a risk factor for the major mental illnesses treated at the hospitals: the majority of patients with schizophrenia, epilepsy, substance abuse disorders, or depression are poor, unemployed, and/or unskilled. Often families abandon a patient because of the family's poverty. For example, a key reason for family abandonment among families living in compound houses in Accra is that the family rents out the rooms of mentally ill relatives when they are admitted to a hospital for long periods.[9] The common rental practice in Accra and other cities is to require tenants to pay rent for at least one year. Families often claim—if a hospital wants to discharge a patient when his or her room has been rented for a period of long-term tenancy—to need extra time to arrange alternative accommodation for the discharged patient.

On the other hand, mental illness causes poverty. Individuals who are diagnosed with debilitating conditions (such as epilepsy) early in life, and whose lives become circumscribed by institutional care, lose opportunities for schooling as well as skills training and employment (Thompson et al. 2008). Furthermore, mental illness is highly stigmatized in Ghanaian society. This undermines the ability of discharged and/or rehabilitated patients to secure new employment or return to their old jobs. It also suggests that in addition to improving treatment and rehabilitation, poverty reduction strategies have to be central to addressing the relationship between mental illness and destitution.

INTERVENTIONS

There have been concrete attempts by mental health professionals, religious leaders, and ordinary community members to provide solutions to the problem of destitution among the mentally ill in Ghana. At least three approaches can be identified: village settlements, Pentecostal Christian outreach interventions, and humanitarian and rights-based interventions.

Village Settlements

The village system has roots in traditional forms of mental health care in Ghana. In the 1950s Field noted how householders in the shrine villages she visited took in patients and their relatives as lodgers, as relatives usually accompanied patients in search of healing. This arrangement enabled the patient to access the services of the healer while remaining a part of the village community (Field 1960, 163–199). Recent anthropological work suggests that the model of the shrine village is still followed in some parts of Ghana (Read 2005; Doku et al. 2007). Beyond these largely anthropological descriptions, there are no data on how many shrine villages exist, how many clients they serve, and what their treatment outcomes are.

Psychiatrists began experimenting with the village model two decades after the establishment of the Accra Psychiatric Hospital in 1906, but early suggestions for establishing a village for harmless deviants did not lead to any concrete developments. The hospital was experiencing overcrowding, a situation that persists to date. Between 1930 and 1932, Dr. F. MacLagan, the British alienist, made a number of recommendations for addressing the problem, including establishing a bush camp for harmless patients, building an additional dormitory at the hospital, and returning patients to their relatives to relieve congestion (Public Records and Archives Administration Department, Accra, cso 11/8/11). In these professional accounts there was a clear demarcation between harmless and harmful lunatics and the implicit idea that the harmless ones could be reintegrated into society. But there was also professional recognition of the difficulties involved in reintegrating into their families both categories of lunatics, as the earlier discussion on legitimation processes suggested. This explains the suggested establishment of a bush camp as a first resort, which would allow patients to live outside the institution as well as away from family members, who might not want their mentally ill relative back. It appears that this first suggestion of establishing a village for harmless deviants did not lead to any concrete developments. Although overcrowding persisted at Accra Psychiatric Hospital in the decades that followed, a village settlement system was not fully implemented until the 1950s. In 1957, the year when Ghana became independent from the British, a hospital annex was opened in Adomi, sixty miles outside of Accra (Forster 1958). This was a village settlement that was modeled after Nigeria's Aro system (Asuni 1967). To minimize overcrowding at the main hospital, 300 patients were transferred to this facility, but there are no records of what became of these patients. However, Dr. Albert Boohene, the Ghana Medical Association representative of the 1966 national health review committee, recalls a "shocking number of dead bodies lying in the bushes" when the committee visited the settlement.[10] Inhabitants had been left to fend for themselves with no supervision or psychosocial support. They suffered malnutrition and a lack of appropriate shelter and clothing and the deaths were attributed to a lack of food and cold weather conditions. Essentially, these psychiatric initiatives did not take root, unlike the more famous Aro system. This may have been due to Ghana's sociopolitical turmoil in the 1960s and 1970s, and the economic downturn that resulted in the imposition of structural adjustments on the country by the World Bank and the International Monetary Fund during the 1980s and 1990s. The withdrawal of government subsidies for social services led to the collapse of several institutions—including the country's health and mental health system.

Pentecostal Christian Outreach Interventions

Christian healing services, both in the past and today, generally take place in churches or prayer camps. The mental health services provided by prayer camps have been discussed in the previous section of this chapter. In recent times this largely institution-based service has turned its attention to outreach work with the mentally ill destitute. The work of Christian faith healers has been featured in newspapers and on television. In September 2007 the quiet town of Kintampo, in Ghana's Brong Ahafo region, was treated to a surprise Pentecostal deliverance crusade.[11] Two religious healers from Kumasi, in the Ashanti region, appeared in town, recruited local assistants, and rounded up as many vagrants as they could into a small arena. There the healers and their assistants bathed the vagrants in public, gave them haircuts and a change of clothes, and performed healing prayers. Adults and children gathered to watch, some laughing and jeering at the vagrants. Some vagrants, appearing visibly shaken, attempted unsuccessfully to resist the exercise. The religious healers claimed to have cured these vagrants and announced future deliverance sessions in neighboring towns.

These Christian outreach interventions are largely informed by and modeled on the biblical story in which Jesus cast demons out of a mad man (Matthew 8:28–34). This approach is problematic in a number of ways. First, the healers assume that all vagrants are mad, but this—as shown above in this the chapter—is often not correct. Second, like prayer camp healers, outreach healers attribute madness to spiritual forces (because differentiation is not salient in their discourses), especially parasitic demons, and claim that healing prayers can effect cures. These claims are often untrue. For example, days after the Kintampo deliverance crusade, at least two vagrants who occupied particular spots in the town had returned to their spots, minus their new clothes and back to their usual (and possibly preferred) unkempt appearance.[12] These new methods hold both salvation and risk for their target population, in the same way that prayer camps do for their clients. It is difficult to know whether these intervention approaches are informed by genuine concern for the welfare and rehabilitation of vagrants, or whether they are informed by the healers' need to expand their public activities to shore up their spiritual relevance and legitimacy in a highly religious Ghanaian public sphere. More research is required to follow trends in this area and their impact on the welfare of destitute individuals.

Humanitarian and Rights-Based Interventions

Humanitarian interventions for the destitute have coexisted with village systems and religious healing approaches for a considerable length of time. Ray Kea (1982, quoted in Iliffe 1987) provides an account of the marginalized status of the poor and destitute in seventeenth-century Gold Coast. He notes that these groups survived on "institutional poor relief"—charity provided by benevolent local people and established European communities. The profile of the destitute during this period was of the disabled or of the able-bodied who lacked "access to land and to the labour of themselves" (quoted in Iliffe 1987, 64). Although there is no mention of mental illness in these destitute communities, there is a recognition that psychological distress is a common everyday experience. Jerome Destombes discusses official concern and interventions during the colonial era for northern migrants who become destitute in the southern towns in which they sought seasonal or permanent work. Interventions included "the establishment of 'refuges' or '*poor home*[s]' along the main migration roads and of a fund for the repatriation of '*sick and derelict*' labour and the provision of 'rest houses'" (1999, 29). These interventions ceased in postcolonial Ghana due to a lack of government funding. Acquah describes a destitutes' hostel that was established in the 1950s in Chorkor, a neighbourhood in Accra, with accommodation for twenty inmates, which aimed to provide rehabilitation and reintegration into society for destitutes, including those who had been abandoned at the Accra Psychiatric Hospital by their relatives. Most inmates had a "serious disability and [were] unfit for work" (1958, 81). Although the services provided by the Chorkor hostel were urgently needed, it was not large enough to accommodate the growing number of destitutes in Accra. As mentioned above, the 1953 survey recorded 170 vagrants (Acquah 1958, 81). In recent years two retired psychiatrists have made independent attempts to establish humanitarian services in Accra and Tamale, in northern Ghana, for the mentally ill destitute.[13] These initiatives are modeled on Western community-based mental health support and rehabilitation centers (Stickley, Hitchcock, and Bertram 2005) and offer similar services: a drop-in space for counseling and feeding, soup kitchens, and some outreach work.

The establishment of mental health NGOs in the late 1990s has introduced a rights-based intervention approach to mental health advocacy, care, and rehabilitation that builds on the principles of the traditional humanitarian approach. There are now three major mental health NGOs in Ghana that are concerned with mentally ill destitutes. BasicNeeds is an international mental health NGO that assists thousands of people with severe mental illness together their families and carers in Africa and Asia (Bates 2007; see also www.basicneeds.org). Starting in 2002 in Tamale, and in 2004 in Accra, BasicNeeds provides community-oriented, rights-based support to about 14,000 mentally ill Ghanaians and their families (Bates 2007). It focuses on four main areas of activity: providing community mental health services (including education) for mentally ill individuals, their families, and traditional healers; funding and supporting sustainable livelihoods; conducting research; and building capacity in the mental health care system. Its focus on sustainable livelihoods—a poverty reduction approach that facilitates training and employment opportunities and provides income-generating activities—is particularly relevant to the mentally ill destitute, since poverty appears to be both a risk factor and an outcome of mental illness in Ghana. The second NGO, MindFreedom (Ghana) works largely in the area of advocacy. It organizes marches and demonstrations and advocates for mental health in the mass media. The official attempt to clear the streets of Accra of vagrants during Ghana's celebration of the fiftieth anniversary of its independence was criticized in the strongest terms by MindFreedom. In a full-page advertisement in a national newspaper, the NGO challenged the government's decision, calling it a violation of human rights. A third NGO, Psycho Mental Health Foundation was established in 2006. It focuses largely on the problem of substance abuse disorders among school-age youth and provides education and advocacy in schools, colleges, and religious spaces in Greater Accra and the central region of the country.

Rights-based interventions have become the gold standard of global mental health care, since the publication of the *The World Health Report* (World Health Organization 2001). Ghana has introduced a new mental health bill that underscores the need for rights-based mental health care. An important component of this approach is the involvement of patients in advocacy, support, and policy formulation. Until the new bill is implemented, mental health NGOs in Ghana will be instrumental in promoting mental health care that is dynamic, patient-centered, and community-based. They present the best hope for providing sustainable support to marginalized individuals and groups with mental illness, including those living with or at risk of destitution. However, they have two key limitations. First, they have not as yet fully integrated patients into the broad spectrum of their activities. Second, they reach only a minority of needy communities at present, as most of the organizations are located and operate in the Greater Accra area. The NGOs recognize both limitations and are working to overcome them. For example, BasicNeeds seeks to give voice to the mentally ill so that they can represent their own needs to national bodies (Bates 2007). And Psycho Mental Health Foundation is seeking funding to strengthen its advocacy activities and expand them to the Ashanti, eastern, and western regions.

CONCLUSION

By using "the mentally ill destitute" as a conceptual lens, I have identified a broad range of mentally ill groups whose members may choose a life of vagrancy or have that life imposed on them. The local literature suggests that in addition to individuals with psychosis or schizophrenia, elderly women with witchcraft-related depression, young men with substance abuse disorders, elderly people with neurodegenerative disorders such as dementia, and individuals with epilepsy risk becoming destitute. Destitution may be characterized by vagrancy or by sequential institutionalization in psychiatric hospitals, traditional healing centers, and prayer camps.

The risk of destitution is mediated by intrasubjective, intersubjective, social, and structural factors (see table 4.1). The concept of biographical disruption facilitates an examination of intrasubjective (the self-illness relation) and intersubjective (the self-society relation) processes. The symptoms of some mental illnesses highlight the ways the self-illness relation could place sufferers at risk of destitution. The local data suggest that the auditory hallucinations that accompany schizophrenia, for instance, may lead to voluntary destitution. Witchcraft-related depression among elderly women in the Ashanti and northern regions demonstrate the role that intersubjective processes play in destitution risks. A key symptom of depression is discrediting definitions of self, or self-stigmatization. In cultural contexts where elderly women are likely to be labeled and stigmatized as witches, there is a coexistence of witchcraft consciousness and actual witchcraft-related stigma that structure the contents of discrediting definitions of the depressed self. Evidence suggests that this intersubjective process informs the choice of elderly women to live lives of isolation and destitution in shrines or at witch camps (Field 1960; Kirby 2006). These examples underscore the importance of understanding the relationship between self and illness and between the ill self and society, as well as how both may lead to voluntary or enforced destitution for mentally ill individuals.

In terms of the social and structural contexts of destitution, the literature on differentiation and legitimation in Ghana provides important insights. The literature suggests that people with mild conditions—especially those granted conditional legitimacy, such as depression—are often kept at home and in the community. People with severe illnesses deemed illegitimate—especially those that pose a threat or danger to the mentally ill individuals and their significant others, such as psychosis and schizophrenia—receive custodial care. Individuals with severe mental illnesses are most likely to end up at shrines, prayer camps, and/or hospitals, and their families are likely to initiate and enforce shopping for healers within and across these systems, for extended periods. The psychiatric literature suggests that the longer a patient remains at hospital, the greater his or her risk of family neglect, abandonment, and destitution.

Ultimately, the relationship between mental illness and destitution is mediated by a complex interaction of intrasubjective (symptoms that mediate self-imposed social exclusion), intersubjective (discrediting definitions of self influenced by sociocultural norms, including differentiation and legitimation processes), social (family neglect and social stigma), and structural (poverty and poor institutional care) factors. It may be difficult to identify the most salient factor in some cases.

As noted above, Iliffe defines structural poverty as the "long-term poverty of individuals due to their personal or social circumstances" (1987, 4). The profile and experiences of vagrant and revolving-door patients suggest that structural poverty shapes the relationship between mental illness and destitution. For example, 59 percent of vagrant patients surveyed at Accra Psychiatric Hospital in 2006 were unskilled or unemployed. The majority of long-stay patients at the same hospital come from poor migrant communities. Mental illness results in either long-term disability or missed opportunities for work, particularly for long-stay patients: both affect income and social status. Thus, the relationship between mental illness and destitution must be understood in the context of structural poverty.

Mental health experts make strong associations between mental illness and poverty. In low-income countries it is reported that mental illness and impoverishment mutually reinforce each other (Patel and Kleinman, 2003; see also, for example, Gureje and Bamidele 1999 on Nigeria). In these countries, chronic physical and mental ill health caused by extreme poverty undermine productivity and social cohesion; low or no productivity and social exclusion in turn exacerbate poverty (Desjarlais et al. 1995; World Health Organization 2001). It is estimated that 5.4 million Ghanaians live in structural poverty in slum and squatter settlements (de-Graft Aikins and Ofori-Atta 2007). The members of these largely migrant communities are employed in transient and poorly paid work; they live in temporary illegal settlements, facing an ever-present threat of eviction; and many, like those in slum communities throughout Africa, experience a triple threat of urban poverty, social exclusion and deprivation. A recent study exploring the experiences of migrant squatters in Accra supports these discussions (de-Graft Aikins and Ofori-Atta 2007). The study showed that although the squatters lived in overcrowded settlements and suffered from daily food insecurities and physical exhaustion as a result of strenuous manual work, physical illness did not feature explicitly in the list of everyday problems that participants were asked to produce. In contrast, "the link between homelessness and poor mental health was compelling" (ibid., 773). Individuals lived with daily financial, legal, and psychosocial insecurities that "caused chronic worry and anxieties and there was some evidence of psychosomatic disorders" (ibid.). This suggests that strategies to prevent destitution or minimize its impact on the mentally ill will need to be implemented in the context of broader poverty-reduction policies and interventions, such as the government's Growth and Poverty Reduction Strategy (GPRS). In its current formulation, this strategy aims to bring issues of vulnerability and social exclusion into mainstream strategies of human resource development (Ghana National Development Planning Commission 2005). This goal is applicable to mental health care.

This chapter has discussed three sets of interventions for the mentally ill destitute—village systems, Christian outreach healing, and humanitarian and rights-based approaches—and described the strengths and limitations of each. I argue that the humanitarian and rights-based approaches offer the best hope for the future in terms of empirical reach, efficacy, and alignment with current global mental health practice. I will discuss two examples here to support this argument. Current humanitarian initiatives in Accra and Tamale focus on providing temporary accommodation, counseling, and food for vagrants. These initiatives follow Western approaches and incorporate the growing recognition by mental health experts that some individuals choose a life of vagrancy and may not respond to medicosocial rehabilitation. Basher and coauthors note: "Vagrants have conspicuously opted out of their contractual obligations to local communities in return for freedom to wander and release from certain social obligations. . . . They are likely to prefer retaining their state of social deviance, albeit with some marginal medical intervention, to undergoing an extensive personal reorientation and rehabilitation" (1983, 40). The humanitarian approach exists in sharp contrast to the Pentecostal outreach approach that, by equating all forms of vagrancy to spiritually caused madness, aims to effect "extensive personal reorientation and rehabilitation."

Within the range of mental health activities currently provided by NGOs in Ghana, the multifaceted model provided by BasicNeeds offers the best chance for mentally ill individuals in their communities or in institutions to avoid destitution. The sustainable livelihood component of this model is particularly significant, because it sets an important precedent for addressing the role of structural poverty in the onset and outcome of mental illness and the impact of that poverty on sufferers and their families. Family support is crucial to patients' recovery and rehabilitation (Asuni 1967; Ohaeri and Fido 2001; Read 2005; World Health Organization 2001). However, mental illness not only disrupts the lives of sufferers, it also disrupts the lives of their families. In Africa the medical, psychological, psychosocial, and financial burdens resulting from the experience of mental illness are often borne by family members (Akpalu et al. 2007; Doku et al. 2007; Ohaeri and Fido 2001). These multiple burdens contribute to family distancing from and abandonment of the patient. There is a strong association in Ghana between the risk of family abandonment and the family's structural poverty status. Because mental health care in Ghana is grossly short of funds and other resources, the initiatives provided by mental health NGOs are a crucial resource. It will not be enough to provide and strengthen treatment, advocacy, and psychosocial support services for the mentally ill. It is also crucial to establish initiatives that create and sustain wealth for individuals and families affected by mental illness.

NOTES

1. Baasher and colleagues assert, for example, that vagrants in Ethiopia "formed a reservoir for malaria, relapsing fever, typhus, etc." (1983, 37). There is a general view that homeless and destitute individuals face greater physical, sexual, and mental health risks (Kalipeni et al. 2004; Parry-Jones and Queloz 1991; World Health Organization 2001; United Nations Habitat and Human Settlements Foundation 2003), although counter-evidence suggests that physical and mental illnesses are not a given in these populations (Allen 2000; Beiser and Collomb 1981; de-Graft Aikins and Ofori-Atta 2007). Morton Beiser and Henri Collomb, writing on the mental health of rural Senegalese migrating to the capital, Dakar, note that the mental health outcome "is determined not by change per se but by social contingencies which modify the situation" (1981, 455). These social contingencies include "the persistence of familiar cultural norms within the new environment and skills such as literacy and the ability to creatively integrate elements of the old and new cultures" (ibid.).

2. Alan Radley defines *impairments* as "loss or abnormality of physiological or anatomical function" and *disabilities* as "restrictions in the ability to carry out or to fulfil a role in a normal way" (1994, 141).

3. "Handicap" has been defined as the (mainly negative) "assumptions that others make about the sick and their reactions to them" (Radley 1994, 148).

4. Jon Kirby distinguishes between permanent and transitory witch camps in northern Ghana. He notes that the camps "of East Dagbon (and Nanung)—Ngani, Kukuo, Kpatinga—are more or less permanent. The 'witches' cannot go back. But the camp at Gambaga has a fairly good rate of success: it 'effectively reintegrates women back into their communities'" (2006, 14).

5. It is important to note that this is possible only if the course and impact of these conditions are known publicly and accepted as conditions arising from external factors.

6. This shift is clear in published observations of vagrants on the streets. Ione Acquah noted only men wandering the streets of Accra "semi-clothed or naked, their hair and skin caked with dirt." These men were largely "left in the town where they sleep in the open, begging or stealing food," until they became dangerous—when they would, presumably, be forced into hospital care (1958, 143). Fifty years later, media discourses on vagrants focus on the presence of vagrant men and women on major city streets (Munko, 2006, Osabutey, 2006).

7. Personal communication from L. Essuman, co-director of Psychomental Health Foundation, a Ghanaian mental health NGO, April 2008.

8. Based on informal interviews conducted with hospital psychiatrists and nurses in the summer of 2006 for a study on homelessness and mental health among Accra's migrant squatters (de-Graft Aikins and Ofori-Atta 2007).

9. Personal communication from Dr Akwasi Osei, Chief Psychiatrist, Accra Psychiatric Hospital, April, 2007.

10. Personal communication from Dr Albert Boohene, faculty member, Department of Child Health, University of Ghana Medical School, September 2011.

11. This account is based on conversations in October 2007 with Ursula Read, at that time a PhD candidate in anthropology who was conducting research on mental illness experiences in Kintampo and the surrounding villages.

12. Personal communication from Ursula Read, PhD candidate in anthropology, October 2007.

13. Personal communication from Humphrey Cofie, BasicNeeds, April, 2007; Personal communication from Peter Yaro, BasicNeeds, August 2007.

REFERENCES

Acquah, I. 1958. *Accra Survey.* London: University of London Press.

Adinkra, M. 2004. "Witchcraft Accusations and Female Homicide Victimization in Contemporary Ghana." *Violence against Women* 10 (4): 325–56.

Adomakoh, C. C. 1972. "Mental Hospital Patients: A Castle Road Profile." *Ghana Medical Journal* 11 (2): 65–71.

Adrah, R. T., D. Adzosh, P. Afulani, L. L. Afutu, J., Aggrey-Orleans, K. Agyei-Kuffour, F. Akoto, and I. Aja. 2006. "Social Work in Psychiatric Care: The Accra Psychiatric Hospital Situation." University of Ghana Medical School Senior Clerkship Project in Psychology; Department of Psychiatry.

Agyei-Mensah, S., and A. de-Graft Aikins, A. 2010. "Epidemiological Transition and the Double Burden of Disease in Accra, Ghana." *Journal of Urban Health* 87 (5): 879–97.

Akpalu, B., D. Awenva, V. Doku, K. Ae-Inibise, S. Owusu-Agyei, and P. Martin. 2007. "Psychiatric Disorders among the Elderly in Rural Ghana: Preliminary Findings from the Kintampo Demographic Surveillance Site (KDSS)." Paper presented at the First Annual Scientific Conference of the College of Health Sciences, University of Ghana, Accra, Ghana, September 27.

Akrong, A. 2007. "A Phenomenology of Witchcraft in Ghana." In *Imagining Evil: Witchcraft Beliefs and Accusations in Contemporary Africa,* edited by G. ter Haar, 53–66. Trenton, NJ: Africa World.

Akyeampong, E. 2006. "Cannabis and Madness in Ghana." Paper presented at the African Psychiatry Workshop, Harvard University, December 14.

———. 2007. "Slave Routes, Slave Roots and Nation-Building: Ghana, Ghanaians Abroad and the African Diaspora in the 21st Century." Inaugural Lecture, Launch of the International Institute for the Advanced Study of Cultures, Institutions and Economic Enterprise, International Conference Center in Accra, Ghana, August 21.

Allen, C. 2000. "On the 'Physiological Dope' Problematic in Housing and Illness Research: Towards a Critical Realism of Home and Health." *Housing, Theory and Society* 17 (2): 49–67.

Allotey P, and D. Reidpath. 2007. "Epilepsy, Culture, Identity and Wellbeing: A Study of the Social, Cultural and Environmental Context of Epilepsy in Cameroon." *Journal of Health Psychology* 12 (3): 431–43.

Asuni, T. 1967. "Aro Hospital in Perspective." *American Journal of Psychiatry* 124: 763–77.

———. 1971. "Vagrant Psychotics in Abeokuta." *Journal of the National Medical Association* 63 (3): 173–80.

Baasher, T., A. S. E. D. Elhakim, K. El Fawal, R. Giel, T. W. Harding, and V. B. Wankiri. 1983. "On Vagrancy and Psychosis." *Community Mental Health Journal* 19 (1): 27–41.

Banson, M., O. Boadum, M. Boamah, G. Bonsanna, C. Brew-Daniels, V. Caesar, E. K. Coomson, and F. Dapaah. 2006. *Functions, Challenges and Future of the Vagrant Ward of the Accra Psychiatric Hospital.* University of Ghana Medical School Senior Clerkship Project in Psychology.

Barnor, M. A. 2001. *A Socio-Medical Adventure in Ghana: Autobiography of Dr. M. A. Barnor.* Mampong-Akuapem. Ghana: Viesco Universal.

Bartlett, F. 1932. *Remembering.* Cambridge: Cambridge University Press.

Bates, T. 2007. "Empowering Communities to Tackle Mental Health." *Irish Times, Health Supplement,* May 15. www.irishtimes.com/news/health/empowering-communities-to-tackle-mental-health-1.1205980.

Beiser, M., and H. Collomb. 1981. "Mastering Change: Epidemiological and Case Studies in Senegal, West Africa." *American Journal of Psychiatry* 138 (4): 455–59.

Bell, L. V. 1991. *Mental and Social Disorder in Sub-Saharan Africa: The Case of Sierra Leone, 1787–1990.* New York: Greenwood.

Bury, M. 1982. "Chronic Illness as Biographical Disruption." *Sociology of Health and Illness* 4 (2): 167–82.

———. 1997. *Health and Illness in a Changing Society.* London: Routledge.

Charmaz, K. 1983. "Loss of Self: A Fundamental Form of Suffering in the Chronically Ill." *Sociology of Health and Illness* 15 (2): 168–95.

———. 1991. *Good Days, Bad Days: The Self in Chronic Illness and Time.* New Brunswick, NJ: Rutgers University Press.

Deacon, H., I. Stephney, and S. Prosalendis. 2005. *Understanding HIV/Stigma: A Theoretical and Methodological Analysis.* Cape Town: HSRC Press.

de-Graft Aikins, A. 2004. "Strengthening Quality and Continuity of Diabetes Care in Rural Ghana: A Critical Social Psychological Approach." *Journal of Health Psychology* 9 (2): 295–309.

———. 2006. "Reframing Applied Disease Stigma Research: A Multilevel Analysis of Diabetes Stigma in Ghana." *Journal of Community and Applied Social Psychology* 16 (6): 426–41.

de-Graft Aikins, A., and A. Ofori-Atta. 2007. "Homelessness and Mental Health in Ghana: Everyday Experiences of Accra's Migrant Squatters." *Journal of Health Psychology* 12 (5): 761–78.

Desjarlais, R., L. Eisenberg, B. Good, and A. Kleinman. 1995. *World Mental Health: Problems and Priorities in Low-Income Countries.* Oxford and New York: Oxford University Press.

Destombes, J. 1999. *Nutrition and Economic Destitution in Northern Ghana, 1930–1957. A Historical Perspective on Nutritional Economics.* Department of Economic History, London School of Economics Working Paper No. 49/99. http://eprints.lse.ac.uk/22388/1/wp49.pdf.

Doise, W. 1986. *Levels of Explanation in Social Psychology.* Cambridge: Cambridge University Press.

Doku, V., A. Ofori-Atta, B. Akpalu, and A. Osei. 2007. *Country Report of Mental Health Policy Development and Implementation in Ghana.* Unpublished report for the Ghana Mental Health and Poverty Project.

Dovlo, E. 2007. "Witchcraft in Contemporary Ghana." In *Imagining Evil: Witchcraft Beliefs and Accusations in Contemporary Africa,* edited by G. ter Haar, 67–92. Trenton, NJ: Africa World.

Edgerton, R. B. 1966. "Conceptions of Psychosis in Four East African Societies." *American Anthropologist* 68 (2): 408–25.

Ewusi-Mensah, I. 2001. "Post-Colonial Psychiatric Care in Ghana." *Psychiatric Bulletin* 25 (6): 228–29.

Field, M. J. 1958. "Mental Disorders in Rural Ghana." *Journal of Mental Science* 104: 1043–51.

———. 1960. *Search for Security: An Ethno-Psychiatric Study of Rural Ghana.* New York: W. W. Norton.

Fondation d'Harcourt. 2014. "We Have a Right to a Normal Life." Accessed November 3. http://www.fondationdharcourt.org/stories/we-have-the-right-to-a-normal-life.

Forster, E. F. B. 1958. "A Short Psychiatric Review from Ghana." In *Mental Disorders and Mental Health in Africa South of the Sahara*, CCTA/CSA-WFMH-WHO *Meeting of Specialists on Mental Health, Bukavu, Belgian Congo*, 37–41. London: CSA.

———. 1962. "A Historical Study of Psychiatric Practice in Ghana." *Ghana Medical Journal* 1 (1): 25–29.

Forster, E. B., and S. A. Danquah. 1977. "Chronic Mental Illness as Seen in Ghana." *Ghana Medical Journal* 17: 109–117.

Foster, J. 2001. "Unification and Differentiation: A Study of the Social Representations of Mental Illness." *Papers on Social Representations* 10 (3): 1–18.

Freidson, E. 1970. *Profession of Medicine: A Study of the Sociology of Applied Knowledge.* Chicago: University of Chicago Press.

Gervais, M. C., N. Morant, and G. Penn. 1999. "Making Sense of 'Absence': Towards a Typology of Absence in Social Representations Theory and Research." *Journal for the Theory of Social Behaviour* 29 (4): 419–44.

Ghana Ministry of Health. 1994. *1993 Annual Report.* Accra, Ghana: Ministry of Health.

Ghana National Development Planning Commission. 2005. *Growth and Poverty Reduction Strategy (GPRS II) (2006–2009).* Accra, Ghana: Assembly Press. http://www.ndpc.gov.gh/GPRS/GPRS%20I%20Vol%202.pdf.

Human Rights Watch. 2012. "Ghana: Abuse of People with Disabilities." Accessed November 4, 2014. https://www.youtube.com/watch?v=n7HRnXxY_g0#t=28.

Iliffe, J. 1987. *The African Poor: A History.* Cambridge: Cambridge University Press.

Jahoda, G. 1961. "Traditional Healers and Other Institutions Concerned with Mental Health in Ghana." *International Journal of Social Psychiatry* 7 (4): 245–68.

Jilek-Aall, L., M. Jilek, J. Kaaya, L. Mkombachepa, and K. Hillary. 1997. "Psychosocial Study of Epilepsy in Africa." *Social Science and Medicine* 45 (5): 783–95.

Jodelet, D. 1991. *Madness and Social Representations: Living with the Mad in One French Community.* Translated by Tim Pownall. London: Wheatsheaf.

Kabir, M., Z. Iliyasu, I. S. Abubakr, and M. H. Aliyu. 2004. "Perception and Beliefs about Mental Illness among Adults in Karfi Village, Northern Nigeria." *BMC International Health and Human Rights* 4 (3). doi:10.1186/1472-698X-4-3.

Kalipeni, E., S. Craddock, J. R. Oppong, and J. Ghosh, eds. 2004. *HIV & AIDS in Africa: Beyond Epidemiology.* Malden, MA: Blackwell Publishing.

Kirby, J. 2006. "Ghana's 'Witch Camps': Prison or Sanctuary?" Paper presented at the African Studies Association Conference, San Francisco, CA, November 16–19.

Kleinman, A. 1988. *Rethinking Psychiatry: From Cultural Category to Personal Experience.* New York: The Free Press.

Link, B. G., and J. C. Phelan. 2001. "Conceptualising Stigma." *Annual Review of Sociology* 27: 363–85.

Markova, I. 2003. *Dialogicality and Social Representations: The Dynamics of Mind.* Cambridge: Cambridge University Press.

Munko, K. 2006. "Building the Capacity of Community Psychiatry Nurses." *Daily Graphic*, July 26.

Nettleton, S. 1995. *The Sociology of Health and Illness.* Cambridge: Polity Press.

Odejide, A. O., M. O. Olatawura, A. O. Sanda, and A. O. Oyeneye. 1977. "Traditional Healers and Mental Illness in the City of Ibadan." *African Journal of Psychiatry* 3 (4): 99–106.

Ohaeri, J. U., and Fido, A. A. 2001. "The Opinion of Caregivers on Aspects of Schizophrenia and Major Affective Disorders in a Nigerian Setting." *Social Psychiatry and Psychiatric Epidemiology* 36: 493–99.

Osabutey, P. D. 2006. "Prayer Camps: Saviour or Danger?" *Accra Chronicle,* September 6.

Parry-Jones, W. L. L., and N. Queloz, eds. 1991. *Mental Health and Deviance in Inner Cities.* Geneva: World Health Organization.

Patel, V., and A. Kleinman. 2003. "Poverty and Common Mental Disorders in Developing Countries. *Bulletin of the World Health Organization* 81: 609–15.

Public Records and Archives Administration Department, Accra. CSO 11/8/02. Medical Officer F. MacLagan, May 12, 1930. "Persons certified to be Insane—Refusal of the Police Magistrate to Issue Warrants for the Confinement of."

Public Records and Archives Administration Department, Accra. CSO 11/8/11. Medical Officer F. MacLagan. "Congestion in Lunatic Asylum: Proposals for Relief" (1930–1932).

Radley, A. 1994. *Making Sense of Illness: The Social Psychology of Health and Disease.* London: Sage.

Read, U. M. 2005. "Feeling Part of the Outside World: An Ethnographic Study of Recovery from Mental Illness in Ghana." MSc thesis, University College, London.

Sadowsky, J. 1999. *Imperial Bedlam: Institutions of Madness in Colonial Southwest Nigeria.* Berkeley: University of California Press.

Stickley, T., R. Hitchcock, and G. Bertram. 2005. "Social Inclusion or Social Control? Homelessness and Mental Health." *Mental Health Practice* 8 (9): 26–30.

Thomas, A., and S. Sillen. 1993. *Racism and Psychiatry.* New York: Carol.

Thompson, M. et al. 2008. "Living with Mental Illness in Ghana: The Stigma Study." Clinical Psychology Senior Clerkship Project Report, Department of Psychiatry, University of Ghana.

Tooth, G. 1950. *Studies in Mental Illness in the Gold Coast.* London: Her Majesty's Stationery Office.

Twumasi, P. A. 2005. 2nd ed. *Medical Systems in Ghana.* Accra: Ghana Publishing.

United Nations Habitat and Human Settlements Foundation. 2003. *The Challenge of Slums: The Global Report on Human Settlements 2003.* London: Earthscan.

Wagner, W., G. Duveen, M. Themel, and J. Verma. 1999. "The Modernisation of Tradition: Thinking about Madness in Patna, India." *Culture and Psychology* 5 (4): 413–446.

Wagner, W., G. Duveen, J. Verma, and M. Themel. 2000. "'I Have Some Faith and at the Same Time I Don't Believe in It': Cognitive Polyphasia and Culture Change." In *Health, Community, and Development,* edited by C. Campbell and S. Jovchelovitch, special issue, *Journal of Community and Applied Social Psychology* 10 (4): 301–314.

Weinberg, S. K. 1965. "Cultural Aspects of Manic-Depression in West Africa." *Journal of Health and Human Behavior* 6 (4): 247–53.

World Health Organization. 2001. *The World Health Report: Mental Health: New Understanding New Hope.* Geneva: World Health Organization.

World Health Organization. 2005. *Preventing Chronic Disease. A Vital Investment.* Geneva: World Health Organization.

5 CHILDREN AND ADOLESCENT MENTAL HEALTH IN SOUTH AFRICA

ALAN FLISHER, ANDREW DAWES, ZUHAYR KAFAAR,
CRICK LUND, KATHERINE SORSDAHL, BRONWYN
MYERS, RITA THOM, AND SORAYA SEEDAT[1]

*This essay is dedicated by the remaining authors to the memory
of Alan Flisher, our colleague, friend, and mentor,
who passed away prior to its publication.*

EPIDEMIOLOGY

Prevalence studies of psychiatric disorders among children and adolescents in South Africa are characterized by small and unrepresentative samples and/or the use of diagnostic instruments that have not been validated in the local context. Nonetheless, estimates are necessary to inform the development of policies and plans for child and adolescent mental health services. In an effort to fill this information gap, Sharon Kleintjies and coauthors (2006) produced a set of prevalence estimates for children and adolescents in the Western Cape Province. The estimates were based on the results of relevant epidemiological studies, with greater weight being given to studies that were methodologically superior and more proximal geographically. Prevalence rates were adjusted to take into account risk factors particularly present in the South African environment: exposure to violence, maltreatment, and the stresses associated with living in households affected by HIV/AIDS.

Significant numbers of South African children and adolescents are exposed to violence in the community, in schools, and at home (Burton 2008; Leoschut and Burton 2006; M. Seedat et al. 2009). South African studies indicate that exposure is associated with psychological disorder in children and adolescents (Ensink et al. 1997; Peltzer 1999; S. Seedat et al. 2004; S. Seedat et al. 2000; Ward et al. 2001).

Although the prevalence of child maltreatment (both physical and sexual abuse) in South Africa is not established, indications are that the rates are high (Dawes and Ward 2008; Jewkes et al. 2002). Maltreatment is known to be associated with negative psychological outcomes during childhood (English 1998), particularly when chronic. As demonstrated by the Adverse Childhood Experiences studies, the effects persist into adulthood (Chapman et al. 2004; Felitti et al. 1998).

The HIV epidemic affects many South African children (Shisana et al. 2010). Exposure to the stresses associated with living in households affected by HIV/AIDS is a risk factor for psychological disorders in childhood and adolescents (Richter, Stein, Cluver, and de Kadt, 2009), particularly where children are already coping with other adverse experiences such as poverty (Bauman et al. 2009; Cluver and Gardner 2006; Forehand et al. 2002; Wild 2001). Furthermore, HIV infection in children results in a number of neuropsychiatric syndromes, including cognitive impairment; developmental delay; attention and concentration problems; serious mental illness; and common mental disorders, including depression, anxiety, and substance abuse (Rao et al. 2007).

Kleintjies and colleagues (2006) took these risk factors into account and adjusted for comorbidity to provide a more accurate picture of the likely service needs; the overall adjusted prevalence rate they found was 17 percent. Unadjusted and adjusted rates, respectively, for selected disorders were as follows: oppositional defiant disorder, 6.0 percent and 1.50 percent; enuresis, 5.0 percent and 1.25 percent; separation anxiety disorder, 4.0 percent and 1.0 percent; depressive disorder and dysthymia, 8.0 percent and 2.00 percent; agoraphobia, 3.0 percent and 0.75 percent; simple phobia, -3.0 percent and 0.75 percent; social phobia 5.0 percent and 1.25 percent; generalized anxiety disorder, 11.0 percent and 2.75 percent; and post-traumatic stress disorder, 8.0 percent and 2.00 percent. The unadjusted rates for schizophrenia and bipolar affective disorder were 0.5 percent and 1.0 percent, respectively.

The South African rate appears to be somewhat higher than those reported in other low- and middle-income countries such as Brazil, Bangladesh, and India (Patel et al. 2008). Besides the methodological factors that could account for such a finding, the elevated rate could also be attributable to the high levels of exposure to the risk factors outlined above. South African epidemiological studies are required to validate the estimates provided by Kleintjies and colleagues (2006).

The prevalence of substance use disorders among South African adolescents is unknown, but a high proportion of patients attending substance abuse clinics are under twenty years of age (Plüddermann et al. 2007). Substance abuse disorders tend to occur in conjunction with other mental health disorders (Armstrong and Costello 2002; Lubman et al. 2007; Roberts, Roberts, and Xing, 2007). This is important because early problems in both domains are associated with greater functional impairment (Lubman et al. 2007; Rowe, Liddle, and Dakof 2001) and poorer treatment outcomes (Ramo et al. 2005), compared to adolescents with problems in a single domain. Findings from a South African study suggest that use of crystal metamphetamine (known as *tik*), which has reached epidemic proportions in Cape Town, is a risk factor for aggression and depression (Plüddermann et al. 2007).

The above data indicate the burden of mental illness among children and adolescents in South Africa but also highlight what we don't know. There is a striking absence of representative epidemiological data on the burden of child and adolescent mental disorders in South Africa. Because prevalence estimates are essential for service planning, it is vital that such studies be conducted as a matter of priority.

LEGAL AND POLICY CONTEXT

In recent years the South African government has taken significant steps to establish the legal and policy framework for the provision of comprehensive and community-based services for children, adolescents, and adults. A pivotal development that occurred in 1997, soon after the installation of the first democratic government, was the publication of the *White Paper for the Transformation of the Health System in South Africa* (Republic of South Africa Department of Health 1997). A chapter on mental health proposed the planning of a comprehensive, community-based mental health service that would operate at national, provincial, district, and community levels and would be integrated with other health services. In the same year, the department released a set of policy guidelines for improved mental health care. These guidelines were consistent with and informed by the provisions of the white paper, and they identified services for children and adolescents as one of the priority areas for intervention. The guidelines were approved by the national and provincial governments but were formally published or extensively distributed. Nor were implementation guidelines developed to implement the white paper's policy recommendations (Draper et al. 2009).

In 2001 and 2003 the government released policy guidelines for adolescent and youth health and for child and adolescent mental health (Republic of South Africa Department of Health 2001, 2003). Each set of guidelines proposed five general intervention strategies: the promotion of a culturally sensitive, safe, and supportive environment; provision of information; skills development; provision of counseling; and ensuring access to health services. The guidelines for child and adolescent mental health referred to the need to transform and make services more accessible to this population through the implementation of a community-based model with three service tiers, from primary to super specialist levels of care. Although not dealing specifically with child health services, the Children's Act (No. 35 of 2005) has a number of implications for preventive services for children and adolescents in vulnerable circumstances (Dawes 2009; Dawes and Ward 2011).

A MODEL FOR CHILD AND ADOLESCENT
MENTAL HEALTH SERVICES

In 2003 the government commissioned a research project to develop norms and standards and to lay the foundation for integrated child and adolescent mental health services (CAMHS) that would ensure accessibility to health services (Dawes et al. 2004; Lund et al. 2009). The next three sections of this essay draw on that research.

Andrew Dawes et al. (2004) proposed a framework for CAMHS that was informed by a set of standards referring to the quality that service users could expect to characterize the services they received (see also Lund et al. 2009). The standards were derived from three main sources: those developed for the National Health Service in the United Kingdom (UK Department of Health National Child and Adolescent Support Service and the University of Durham 2004), recommendations of the World Health Organization (2004 and 2005), and a volume by Robert Desjarlais and coauthors (1995) that addressed mental health in developing countries. The standards statements were divided into three categories.

First were those standards applicable to the core features of CAMHS. According to these, the South African Department of Health should include mental health in primary health care settings; provide a continuum of services; balance prevention, promotion, treatment, and rehabilitation; and prioritize children most at risk. The second group included standards that addressed evidence and service planning, which recommended that the Department of Health should conduct regular assessments of levels of service provision and need; use this information to plan and commission comprehensive services; and involve parents, other family members, and communities in service planning.

Finally, there were standards that concerned the range of services, staffing, and facilities. According to these, the government should offer early intervention and mental health promotion in all locations; coordinate and integrate services across health, education, social care, youth justice, and voluntary sector agencies; use a multidisciplinary team approach; train, supervise, and support all staff to provide a full range of interventions; ensure that care is developmentally appropriate; keep children's and adolescents' mental health care facilities separate from adults if appropriate—for example, in in-patient facilities; offer services as near to home as possible and in child-centered settings, such as schools, youth clubs, and the family; and offer twenty-four-hour care.

These standards are all compatible with the national policy guidelines that were referred to earlier (Republic of South Africa Department of Health 2003). However, the policy guidelines for child and adolescent mental health went further, proposing a three-tiered system of service organization that was modeled on the work of Dawes and coauthors (1997). According to this system, generic health workers in the first tier aim to identify children or adolescents with mental health problems; provide basic interventions, such as crisis intervention and other forms of counseling, when they are able to and refer patients to higher tiers when they are not. Specialists and super specialists in the second and third tiers, respectively, provide supervision, consultation, and training to those at lower levels and provide some services directly.

Although such schemes are extremely useful in providing a broad direction forward, they are less appropriate when it comes to indicating what components a new system should include, and where those components should be located in the broader health system. For example, mental health services at the third tier could be situated in general hospitals, psychiatric hospitals, or free-standing units such as a substance abuse unit.

SERVICE STRUCTURE

For these reasons, it is preferable to have a service structure with two broad divisions—general health services (type A), and specialist child and adolescent mental health facilities (type B). The former can be subdivided into hospital-based services (at the primary, regional, and provincial levels, which would be type A1) and services provided at primary health care facilities (clinics and community health centers, which would be type A2). Type B services can be subdivided into child and family units, child therapy centers, adolescent units, substance abuse units, eating disorders units, and other specialist facilities (which could include psychiatric hospitals, although we would not recommend that young people receive services in such hospitals). Ideally, there is also a regional child and adolescent mental health team (type C) that provides consultation to all the facilities listed above and that coordinates and supports services (see figure 5.1).

This structure can serve at least two purposes. First, it can be used as a scaffold to assess existing services. Second, it can be used to indicate the direction in which services should be headed—that is, what norms for staffing service provision should we have? These matters will be dealt with in the following two sections.

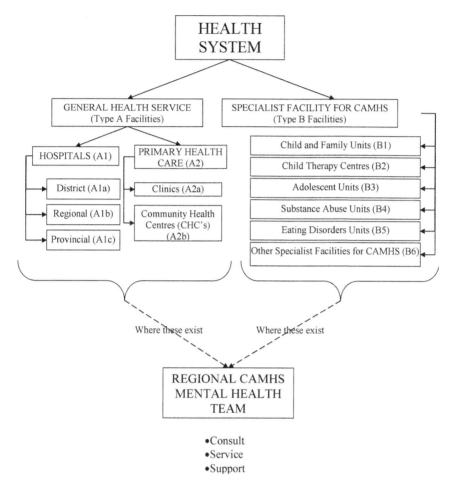

Figure 5.1. A Framework for Integrated Child and Adolescent
Mental Health Services (CAMHS) in South Africa

ESTABLISHING STAFFING LEVELS

Dawes and coauthors (2004) collected data for public-sector services such as the
numbers and levels of staff members in each component of the specialist CAMHS
and general health services from the mental health coordinators in all nine provincial health departments (following the typology outlined in figure 5.1). Interviews were also conducted with provincial coordinators. In addition, the exercise
sought to establish the support structures that were available for CAMHS in each
province; the existence, composition, degree of integration, and level of support

offered by CAMHS teams; and what mental health services were actually provided for children and adolescents by the department of health as well as other government departments, nongovernmental organizations, and community-based organizations in each province.

Before discussing staff numbers, Dawes and coauthors presented some general observations that emerged during their provincial visits. First, referral patterns followed the same pathways as had been the case under apartheid, when there had been four provinces. The provinces that had been created after the end of apartheid had no specialist facilities and referred patients to the existing facilities in other provinces. Second, the integration of CAMHS into primary health care services had not been achieved to any significant extent in any of the provinces. Third, service providers at the primary health care level had generally received insufficient training to offer meaningful mental health services. Fourth, no province had a formally constituted team that offered consultation, coordination, and support. And finally, those who lived outside the capital cities of the four apartheid-era provinces had very limited access to specialist CAMHS. These data were collected in 2004; because no national study has since been conducted on CAMHS, it is difficult to assess whether there have been any significant changes since then.

Assembling accurate data from the provinces was a challenge. For six provinces, there was no information for at least one aspect of their services. This lack cannot be ascribed entirely to insufficient resources. For example, in the case of the Western Cape, which is a province with abundant resources by South African standards, information was not available for general hospital outpatient and general hospital inpatient services (type A1), primary health care services (type A2), or specialist facilities (type B).

One reason for this situation was the lack of systems needed to generate the information. For example, it was difficult to estimate the number of full-time equivalent staff owing to the integration of CAMHS indicators into those for general health services, and the integration of mental health care service indicators into those for general health services. Details were not available on the proportion of time that staff members devoted to providing CAMHS. Similarly, details were not available regarding the proportion of children and adolescents who presented with mental health problems, or who presented with other problems but were also suffering from a mental health problem. Another critical reason was the lack of personnel with the capacity, motivation, and time to ensure that, when data were available, they were of good quality, appropriately analyzed, and used for decision making.

Dawes and coauthors (2004) found that CAMHS were almost entirely general health services (type A). This was particularly evident for Limpopo, Mpuma-

Table 5.1. Ratios of Mental Health Practitioners to
Children in All South African Provinces

PROVINCE	RATIO
Gauteng	1:19,355
Mpumalanga	1:5,099
North West	1:5,388
Free State	1:103,276
Limpopo	1:58 9861
Northern Cape	No data
Eastern Cape	1:22,565
KwaZulu-Natal	1:9,881
Western Cape	1:34,702

Source: Adapted from Dawes et al. 2004.
Note: The data were provided by the provincial departments of health and include
all categories of mental health professionals employed in the public service.

langa, Northern Cape, North West, and Eastern Cape, where there were no specialist CAMHS at the time of the study. It is likely that this situation existed more
by default than by design. Although South African and international guidelines
stipulate that CAMHS should be provided in the general health service, it is necessary that there be a balance in the suite of available services. In the absence of
specialist mental health services, it is not possible to provide training, support,
supervision, consultation, or liaison for practitioners delivering CAMHS in the
general health sector, nor is it possible to provide suitable referral destinations
for problems that cannot be managed in the general health system. The quality
of services is thus likely to be substantially compromised, and indeed it became
evident that this was the case when Dawes's team visited the provincial health
departments. Finally, the absolute levels of service provision were very low. The
ratios of all mental health practitioners in the public health service to the number
of children and adolescents are presented in Table 5.1.

The reliability of the figures in Table 5.1 cannot be guaranteed due to the
limited information provided, its poor quality, and the uneven quality of data
across provinces. For this reason, it was not possible to provide ratios of the various professional groups to the child and adolescent population in the country as
a whole. However, the extent of the low levels of service provision can be inferred
from the numbers of staff members in the three provinces for which data were
available for the types of services they delivered. These provinces were Mpumalanga, North West, and KwaZulu-Natal, which had populations of children and

adolescents nineteen years or younger of 1,463,396, 1,537,458 and 4,397,236 respectively (based on the 2001 census). At the time, therefore, the total population of children and adolescents in these three provinces was 7,398,090. The total numbers of staff in the various categories (with the equivalent number per million population of children and adolescents) are provided in Table 5.2 (see below for a discussion of how the norms were developed and of the implications of these numbers).

These numbers and the staff per million population of children and adolescents may underestimate the situation for the country as a whole because the provinces with the most resources (Gauteng and Western Cape) are excluded owing to incomplete data. However, the numbers serve to illustrate the challenges for the development of CAMHS in South Africa, given that the majority of the country's population lives outside the best-off provinces.

When one considers the prevalence rates of psychiatric disorders among children and adolescents in South Africa, it is quite obvious that only a minute fraction of the need can be addressed by the current levels of service provision. This raises the question of what norms should be used to address the needs of children and adolescents with mental health problems.

DEVELOPING NORMS FOR MENTAL HEALTH SERVICES

Building on previous work in which South African service norms were developed for adults with severe psychiatric disorders and for community mental health services (Flisher et al. 2003; Lund and Flisher 2006), Dawes and coauthors (2004) developed a model to calculate service norms for children and adolescents with mental health problems in South Africa (see also Lund et al. 2009). The model was developed using Microsoft Excel and can be adapted by adjusting any of the following parameters: population size, age distribution, prevalence, comorbidity, levels of coverage, attendance at ambulatory care facilities, ambulatory care use rates, ambulatory care workloads, duration of consultations, and number of staff members.

There were five stages in the modeling process. First, based on 2001 census data, the number of children and adolescents in each province was calculated.

Second, the prevalence of psychiatric disorders reported in the article by Kleintjies and coauthors (2006) informed the model. These prevalence rates were adjusted for comorbidity to prevent inflated service needs and were used to calculate a minimum level of service coverage, based on the proportion of children and adolescents with each disorder that would receive CAMHS.

Third, the likely use of services by the identified cases according to each level of the service framework described above was calculated. The measures of ser-

Table 5.2. Staffing Numbers and Minimum Staffing Norms for Selected Provinces in South Africa, per Million Population < 19 in 2004

	MPUMALANGA POPULATION <19* = 1,463,396		NORTH WEST POPULATION <19* = 1,537,458		KWAZULU-NATAL POPULATION <19* = 4,397,236	
	CURRENT	NORM	CURRENT	NORM	CURRENT	NORM
Type A1 (general hospital outpatients)						
General nurses	7.0	3.4	5.1	8.9	1.0	25.5
Psychiatric nurses	0.0	1.3	9.3	3.6	92.0	10.2
Occupational therapists	0.1	2.5	2.1	1.3	3.0	3.8
Occupational therapy assistants	0.0	1.7	1.1	2.7	1.0	7.6
Social workers	0.1	1.7	1.1	1.8	11.0	5.1
Psychologists	0.0	1.7	1.1	1.8	0.0	5.1
Psychiatrists	0.0	0.0	0.0	0.0	1.0	0.0
Registrars (residents) and medical officers	12.2	1.3	7.3	1.3	6.0	3.8
TOTAL	**19.5**	**20.4**	**27.1**	**21.4**	**115.0**	**61.2**
Type A1 (general hospital inpatients)						
General nurses	77.5†	1.6	14.0†	1.7	1.0	4.7
Psychiatric nurses	18.7†	0.2	0.0	0.2	92.0	0.5
Social workers	1.2†	0.1	3.0†	0.1	11.0	0.3
Registrars (residents) and medical officers	12.9†	0.1	0.0	0.1	6.0	0.2
TOTAL	**109.5†**	**1.9**	**17.0†**	**2.0**	**110.0**	**5.7**
Type A2 (primary health care)						
General nurses	46.4	81.3	166.0†	85.4	12.0	244.2
Psychiatric nurses	12.5	32.5	7.0	34.2	75.0	97.7
Occupational therapists	1.3	8.1	0.0	8.5	3.0	24.4
Occupational therapy assistants	0.8	24.4	0.0	25.6	22.0	73.2

Table 5.2. (*continued*) Staffing Numbers and Minimum Staffing Norms for Selected Provinces in South Africa, per Million Population < 19 in 2004

	MPUMALANGA POPULATION <19* = 1,463,396		NORTH WEST POPULATION <19* = 1,537,458		KWAZULU-NATAL POPULATION <19* = 4,397,236	
	CURRENT	NORM	CURRENT	NORM	CURRENT	NORM
Social workers	3.2	16.3	4.0	17.1	0.0	48.8
Psychologists	0.0	16.3	0.0	17.1	1.0	48.8
Registrars (residents) and medical officers	1.2	16.3	3.0	17.1	23.0	48.8
TOTAL	**65.4**	**195.0**	**180†**	**204.9**	**136.0**	**586.0**
Type B (specialist CAMHS outpatients)						
General nurses	0.0	4.6	0.0	4.8	0.0	13.8
Psychiatric nurses	0.0	9.2	0.0	9.6	0.0	27.6
Occupational therapists	0.0	2.3	0.0	2.4	0.0	6.9
Occupational therapy assistants	0.0	6.9	0.0	7.2	0.0	20.7
Social workers	0.0	4.6	0.0	4.8	0.0	13.8
Psychologists	0.0	4.6	0.0	4.8	0.0	13.8
Psychiatrists	0.0	1.1	0.0	1.2	0.0	3.4
Registrars (residents) and medical officers	0.0	3.4	0.0	3.6	0.0	10.3
TOTAL	**0.0**	**36.7**	**0.0**	**38.6**	**0.0**	**110.0**
Type B (specialist CAMHS inpatients)						
General nurses	0.0	4.3	0.0	4.5	0.0	12.8
Psychiatric nurses	0.0	8.5	0.0	8.9	0.0	25.6
Social workers	0.0	2.2	0.0	3.0	0.0	8.5
Psychologists	0.0	2.8	0.0	2.2	0.0	6.4

Table 5.2. (*continued*) Staffing Numbers and Minimum Staffing Norms for Selected Provinces in South Africa, per Million Population < 19 in 2004

	MPUMALANGA POPULATION <19* = 1,463,396		NORTH WEST POPULATION <19* = 1,537,458		KWAZULU-NATAL POPULATION <19* = 4,397,236	
	CURRENT	NORM	CURRENT	NORM	CURRENT	NORM
Psychiatrists	0.0	2.1	0.0	2.2	0.0	6.4
Registrars (residents) and medical officers	0.0	1.4	0.0	1.5	0.0	4.3
TOTAL	**0.0**	**21.3**	**0.0**	**22.3**	**0.0**	**63.9**
Type B (specialist CAMHS day services)						
General nurses	0.0	5.5	0.0	5.8	0.0	16.6
Psychiatric nurses	0.0	5.5	0.0	5.8	0.0	16.6
Psychologists	0.0	3.7	0.0	3.9	0.0	11.1
Psychiatrists	0.0	3.7	0.0	3.9	0.0	11.1
TOTAL	**0.0**	**18.4**	**0.0**	**19.3**	**0.0**	**55.3**
Type C (CAMHS teams)						
Psychiatric nurses	0.0	0.8	0.0	0.9	0.0	2.1
Social workers	0.0	0.8	0.0	0.9	0.0	2.1
Psychologists	0.0	0.8	0.0	0.9	0.0	2.1
Psychiatrists	0.0	0.8	0.0	0.9	0.0	2.1
TOTAL	**0.0**	**3.2**	**0.0**	**3.6**	**0.0**	**8.4**

Source: Adapted from Dawes et al. 2004.

*Refers to child and adolescent population.

†Data almost certainly not valid although provided by provincial mental health coordinators; the data may refer to the total numbers of staff as opposed to those who provide mental health services.

vice use were daily patient visits for outpatient services, day service placements for day programs, and beds for inpatient services.

Fourth, the number of clinical staff members required for the services was calculated. Staffing of inpatient facilities and day programs was based on information provided in the provincial consultations. Norms for the CAMHS teams were based on the assumption that each health district should have at least one visit per month from a CAMHS specialist.

On the basis of the above data, it was possible to calculate staffing norms for all facility types. A more detailed explanation of how the norms were calculated (including the formulas used) is available (see Dawes et al. 2004; in Lund et al. 2009).

The minimal norms for the three provinces for which complete data were available are provided in Table 5.2. Although in most instances they are higher than current levels of service provision, in some cases they are lower. However, it is important to keep in mind that the norms represent minimal levels of service provision. Just because a norm has been met does not mean that service levels are sufficient to meet need. Rather, in such cases, it would be necessary to increase current staffing levels so that a larger proportion of children and adolescents with problems could receive services. In addition, where the norms are being met, this is solely the case for type A1 services (those provided in general hospitals). In such cases, it is necessary to develop types A2, B, and C services to provide more comprehensive care and to improve the support for those providing type A1 services.

The implication of this study is that each province should plan for the development of services of all the types described above and should set realistic targets for appropriate levels of staffing of each type. The minimal norms should be used as a basis for planning. And even with the large discrepancies between the current numbers of staff and the norms, it is important to remember that the norms are based on very conservative assumptions. They cover only 15–30 percent of the children and adolescents who are suffering from mental health problems.

The relatively inaccessible and underdeveloped nature of existing mental health services, in the face of the considerable need for them, raises the question of where children and adolescents with mental health problems receive help now. No data are available to answer this question definitively. However, it is probable that a large majority do not receive any help whatsoever. As a result, they and their caregivers experience suffering both as a direct result of the mental health problem and as a result of the associated stigma. Also, they suffer the consequences of mental health problems in childhood and adolescence, such as poor scholastic progress, increased likelihood of dropping out of school, poor peer relationships, and mental health problems later in life.

TRADITIONAL HEALERS

Thus far we have considered services in the public health system. Several studies and our clinical experience confirm that traditional healers are often consulted in sub-Saharan Africa for mental health problems at all life stages. Estimates of the proportion of adult African patients in community samples that have consulted a traditional healer range from 41 percent to 75 percent (Ensink and Robertson 1999; Freeman 1992; Freeman, Lee, and Vivian 1994; Patel, Simunya, and Gwanzura 1997). More recently, Katherine Sorsdahl and colleagues (2009) examined the role of traditional healers in mental health–seeking behavior in a nationally representative community sample of adults. Results revealed that 9 percent of the respondents consulted traditional healers, and 11 percent consulted a religious or spiritual advisor. Children and adolescents with mental health problems are very likely to receive interventions from traditional healers. However, we were not able to locate any studies that document the proportion of children and adolescents in South Africa who receive such interventions.

One important reason why traditional healers are consulted is that they offer interventions that are congruent with the culture of the service user (Freeman, Lee, and Vivian 1994; Mbanga, Niehaus, and Mzamo 2002; Nattrass 2005; Patel, Simunya, and Gwanzura 1997). In many traditional African belief systems, mental health problems are attributed to spiritual sources (including ancestors), and traditional healers are viewed as having the expertise needed to address these causes (Swartz 2008; Dawes and Cairns 1998). Furthermore, traditional healers are often more accessible than Western mental health care. It has been estimated that there are at least 200,000 traditional healers in South Africa, or approximately one per every five hundred South Africans (Sorsdahl, Stein, and Flisher 2010).

Karen Ensink and Brian Robertson (1999) assessed the categories of distress among children and adolescents in Cape Town, according to traditional healers. The categories were *ukuthwasa* (calling to be a healer), *amafufunyane* (possession by evil spirits), *ukuphambana* (madness), *isinyama esikolweni* (bewitchment at school), and *ukuphaphazela* (an episode of fearfulness). The first three categories have been identified in both adults and children and can be characterized as culture-bound syndromes because they do not correspond to specific disorders in the fourth edition of the American Psychiatric Association's *Diagnostic and Statistical Manual of Mental Disorders* (DSM-IV). Although *ukuthwasa* is not necessarily believed to be a disorder or illness, it can progress to another illness, such as *amafufunyane* or *ukuphambana,* if the calling to be a healer is not fulfilled. However, the last two categories can be considered as cultural variations of DSM-IV disorders. *Isinyama esikolweni* meets the DSM-IV criteria for conversion disorder with sensory deficit (similar to brain fag syndrome), and *ukuphaphaz-ela* is similar to sleep terror disorder and may also correspond to other anxiety disorders.

Given the significant support for traditional understandings of children's distress and methods of cure, clinical services that fail to take these understandings into account will fail to understand their patients and hence the provision of uninformed and suboptimal assessments and interventions, as well as deficits in rapport. Future research and policy and service planning initiatives need to ensure that the role of traditional healers does not continue to be overlooked (Sidley 2004; Sorsdahl, Stein, and Flisher 2010).

The focus of this essay has been on the delivery of mental health services that aim to intervene once problems have developed. We have focused on CAMHS, but it is important to be aware of the significant need for specialized substance abuse prevention and treatment efforts to address the needs of significant numbers of South African adolescents, many of whom probably have comorbid substance abuse and mental health problems. As is the case for people with mental health disorders, services for young people with substance abuse disorders remain grossly inadequate and fragmented (Harker et al. 2007; Louw 2004; Myers 2004; Myers and Fakier 2007; Myers, Louw, and Fakier 2008).

We also did not devote attention to mental health promotion or the prevention of mental ill health. This partially reflects the inadequate focus that these aspects of health care receive in South Africa. There is an urgent need to restore the balance between curative and preventive or promotional interventions. A review of child and adolescent risk and protective factors and of evidence for promotion and prevention interventions in low-resource settings has been conducted by Inge Petersen and coauthors (2010). We need strategies to strengthen individuals and families, as well as communities and systems, and to remove societal barriers to mental health (Patel et al. 2008). By implementing such strategies, we will not only succeed in improving the mental health of South African children and adolescents but also contribute to the country's social and economic progress by improving educational outcomes and social functioning in adulthood.

Ultimately, this is a matter of social justice. The UN Convention on the Rights of the Child (in Article 24) and the South African Constitution (in Section 28) enshrine the right of children and adolescents to health and health services. At present the mental health care needs of the vast majority of young people in South Africa are not being met, a clear abrogation of their constitutional rights. It is of great concern that even though they have been made available to the provinces, the norms for CAMHS that were developed for the Department of Health in 2005 remain to be implemented. Basic cost estimates have also been undertaken. What is required is the political will at both national and provincial levels to officially adopt the norms and provide the necessary finances, infrastructure, and human resources to ensure at least a minimal level of service to children and adolescents in every province. Provincial and district health service managers need to be trained in the use of these norms as a planning tool for CAMHS. This development needs to be accompanied by the establishment of provincial intersectoral structures for child and adolescent mental health, to systematically address mental health promotion and prevention needs from infancy to adulthood.

NOTE

1. Reproduced from the *Journal of Child and Adolescent Mental Health* (2012) 24(2): 149–161 with permission ©NISC (Pty) Ltd.

REFERENCES

Armstrong, T. D., and Costello. 2002. "Community Studies on Adolescent Substance Use, Abuse, or Dependence and Psychiatric Comorbidity." *Journal of Consulting and Clinical Psychology* 70 (6): 1224–39.

Bauman, L. J., E. Johnson, R. Berman, and I. Gamble. 2009. "Children as Caregivers to Their Ill Parents with AIDS." In *How Caregiving Affects Development: Psychological Implications for Child, Adolescent, and Adult Caregivers,* edited by K. Shifren, 37–63. Washington: American Psychological Association.

Burton, P. 2008. *Merchants, Skollies and Stones: Experiences of School Violence in South Africa.* Cape Town: Centre for Justice and Crime Prevention.

Chapman, D. P., C. L. Whitfield, V. J. Felitti, S. R. Dube, V. J. Edwards, and R. F. Anda. 2004. "Adverse Childhood Experiences and the Risk of Depressive Disorders in Adulthood." *Journal of Affective Disorders* 82 (2): 217–25.

Cluver, L., and F. Gardner. 2006. "The Psychological Well-Being of Children Orphaned by AIDS in Cape Town, South Africa." *Annals of General Psychiatry* 5 (8): 5–8.

Dawes, A. 2009. "Editorial: The South African Children's Act." *Journal of Child and Adolescent Mental Health* 21 (2): ii–vi.

Dawes, A., and E. Cairns 1998. "The Machel Study: Dilemmas of Cultural Sensitivity and Universal Rights of Children." *Peace and Conflict* 4 (4): 335–48.

Dawes, A., C. Lund, Z. Kafaar, R. Brandt, and A. J. Flisher. 2004. *Norms for South African Child and Adolescent Mental Health Services (CAMHS): Report for the Directorate: Mental Health and Substance Abuse, National DoH (Department of Health).* Cape Town: Human Sciences Research Council and University of Cape Town.

Dawes, A., B. Robertson, N. Duncan, K. Ensink, A. Jackson, P. Reynolds, A. Pillay, and L. Richter. 1997. "Child and Adolescent Mental Health Policy." In *Mental Health Policy Issues for South Africa,* edited by D. Foster, M. Freeman, and Y. Pillay, 193–215. Cape Town: Medical Association of South African Multimedia.

Dawes A., C. L. Ward. 2008. "Levels, Trends, and Determinants of Child Maltreatment in the Western Cape Province." In *The State of Population in the Western Cape Province,* edited by R. Marindo, C. Groenewald, and S. Gaisie S, 97–125. Cape Town: HSRC.

———. 2011. "Violence and Violence Prevention: New Roles for Child and Adolescent Mental Health Practitioners." *Journal of Child and Adolescent Mental Health* 23 (1): 1–4.

Desjarlais, R., L. Eisenberg, B. Good, and A. Kleinman. 1995. *World Mental Health: Problems and Priorities in Low-Income Countries.* New York: Oxford University Press.

Draper, C. L., C. Lund, S. Kleintjes, M. Funk, M. Omar, A. J. Flisher, and the MHaPP Research Programme Consortium. 2009. "Mental Health Policy in South Africa: Development Process and Content." *Health Policy and Planning* 24 (5): 342–56.

English, D. J. 1998. "The Extent and Consequences of Child Maltreatment." *Future of Children* 8 (1): 39–53.

Ensink, K., and B. Robertson. 1999. "Patient and Family Experiences of Psychiatric Services and Indigenous Healers." *Transcultural Psychiatry* 36 (1): 23–43.

Ensink, K., B. A. Robertson, C. Zissis, and P. Leger. 1997. "Post-Traumatic Stress Disorder in Children Exposed to Violence." *South African Medical Journal* 87 (11): 1526–30.

Felitti, V. J., R. F. Anda, D. Nordenberg, D. F. Williamson, A. M. Spitz, V. Edwards, M. P. Koss, and J. S. Marks. 1998. "Relationships of Childhood Abuse and Household Dysfunction to Many of the Leading Causes of Death in Adults: The Adverse Childhood Experiences (ACE) Study." *American Journal of Preventive Medicine* 14 (4): 245–58.

Flisher, A. J., C. D. H. Parry, J. Evans, M. Muller, and C. Lombard. 2003. "Substance Use by Adolescents in Cape Town: Prevalence and Correlates," *Journal of Adolescent Health* 32 (1): 58–65.

Forehand, R., D. Jones, B. Kotchick, L. Armistead, E. Morse, P. S. Morse, and M. Stock. 2002. "Noninfected Children of HIV-Infected Mothers: A 4-Year Longitudinal Study of Child Psychosocial Adjustment and Parenting." *Behavior Therapy* 33 (4): 579–600.

Freeman, M. 1992. "Planning Health Care in South Africa—Is There a Role for Traditional Healers?" *Social Science and Medicine* 34 (11): 1183–90.

Freeman, M., T. Lee, and W. Vivian. 1994. *Evaluation of Mental Health Services in the Orange Free State.* Johannesburg: University of the Witwatersrand Department of Community Health.

Harker, N., T. Carney, B. Myers, C. D. H. Parry, and P. Cerff. 2007. *Technical Report on Audit of Primary Prevention Programmes in Cape Town 2007.* Cape Town: South African Medical Research Council.

Jewkes, R., J. Levin, N. Mbananga, and D. Bradshaw. 2002. "Rape of Girls in South Africa." *Lancet* 359 (9303): 319–20.

Kleintjies, S., A. J. Flisher, M. Fick, A. Railon, C. Lund, C. Molteno, and B. A. Robertson. 2006. "The Prevalence of Mental Disorders among Children, Adolescents and Adults in the Western Cape, South Africa." *South African Psychiatry Review* 9 (3): 157–60.

Leoschut, L., and P. Burton. 2006. *How Rich the Rewards: Results of the National Youth Victimisation Study.* Cape Town: Hansa.

Louw, S. 2004. "Opvoedkundig-sielkundige Criteria vir die Evaluering van Rehabilitasieprogramme vir Dwelafhanklike Adolessente in Suid-Afrika." PhD diss., University of Johannesburg.

Lubman, D., A. B. Allen, N. Rogers, E. Cementon, and Y. Bonomo. 2007. "The Impact of Co-Occurring Mood and Anxiety Disorders among Substance-Abusing Youth." *Journal of Affective Disorders* 103 (1): 105–12.

Lund, C., G. Boyce, A. Flisher, Z. Kafaar, and A. Dawes. 2009. "Scaling Up Child And Adolescent Mental Health Services in South Africa: Human Resource Requirements and Costs." *Journal of Child Psychology and Psychiatry* 50 (9): 1121–30.

Lund, C., and A. J. Flisher. 2006. "Norms for Mental Health Services in South Africa." *Social Psychiatry and Psychiatric Epidemiology* 41 (7): 587–94.

Mbanga, I., D. J. H. Niehaus, and N. C. Mzamo. 2002. "Attitudes towards and Beliefs about Schizophrenia in Xhosa Families with Affected Pro-Bands." *Curationis* 25 (1): 69–74.

Myers, B. 2004. *Technical Report on Audit of Substance Abuse Treatment Facilities in Gauteng 2003–2004.* Cape Town: South African Medical Research Council.

Myers, B., and N. Fakier. 2007. *Audit of Substance Abuse Treatment Facilities in Gauteng and KwaZulu-Natal 2006–7.* Cape Town: South African Medical Research Council.

Myers, B., J. Louw, and N. Fakier. 2008. "Alcohol and drug abuse: removing structural barriers to Treatment for Historically Disadvantaged Communities in Cape Town." *International Journal of Social Welfare* 17 (2): 156–65.

Nattrass, N. 2005. "Who Consults Sangomas in Khayelitsha? An Exploratory Quantitative Analysis." *Social Dynamics* 31 (2): 161–82.

Patel, V., A. J. Flisher, A. Nikapota, and S. Malhotra. 2008. "Promoting child and adolescent mental health in low and middle income countries." *Journal of Child Psychology and Psychiatry* 49 (3): 313–34.

Patel, V., E. Simunyu, and F. Gwanzura. 1997. "The pathways to primary mental health care in high-density suburbs in Harare, Zimbabwe." *Social Psychiatry and Psychiatric Epidemiology* 32 (2): 97–103.

Peltzer, K. 1999. "Posttraumatic Stress Symptoms in a Population of Rural Children in South Africa." *Psychological Reports* 85(2): 646–50.

Petersen, I., A. Bhana, A. Flisher, A. Swartz, and L. Richter. 2010. *Promoting Mental Health in Scarce-Resource Contexts.* Cape Town: HSRC.

Plüddermann, A., A. J. Flisher, C. Parry, and R. McKetin. 2007. "Metamphetamine Use and Mental Health in High School Learners in Cape Town [Abstract]." *Journal of Child and Adolescent Mental Health* 19: 195.

Ramo, D. E., K. G. Andersen, S. R. Tate, and S. A. Brown. 2005. "Characteristics of Relapse to Substance Use in Comorbid Adolescents." *Addictive Behaviors* 30:1811–23.

Rao, R., R. Sagar, S. K. Kabra, and R. Lodha. 2007. "Psychiatric Morbidity in HIV-Infected Children." *AIDS Care* 19:828–33.

Republic of South Africa Department of Health. 1997. *White Paper for the Transformation of the Health System in South Africa.* Pretoria: Government Printer.

———. 2001. *Policy Guidelines on Adolescent and Youth Health.* Pretoria: Government Printer.

———. 2003. *Policy Guidelines: Child and Adolescent Mental Health.* Pretoria: Government Printer.

Richter, L., A. Stein, L. Cluver, and J. de Kadt. 2009. "Infants and young children affected by HIV/AIDS." In *HIV/AIDS in South Africa 25 Years On,* edited by P. Rohleder, S. C., Kalichman, and L. Swartz, 69–87. New York: Springer.

Roberts, R. E., C. R. Roberts, and Y. Xing. 2007. "Comorbidity of Substance Use Disorders and Other Psychiatric Disorders among Adolescents: Evidence from an Epidemiologic Survey." *Drug and Alcohol Dependence* 88 (Suppl. 1): S4–13.

Rowe, C. L., H. A. Liddle, and G. D. Dakof. 2001. "Classifying Clinically Referred Adolescent Substance Abusers by Level of Externalizing and Internalizing Symptoms." *Journal of Child and Adolescent Substance Abuse* 11: 41–65.

Seedat, M., A. Van Niekerk, R. Jewkes, S. Suffla, and K. Ratele. 2009. "Violence and injuries in South Africa: Prioritising an agenda for prevention." *Lancet* 374 (9694): 1011–22.

Seedat, S., C. Nyamai, F. Njenga, B. Vythilingum, and D. J. Stein. 2004. "Trauma exposure and post-traumatic stress symptoms in urban African schools. Survey in Cape Town and Nairobi." *British Journal of Psychiatry* 184 (2): 169–75.

Seedat, S., E. Van Nood, B. Vythlingum, D. J. Stein, and D. Kaminer. 2000. "School Survey Of Exposure To Violence and Posttraumatic Stress Symptoms in Adolescents." *Southern African Journal of Child and Adolescent Mental Health* 12: 38–44.

Shisana, O., L.C. Simbayi, T. Rehle, N. P. Zungu, K. Zuma, N Ngogo, N. S. Jooste, et al. 2010. *South African National HIV Prevalence, Incidence, Behaviour and Communication Survey, 2008: The Health of Our Children.* Cape Town: Human Sciences Research Council.

Sidley, P. 2004. "South Africa to Regulate Healers." *British Medical Journal* 329 (7469): 69–75.

Sorsdahl, K. D. Stein, and A. Flisher. 2010. "Traditional Healer Attitudes and Beliefs Regarding Referral of the Mentally Ill to Western Doctors in South Africa." *Transcultural Psychiatry* 47: 591–609.

Sorsdahl, K., D. J. Stein, A. Grimsrud, A. Seedat, A. J. Flisher, D. R. Williams, and L. Myer. 2009. "Traditional Healers in the Treatment of Common Mental Disorders in South Africa." *Journal of Nervous and Mental Disease* 197: 434–41.

Swartz, L. 2008. *Culture and Mental Health—A Southern African View.* Cape Town: Oxford University Press.

UK Department of Health National Child and Adolescent Support Service and the University of Durham 2004. *Child and Adolescent Mental Health Service Mapping Exercise.* Durham, UK: University of Durham, Centre for Public Mental Health. Accessed October 4, 2013. http://www.childrensmapping.org.uk/results/publications /CAMHS_Atlas_2003.pdf.

Ward, C.L., A. J. Flisher, C. Zissis, M. Muller, and C. Lombard. 2001. "Exposure to Violence and Its Relationship to Psychopathology in Adolescents." *Injury Prevention* 7: 297–301.

Ward, C.L., A. van der Merwe, and A. Dawes, eds. 2012. *Youth Violence in South Africa: Sources and Solutions.* Cape Town: University of Cape Town Press.

Wild, L. 2001. "Review: The Psychosocial Adjustment of Children Orphaned by AIDS." *Southern African Journal of Child and Adolescent Mental Health* 13: 3–22.

World Health Organization. 2004. *Mental Health Policy and Service Guidance Package: Quality Improvement for Mental Health.* Geneva: World Health Organization.

———. 2005. *Mental Health Policy and Service Guidance Package: Child and Adolescent Mental Health.* Geneva: World Health Organization.

6 SOME ASPECTS OF MENTAL ILLNESS IN FRENCH-SPEAKING WEST AFRICA

RENÉ COLLIGNON

Since they first blossomed in Europe in the nineteenth century, two scientific disciplines that take the concept of "difference" as an object of reflection—psychiatry and ethnology—have both been haunted by the question of "otherness." In his study of the history of madness (1961), Michel Foucault showed how the identity of the modern rational subject, as subject of the contract, has been constructed in the West by contrasting it to a backdrop of a series of figures of otherness: the primitive, the savage, the child, the woman, the madman. Since before the period of colonization the African had already been given the role of one of these figures in the Western imagination: that of the primitive. How, then, could one conceive of a mad African, when his difference was already held to be radical on the colonial scene, a realm of power where the fiction of the contract does not hold for the "native" under guardianship? The very nature of the colonial relation helps explain some of the erring ways of colonial psychiatry. Megan Vaughan (1983, 1991) has suggested that the main focus of reflection of colonial physicians was not the construction of a mad African so much as a constant effort to reaffirm the irreducible difference between the African and the colonizer. And this, according to Vaughan, explains the broad consensus enjoyed in the 1930s by the theory of "deculturation," which was believed to explain the mental pathology observed among the colonized who came into contact with civilization. The effects of the change wrought by colonization on the psyche were approached in terms of cultural and racial difference.[1]

In this context, it is easier to understand why it was only during a later period—when growth in social psychiatry and psychoanalysis and developments in medical anthropology made it possible to move beyond the hegemonic Western model of the individual as sovereign autonomous entity—that fresh attention was brought to bear on family discourse, the collective speech of the sick person's entourage, as expressed through the afflicted person. Such an approach to psychic suffering shifts our perspectives and makes it possible to base mental pathology in Africa on new foundations.

THE PSYCHIATRIC CLINIC OF FANN

The "Clinique neuro-psychiatrique de Fann" opened in 1956, shortly before Senegal attained independence in 1960. After the death of Moussa Diop, the first Senegalese psychiatrist, in 1967 it was renamed Clinique Moussa Diop de Fann and again, after the separation of neurology and psychiatry in 1968, Clinique psychiatrique de Fann. It was the first ward or division of a hospital that would later become the University Hospital of Fann, a "Centre Hospitalier Universitaire" (CHU) or University Teaching Hospital (UTH) in Dakar.

In the early 1960s, the first director of neuropsychiatry at the school of medicine, Henri Collomb[2] entrusted the task of studying local representations of mental disorder and its customary forms of control and socialization to András Zempléni.[3] Zempléni's surveys showed that the Wolof and the Lebu shared certain broad stereotypes of madness (the agitated lunatic, or *le fou agité;* the vagrant madman; the woman who becomes mad after childbirth; the village idiot; and so on) that present distorting mirrors of the universe of values of their society. Beyond this popular imagery, however, there exists an indigenous notion of mental disorder with a wider extension, the contours of which include behaviors, states, and pictures that these populations recognize as pathological.

These conceptions of mental illness are markedly different from those of Western psychiatry, both in their approach and in their very foundations. In Senegal there is no clear divide between popular knowledge and a body of learning reserved for specialists: families, therapists, and patients share the same categories of interpretation. The Wolof and the Lebu may be capable of recognizing the recurrence of certain pathological manifestations, but they are not as concerned with naming them or classifying them according to descriptive criteria and symptoms so much as with speculating more generally about the origin and causes of the sickness. The concept of "crises," however, does exist for the Wolof, who differentiate between the epileptic fit, the psychomotor fit of someone possessed by a spirit, the acute anxiety attack of a victim of witchcraft, and the maniac's fit of rage. In keeping with the etiological reasoning mentioned above, these crises are not seen in terms of sets of nosographic signs but rather in terms of causal categories of interpretation that constitute the real principles of classification of disorders.

This emphasis on causal imputation recognizes in pathological behavior the consequences of external aggression perpetrated by malevolent spirits or humans:

1. The torments they inflict on their chosen victims are attributed to ancestral spirits (*rab* or *tuur*), seeking alliance with humans.
2. Encounters with *jinne* and *seytane*, spirits of Islamic origin, in the bush provoke devastating fear that leads to madness (serious psychotic hallucinations and dementia).
3. Witches (*dëmm*), driven by the insatiable desire to devour other people, attack the life force of their victims. Witchcraft attacks are primarily associated with a syndrome characterized by abrupt and massive anguish and fear of imminent death involving suffocation and oppression.
4. A mental disorder can also be ascribed to the action of a rival seeking to harm an envied competitor. This interpersonal magic (*liggeey*, or magic "work"), carried out by the *marabout* (a witchdoctor in the Islamic context) at the request of a third party, is usually presented as a defense against the adverse intentions of an aggressor.

This set of representations is characterized by a "persecutory" model, endowing the patient with the status of victim and exonerating him or her of responsibility for his or her illness. Psychiatrists in Africa have emphasized the importance of persecution in their observations:

> Persecution colors the whole of African psychiatry. Experienced on a delusional, interpretative, or cultural plane, it explains everything that disturbs the order, disorganizes relations, and harms the individual in his physical, mental, or spiritual being. It is felt by the sick person, proposed by his family or entourage, put into form by the healer or the marabout. Themes of persecution, often supported by visual or verbal hallucinations, lie at the centre of all chronic and acute psychoses (including manic states). They are always made explicit in neuroses, often in psychosomatic illnesses and in any kind of situation experienced as being painful and disagreeable. . . . The frequency of the persecution (influence, possession, action on the physical, psychic and social being) contrasts with the scarcity of themes of shamefulness, guilt, self-accusation, and self-deprecation. (Diop et al. 1964, 333)[4]

Within the Fann's team, Marie-Cécile Ortigues and Edmond Ortigues (1966) proposed a psychoanalytical interpretation of the modalities of oedipal positions among the Wolof and the Lebu. In that society, the image of the father as lawmaker and rival tends to get confused with that of collective authority. Its symbolic function remains attached to the figure of the ancestor who, as someone who is already dead, cannot be harmed or equaled. As the father is impervious to the rivalry of the son, the rivalry is displaced in the direction of the brothers, who become the object of polarization of aggressive impulses. Any bad thoughts toward brothers, who are equals (*nawle*), is projected and inverted into persecutory reactions because the individual cannot bear to assume his own aggressive impulses. As this tendency appears to be universal, everyone is quick to feel persecuted and is constantly concerned with protecting himself or herself from the threatening intentions of which he or she is the object, leading to internalization of guilt: "Everything happens as if the individual cannot bear to feel himself divided internally, moved by contradictory desires. The bad is always situated outside the self. . . . Here, the tendency is to project the guilt-inducing impulses onto spirits or other humans" (Ortigues and Ortigues 1966, 128). As a conclusion to their observations, they suggest that the oedipal conflict is resolved in the following terms: "the rivalry between 'brothers' is overcompensated for by very strong solidarity," adding that "it is tempting to say that this is a reaction-formation that can be observed as a sociological constant" (ibid., 142).

For Zempléni, this recognition of the persecutory relation as a normal and current form of relation among the Wolof and Lebu raises two questions:

1. In this context, where a common set of signifiers is available, how is the interpretation of mental disorder organized? Zempléni points out that the search for the meaning of the disorders is left neither to the subjectivity of the sick person nor to the sole judgment of his or her entourage; it constitutes an interactive process that mobilizes the family and the patient in a collective discourse that enables everyone to express the strangeness of a very personal experience and to keep it within the bounds of an intelligibility of which the collective representations provide the keys and the idiom. The active search for agreement about the entities to be blamed for the illness sustains a dialogue in the group—which, once agreement has been reached about the identity of the causal agent, then seeks approval of its agreement through the diagnosis of a traditional therapist. That person's interpretation extends this first familial consensus to the dimensions of the traditional cure by giving it its typical triadic structure, which consists of a combination of the pathological experience of the patient, the voice of family consensus, and the experience of the therapist (Zempléni 1968, 94–95).

2. For the psychiatrist, the delicate question then arises of how to distinguish between delusion and hallucination and the standard persecutory interpretation pertaining to shared beliefs. The entourage is not surprised by the psychosensory experiences associated with the action of different external, malevolent entities—for example, "voices" or visual hallucinations—and does not consider them to be pathological from the start or per se. The comments and descriptions of these experiences given by the sick person rarely enable the psychiatrist to specify the symptoms of the hallucinatory series: vision, hallucinatory vision, persistent idea, dream, hallucination, or something else: "Here, the radical division between reason and unreason established by classical Western psychiatry . . . becomes blurred, giving way to a continuity of interpretative schemas with delusional themes and

parasensory experiences current with the actual hallucinatory experience" (Zempléni 1968, 96). These experiences do not make the mentally ill person a stranger to his or her group, an alienated person. The patient's personal experience remains accessible to his or her entourage—within the limits, however, of a certain collusion maintained between them by this dialogue on the origin and meaning of the disorder.

Just as for the psychiatrist a patient's criticism of his or her own delusional productions and abnormal behavior is one of the signs that healing is under way, in the world of the Wolof and Lebu it is the beginning of the interpretation of these productions and behaviors that is believed to herald a forthcoming healing. "For the presumed victim of the *rab*, beginning to compose intelligible messages out of the visions, dreams and voices that obsessed him up until then by their emotive and fantastical immediacy" means showing that the victim is a social being, that he or she recognizes the symbolic code of the group. "However," Zempléni accurately observes, "this contrast [between the different therapeutic conceptions] is only superficial: in both cases, it is a matter of the compliance, conformity between individual experience and collective rule. Western criticism is a form of interpretation and Wolof-Lebu interpretation is a form of criticism" (Zempléni 1968, 98).

M.-C. Ortigues and E. Ortigues propose an analysis of the traditional formations of persecutory interpretations whereby they correspond to different levels of organization of the personality. According to this analysis, witchcraft corresponds to the pregenital oral level; *maraboutage* (interpersonal magic) corresponds to the phallic genital level; and the subject of the *rab*, by reference to parental images (the superego), can be used at all structural levels of the personality (Ortigues and Ortigues 1966, 225–69). Once they have established these hypotheses, the authors propose a formal analysis of persecutory interpretations, using criteria of internal coherence specific to each system, and they show how these cultural signposts can be used to analyze delusions (ibid., 271–300). They illustrate this approach with the study of acute psychotic reactions (*bouffées délirantes*). In the eyes of the psychiatrist, the speed and depth of the regressions presented by these pathological pictures and the quick reversibility of psychotic episodes, with themes related to the persecutory interpretations supplied by the culture, represent a privileged form of the local pathology that can be considered a specifically African mode of resolving tensions.[5]

Various publications bear witness to the fertility of this confrontation between clinic and cultural signposts. Detailed case studies using the patient's categories illustrate this attention focused on the modalities of expression used by patients to speak of their experience. If persecutory themes are frequently evoked, these observations show that they do not exclude other themes, and that great mobility and a remarkable plasticity are displayed in the manner of calling them into use, according to the possibilities and needs of the patient and his or her entourage within a general context of religious syncretism.

But this is not a culturalist approach seeking to reduce the psychological to the cultural. In Fann in the 1960s, a powerful emphasis was placed on the consideration of professional deontology in an intercultural situation, the lessons of which did not always appear to have been respected elsewhere: "It would be as reprehensible for a doctor to ignore the traditions and their organizing power as it would be to send the patient back into that context as if to confine him" (Ortigues, Martino and Collomb 1967, 145).

What was important in the view of the therapists was to seek to understand the patient's place in what he or she said. Cultural decoding was not an end in itself. In every society, however traditional it may be, personal questioning arises, new constructions are sought through the play of social concepts and through more personal appropriation of cultural references. The therapist's role, then, is to accompany the patient in his or her self-questioning, while respecting his or her choice of means of expression. This receptive attitude about the local point of view by the psychiatrists caused the news to spread through Senegalese families that "the doctors at the Fann hospital believe in *rab!*" With this approach, patients go more or less far down the path of empowerment, accepting their position as the agents of their own lives—the modern course proposed by psychiatrics in hospital settings—to varying degrees. In the context of changing societies, people increasingly find themselves caught between two worlds, where systems of reference become confused, are sought for, and reconstructed as the price of compromise.

FROM THE 1980S TO THE PRESENT

The research launched under the impetus of Collomb in several complementary directions[6] (linking data from psychiatric observation to the cultural and social dimensions, developing institutional psychotherapy practices and social psychiatry, and so forth) required constant efforts to train African mental health workers, including the creation of psychiatric internships in the hospitals of Dakar, a specialist studies diploma in psychiatry, and—for nurses and higher-level health technicians—a diploma of initiation into psychopathology. This set of measures was intended to create a workforce of health workers, each adequately trained for his or her particular level[7]—a necessary condition for the introduction of a differentiated system of care for mental patients.

The efforts made to move away from the hospital and initiate a regionalization of care included many ups and downs. Collomb, inspired by the experience
of therapeutic communities with traditional healers and wishing to integrate patients into a community in which they could live and participate fully, created
"psychiatric villages," where the medical presence was to play second fiddle to the
therapeutic action of nurses and organizers. But the functioning of these villages
steadily deteriorated in the absence of the careful and regular supervision they
needed from psychiatrists, and they have never been revived.[8]

An itinerant system for mental health care called DIAMM (for *Dispositif itinérant d'assistance aux malades mentaux*), composed of a psychiatrist and nurse
or social worker coming from Dakar to provide consultations for patients in the
Thiès region, has succeeded in operating steadily for a number of years, thanks
to the logistical support of a nongovernmental organization and alliances with
external local initiatives such as the Mental Health Center, *Dalal Xel,* created by
the Brothers of Saint John of God in Thiès (Guèye and Seck 1998; B. Seck et al.
1981). The regional hospital of Saint-Louis has opened a psychiatry consultancy
and made a few hospital beds available to psychiatric patients thanks to the recruitment of a psychiatrist by the Association for the Promotion of the Hospital
(in keeping with the measures introduced by the law of July 13, 1986, on the responsible participation of populations in the health effort). In Niakhar, a mental
health hut (or "psychiatric village") has been created on the personal initiative of
a former Serer interpreter who had worked for a long time with the Fann team
during the 1970s.[9] A nongovernmental organization that advocates for the recognition of traditional practitioners has built an experimental center for traditional
medicines that brings together Serer healers in Fatick. Even more recently, the
Brothers of Saint John of God have opened a second *Dalal Xel* center in Fatick,
where young doctors specializing in psychiatry come for periods of training under the supervision of the Fann psychiatric department.

Africanization of Personnel

The period following Collomb's departure from the Fann psychiatric hospital
has been marked by the gradual withdrawal, now completed, of French cooperation aid for development in the field of mental health and the Senegalization of
health care personnel. This process has taken place in the context of a general
economic climate of grave crisis, including the devaluation of the currency and
the imposition of structural adjustment plans by the World Bank and the International Monetary Fund. This particularly difficult situation—the repercussions
of which, in terms of the worsening of working conditions, the material disrepair
of hospital structures, and the impact on the professional motivation of health

workers, among others, are hard to measure[10]—also corresponded to increasing difficulties among local publishing organizations.[11]

Psychiatry in Senegal is at a turning point. After its founding, a period marked by the enthusiasm of the pioneers, has come a time of doubt, of questioning of its heritage, and of reevaluations. In this context of Africanization, with new generations of young doctors, the question of otherness that marked the relationship between therapists and patients of different cultures that has been formulated up until now will shift its focus. The duality that marks the position of African psychiatrists as Africans trained professionally in a tradition foreign to their culture of origin—training that enjoys the prevailing prestige of science in the world—places them in a position of fragility that was not shared by their expatriate European colleagues. This dimension, which had already been noticed during Collomb's tenure,[12] was movingly underlined by Momar Guèye, professor of psychiatry at the hospital at Fann, in his homage to Professor Babakar Diop, Collomb's successor at Fann, whose words Guèye recalled on the occasion of Diop's death: "Meeting the other (the patient) is also heavy with consequences for the African psychiatrist trained in the French school. He commits a transgression by penetrating into the domain of mental illness traditionally reserved for the healer invested with the function of healing." These words were the occasion for Guèye to echo the uneasy questioning of the deceased's colleagues about the sense of destiny of Diop and his broken dream (Guèye 1998–99, 4).

At the time of Diop's death, the professionals in the psychiatric clinic at Fann had felt bereft of effective management for some time. Professor Diop, for health reasons, had spent too much time away from his post without having adequately delegated his powers and responsibilities. When he died in 1998 after a long illness, Diop left behind him a staff whose spirit and ability to function had been damaged. The prospects he had sketched out for closer integration of mental health care into public health services (Diop 1974) were to have been fleshed out by the Senegalese team whose work he directed in the rural Serer region. He had expected great things of a survey, the Senegalese component of a World Health Organization Collaborative Study on strategies for extending mental health in primary health care. The publication of the first results was promising, presenting precious data about the types of psychiatric disorders to be encountered in the health centers of this rural zone, and evaluating the sensitivity of health workers to mental health problems;[13] it appeared possible that healthcare providers would be able to make a rigorous selection of mental health problems for priority action, to define a limited list of drugs for their treatment, and to design brief training courses to allow auxiliary health workers to detect and manage common mental disorders (Diop, Collignon, and Guèye 1976; Diop et al. 1980 and 1982; Harding et al. 1979). However, the impetus was soon lost due to Diop's illness and the lack of a suitable replacement for him, and the enterprise came to a premature end.

A series of publications following Diop's death bears witness to the way the team that gathered around Fann hospital director Momar Guèye got down to the task of critical questioning—sometimes distressed, but always courageous—about the foundations of action,[14] the search for a radical reform, and new dynamic of a collective project needing to be reinvented.

Several contributions by the psychiatrists of Fann to a collective work published by the Association des Chercheurs Sénégalais (1997) undertook a critical reassessment of the Fann clinic and reported the crisis within the institution. These texts clearly argued for the need to bring psychiatry back into a medical context (Ba and Sylla 1997), with an emphasis on scientific training, legal credentials, and pleas for the re-medicalization of psychiatry—a strong reaction against the social psychiatry or ethnopsychiatry introduced by Collomb (Seck and Sarr 1997). A call had already been issued for a return to the clinical rigor of semiology and the increased use of standardized instruments (scales of evaluation, questionnaires, screening instruments, and so forth) for use in quantitative psychopathology and the refinement of differential diagnosis (Ba and Samuel-Lajeunesse 1984; Ba 1987a, 1987b). The need to revaluate biological and medicated therapeutic methods in training, research (Ba and Sylla 1997), and practice (Seck and Sarr 1997) had been asserted, recalling the still-current indications for certain treatments, such as electroconvulsive therapy (ECT), intended to bring those treatments out of the disrepute into which they had been thrown by ideological criticism.[15] This reactive movement questioned the unintended consequences of the separation of neurology and psychiatry, a result of Collomb's more resolutely social orientation to psychiatry in the late 1960s, and was no doubt motivated by considerations on several different levels.

Recent developments in the prevailing paradigms of psychiatry undoubtedly play a role, such as the increasing importance of biological psychiatry and pharmacology and the worldwide distribution of the American Psychiatric Association's *Diagnostic and Statistical Manual of Mental Disorders,* especially after 1980 with the third and subsequent editions. Young Senegalese psychiatrists partly trained in Europe are particularly sensitive to these developments, attracted as they are by the prestige and resources deployed by medical science. This attraction is made all the more powerful by the painful awareness of the loss of reputation of the department of psychiatry at Fann, and the consequent desire to strengthen the prevailing criteria of legitimization in the medical field, in which psychiatry occupies a singular, often rather marginal, position.[16]

The attention of doctors in training is still drawn to a series of manifestations of typical African pathology, including *bouffées délirantes*[17] and puerperal or acute reactive psychosis.[18] Epilepsy, which has a high rate of prevalence in Africa, remains a subject of preoccupation not only for neurologists but also for psychiatrists,[19] in particular because of the prejudices that surround the illness and stigmatize the sick person, and it is not an uncommon reason for psychiatric consultation.[20] Whether the Western construct of clinical depression exists in Africa was long a question of historical debate.[21] Over time, a certain consensus has been reached about the African characteristics of depressive disorders: the importance of somatic signs and symptoms; the almost constant presence of delusional ideas of persecution; and the rarity of ideas of worthlessness, self-accusation, and suicidal behavior. However, retrospective studies of files stored at the Fann hospital[22] appear to highlight an evolution in symptomatology among subjects imbued with Western culture. Although always present, the systematizing of delusions has given way to complex and diffused feelings of persecution that no longer succeed in channeling anxiety. Current economic changes facing Africans and their devastating effects on the traditional family and other solidarity-enhancing groups have forced the individual to face the challenges of competition, including the management of aggressiveness. The development of clinical material over the years seems to emphasize the progressive appearance of guilt in association with increasing modernity.

Collomb's team had introduced institutional improvements in the hospital to make psychiatry more open to a social mission (in this case, the integration of patients into society). A therapeutic community was established: the *pénc* (a meeting of the hospital ward, modeled on a village palaver) was initiated and organized with an open-door policy and the admission of patients' companions, who came to stay on the wards with the patients while they were hospitalized. These hospital practices are still followed. However, the presence of the companion, which is gradually becoming widespread in other health services, is now seen by health care personnel as little more than a palliative to the shortcomings of an understaffed hospital, and as a result the initial goal has been forgotten—that is, the companion's potential as an auxiliary to be mobilized by the medical professionals in their therapeutic project for the patient (Gbikpi 1981; Collignon 2001). However, a survey carried out at the psychiatric hospital of Thiaroye (Franklin et al. 1996a and 1996b), based on the analysis of a systematic sample of 935 records of initial outpatient visits, highlights the strong attachment of populations to this local practice of accompanying patients as a cultural response to mental illness. Patterns of patient companionship were found to correlate strongly with specific sociodemographic and clinical characteristics of patients and their companions. Interpretations of these findings helped clarify both prevailing attitudes toward the mentally ill and the social response to and management of mental illness.[23] As for the *pénc*, the dimension of normative speech of the group, or the words of order, appears to have gradually prevailed over listening to the expression of personal suffering, or the words of the sick person conveying his subjective drama. I. Sow et al. (1986) and J. Selguetia (1997) report the steady deterioration of this practice of institutional psychotherapy, which has been reduced to a sort of routine custom stripped of its profound sense of opening to and reception of the words of the patients and their families.

Another element in recent critiques of past psychiatric practices is the repudiation of a certain drift that led to the presence of healers being tolerated in the hospital, despite the lessons to be learned from ethnological research into the foundations of the healer's effectiveness in his own environment, which cannot be reduced to a situation of paramedical dependence (Zempléni 1980). This last point stems from a desire to clarify the specific areas of response to the phenomenon, now fully recognized, of the twin demands for health care (Picard 1985; Picard and d'Almeida 1985): the families of psychiatric patients call for two systems of care—hospital and biomedicine on the one hand and traditional indigenous practices on the other. Local people resort to biodmedicine or indigenous therapies, successively or independently, or use them simultaneously in a complementary manner. Feeling that they lack the necessary training in the methods of psychotherapy, some psychiatrists in the clinic of Fann tend to confirm the popular social division of labor, in which the hospital has the power to calm and only the healer has the power to heal. This causes them to adopt a position of relative withdrawal, resigning themselves in a way to their limited power but fully recognized by the population, who are grateful to them for using the sedative power of psychotropic drugs during periods of crisis.

However, such a position is clearly not fully satisfactory, and this is confirmed by the way psychiatric texts call for training that is more diversified in its theoretical foundations and more attentive to recent developments in psychiatry. In the last few years, initiatives to introduce training in techniques such as behavioral therapy and family therapies have been offered to health care personnel wishing to widen their perspectives and their levels of intervention with regard to both outpatients and inpatients.[24] These have enjoyed enough of a success that practitioners and teachers, trained locally in these techniques by specialists visiting regularly from France and Belgium, are now capable of transmitting their skills in turn to people in other African countries.[25]

An article by Moussa Ba, Omar Ndoye, and Momar Guèye (1998–1999) serves as a reminder that the appeals of some patients are insistent enough to cause health workers to question their Western approach to psychiatry in the face of the symptoms patients present and their demands for help as they question their own identity and seek a compromise that is culturally acceptable to them and their community. Ba, Ndoye, and Guèye demonstrate that the major advances made in integrating Western and indigenous approaches to psychiatry since the 1960s in Fann[26] have not been forgotten, and that they still profoundly inspire young African psychiatrists and clinical psychologists in their approach to patients today. The enduring force of Collomb's approach is illustrated in a particularly striking way in numerous remarkable clinical case studies of young adults, adolescents, and children (Mbodji 1997a and 1997b; Ly 1997 and 2003–2004; Ouedraogo and Siranyian 2003–2004; Siranyian 2003–2004). The field of child psychiatry has undergone new growth fostered by the teams of Birama Seck at the day hospital for children called Kër Xaleyi "(the house of children")" at Fann hospital; Thérèse Agossou in Bénin; and by S. Siranyan and A. Ouedraogo in Burkina Faso, among others. These pediatric psychiatry clinics demonstrate a continuing commitment to sensitive and integrative approach, always trying to get as close as possible to the problem facing the person who is questioning his or her destiny.[27]

Domains hitherto little explored by psychiatrists, and to which current world developments have brought attention, are opening up most notably in the direction of pathologies related to migrations (Collignon and Guèye 1989; Ebin 1990–1991; O. Sylla and Mbaye 1990–1991); problems related to aging populations (Guèye, Loum, and Sylla,1995); liaisons between psychiatry and other medical specializations (Fall, Seck, and Charlier 2001–2002); evaluations of outpatients' compliance within the framework of the relation between the psychiatrist, the patient, and his or her family (Thiam, Ndiaye, and Guèye 2001–2002); hospitalism and chronicity (Guèye 1998; Ndiaye 1989); psychopathy (A. Sylla, Ndoye, and Guèye 2001); sexuality disorders (Ndoye 2003); and counseling and psychological consultation for people living with HIV/AIDS (Dago-Akribi 2001–2002; d'Almeida, Diop, and Apovo 1989; Réseau de Recherche en Santé de la Reproduction en Afrique 1991; Collignon, Gruénais, and Vidal 1994; Ouedraogo, Ouedraogo, and Sanou 2001–2002).

Elsewhere in French-Speaking Africa

The legacy of Henri Collomb and the works of the Department of Psychiatry at the University Hospital of Fann extend far beyond Senegal. Over the last few years, as professors and students from other countries have trained in Dakar and gone on to establish training institutions in their countries of origin, the dynamic transmission of knowledge and the exacting nature of research in psychiatry have gained more solid foundations across Africa. Among those responsible for these developments are René Gualbert Ahyi and Thérèse Agossou,[28] who have established a training center for psychiatrists in Cotonou, Benin, that has passed on the torch to young Africans from the countries of this region; Baba Koumaré, who presides over the destiny of psychiatry in Mali; Arouna Ouedraogo, who is developing psychiatry in Burkina Faso with colleagues from that country who have been trained in Dakar or Cotonou; Mathias Makang Ma M'Bog, in Cameroon; and Dr. Sadyo Barry, in Niger.

I am not in a position to give accounts of the wealth of developments in all these different countries because of difficulties in accessing widely dispersed documentation, but I mention work carried out in Mali as an example which, on its own, shows how necessary it is to pursue specialized research and update the literature on mental health in these emerging countries. A remarkable body of work has been produced since 1982 under Baba Koumaré in the psychiatry department of the Point G Hospital in Bamako (Coulibaly, Koumaré, and Coudray 1983; Uchôa 1988; Keita, Miquel-Garcia, and Koumaré 1994), in particular a special issue of *Psychopathologie africaine* devoted entirely to mental health in Mali (Koumaré 1992[29]). These works lead to fundamental reflection on the place of culture in modern African psychiatry, on ways of linking traditional and conventional systems of care, and on the realistic development of collaboration between psychiatrists and healers. Clinical, therapeutic, epidemiological, and anthropological perspectives have been explored by the Mali team. Psychiatric researchers from Mali have also engaged in collaborations with Canadian researchers from the Douglas Research Centre—which is affiliated with McGill University in Montreal and is a World Health Organization Collaborating Center for Research and Training in Mental Health—and from the Department of Anthropology of the Université de Montréal, whose researchers specialize in cultural approaches to psychiatry.[30] In the fields of epidemiology and anthropology, one notable contribution from a multidisciplinary Italian team—made up of psychiatrists, psychologists, and ethnologists under the direction of Piero Coppo—working on the plateau of the Dogon country under the auspices of the Regional Center of Traditional Medicine of Bandiagara, has also enriched the list of achievements in Mali.[31]

Local and international organizations and professional associations are cooperating on mental health care initiatives in Africa and psychiatric hospitals and clinical teams from the North and from African countries are working together on research and workshops. However, the work produced or presented often remains very difficult to access. A list of meetings (Collignon and Guèye 2003, 106–7) clearly emphasizes the difficulty in establishing real continuity among international meetings held in Africa.[32] Yet such continuity is absolutely necessary to lay the foundations for a dynamic, collective accumulation and dissemination of knowledge and practical skills; no doubt it would also be very helpful in making African mental health professionals feel less isolated in their respective countries. At the First Pan African Conference on Mental Health, held in Dakar in 2002, participants were urged to pool their resources to create a document library in the psychiatric clinic of Fann hospital dedicated to psychiatry and medical anthropology in Africa. A website and a network based around the journal *Psychopathologie africaine*[33] are in the process of being set up, and both should help improve the circulation of information.

NOTES

1. For a brief look at the history of French colonial psychiatry in Africa, see Collignon (1995–1996, 2002).

2. An annotated bibliography lists all the works of the pluridisciplinary team gathered around Collomb between 1959 and 1978 (Collignon 1978). See also Collignon (1982); Collignon and Guèye (1995).

3. Here I closely follow chapter 2 of the thesis that Zempléni devoted to the interpretation and traditional therapy of mental disorder among the Wolof and the Lebu (Zempléni 1968).

4. Unless otherwise noted, all translations are my own.

5. Collomb (1965, 214) characterizes the local semiology of the *bouffées délirantes* as follows:

> It frequently occurs among apparently healthy and well-integrated personalities presenting no evident psychopathological structure; the patient and his or her entourage are familiar with the psychotic, delusional event, which is integrated from the start into the cultural systems; the patient's emotional state shows little change, and there is little anxiety; the state of consciousness shows little change, and it is rare for the delusion to be accompanied by a state of confusion; themes of persecution predominate in the content of the delusion; visual hallucinations are usual; a small proportion of cases evolve into chronic disorders with regard to the repetition of delusional attacks. These episodes respond remarkably well to neuroleptics and electroconvulsive therapy (ECT); a traditional treatment is always followed concurrently. When cured, the patient does not bear witness to a personal experience of a radical transformation of the world.

6. See the annotated bibliography over 20 years (1979–1999) of psychiatry in Senegal: Collignon (2001).

7. In addition to the Senegalese, Africans from several other francophone countries —such as Benin, Burkina Faso, Gabon, Mali, Mauritania, and the Central African Republic—have been able to take advantage of this training. Between 1979 and 2000 there were about fifty doctoral theses in medicine on subjects involving psychiatry and mental health, forty theses written for the specialist studies diploma in psychiatry, and nearly twenty diplomas of initiation into psychopathology awarded to higher-level health technicians.

8. For a comparative study of the design and realization of psychiatric villages by T. Adeoye Lambo in Nigeria and Henri Collomb in Senegal, see Collignon (1983). The gradual decline into disrepute of this model of care in Senegal is charted in studies of two villages that have always had a precarious existence: Kenia, in Casamance (Kane 1979), and Botou, in eastern Senegal (Ouango 1987), although the creation of such structures in each region was written into the program of law: decree 75–80 on July 9, 1975, "Relative au traitement des maladies mentales" ["On the treatment of mental illnesses"] and decree 75–1093 of October 23, 1975, defined the conditions of organization and op-

eration (in *Journal officiel de la République du Sénégal,* 1975, no. 4436: 1008–1009; *Journal officiel de la République du Sénégal,* 1975, no. 4456: 1063–1064). Note that the experiment launched by Lambo in the 1950s at the Aro Mental Hospital in Abeokuta enjoyed only lukewarm support from his colleagues and has gradually lost its impact in Nigeria.

9. This nursing assistant, solicited by the Mourid authorities of the holy city of Touba, holds regular consultations for the mentally ill of the region. A psychiatrist from the psychiatric hospital of Thiaroye (in the suburbs of Dakar) also holds a weekly psychiatric consultation in Touba.

10. For many years, low recruitment in the public sector has favored the exodus of young Senegalese psychiatrists trained in Dakar to the developed countries, especially France.

11. For example, there was the disappearance of the *Bulletins et mémoires de la faculté de médecine et de pharmacie de Dakar,* which had given an annual account of the work carried out by the different chairs in the department of medicine and pharmacy since its creation. One of the rare inter-African publications dedicated to psychiatry, the *African Journal of Psychiatry*—created in 1975 by the Association of Psychiatrists in Africa—has not appeared since the early 1980s. The only survivor, at the cost of enormous difficulties, is the journal founded by Collomb and his colleagues in Dakar in 1965, *Psychopathologie africaine*—which adopted a bilingual subtitle in 1980 reaffirming its original editorial policy: *Social Sciences and Psychiatry in Africa/Sciences sociales et psychiatrie en Afrique.*

12. Collomb (1973) presents reflections on the uneasy and ambiguous position of African health care personnel in a hospital environment caught between two worlds of reference and the ambivalence specific to the cooperation between the now independent Senegal and France in medical matters.

13. Health workers diagnosed 9 percent of the patients as suffering from a mental health problem, usually associated with a physical problem. It was found that psychotic and suicidal symptoms (such as hallucinations and delusions) were more likely to be recognized by health workers as diagnostic of a mental disorder, whereas psychophysiological symptoms (such as anorexia, insomnia, and headache) and psychological symptoms (such as anxiety and depression) were less frequently recognized as diagnostic of such a disorder.

14. See, among others, d'Almeida et al. (1986); d'Almeida and Ouango (1997); Ba and Sylla (1997); Guèye (1995); Ndoye, Devos, and Guèye (2000); Sarr and Guèye (1994); Seck and Sarr (1997).

15. M. Baldé (1989), on the strength of his experience at the Sainte-Anne Hospital [Centre hospitalier Sainte-Anne] in Paris, argues that the classic techniques should be abandoned by African psychiatrists, in favor of ECT [electro convulsivo therapy] under short narcosis and curarization. He shows the usefulness of this technique in the African environment when the indications are well specified: major depression, an acute manic episode resistant to chemotherapy, certain puerperal psychoses, catatonic states, schizophreniform disorders, and especially serious catatonic forms.

16. See generalist medical journals such as *Afrique médicale, Dakar médical,* and *Médecine tropicale.*

17. In addition to the classic article by Collomb (1965), see Chirara (1984); Ouango (1984).

18. See Ouango (1984); Dupont and Ouedraogo (1989); Badji (1993).

19. See Karfo (1991); Karfo et al. (1993 and 1997); Uchôa et al. (1993).

20. A. Danfa (1998) points out that it comes in fourth place (15 percent) after schizo-phrenia (23.75 percent), *bouffées délirantes* (17.75 percent) and the misuse of drugs (15.75 percent) in the reasons for consultation in Division III of the psychiatric hospital of Thiaroye during 1997.

21. This question took up a very great deal of space in contributions to the regional symposium of the World Psychiatric Asoociation held in Dakar in April 1981 (Collignon 1981).

22. See Guèye, Collignon, and M'Boussou (1981); Guèye and M'Boussou (1981). In addition, there have been therapeutic recommendations in general medical practice (Ba and Guèye 1984; Guèye et al. 1994; Faye et al. 1994), as well as more recent interest in depression among the aged (Guèye, Loum, and Sylla 1995).

23. The first article in this series (Franklin et al. 1996a) presented the study set-ting, methods, sociodemographic and clinical characteristics of the patients, and the characteristics of the companions. The second examined the statistical associations of companion number, gender, and kinship relationship with the sociodemographic and clinical characteristics of the patients. (Franklin et al. 1996b).

24. These approaches are beginning to stimulate a fresh look at disorders in conjugal and other family situations (see Mbassa Menick and Sylla 1995; A. Sylla 2002).

25. Moreover, French psychoanalysts inspired by Lacan have formed a group to re-search and apply psychoanalytical concepts in Africa (Groupe de recherché et d'applica-tion des concepts psychanalytiques à la psychiatrie en Afrique francophone [Group for the research and application of psychoanalytical concepts to psychiatry in French-speaking Africa] or GRAPPAF). The group regularly proposes seminars offering reflec-tion and training for psychiatrists in Dakar and Ouagadougou, and it has published eight collections called *Les cahiers du GRAPPAF* by l'Harmattan in Paris.

26. Zempléni (1983) affirmed that the linking of medical observation and ethnologi-cal approach as implemented in Fann reached beyond the Freudian anthropology of the indefinite subject of the culture (for example, the Wolof of whom we speak) for a clinical approach that listens to the patient who speaks—to the person who, in his or her existence in society, has to choose from among various possible positions to adopt with regard to the institutions and expectations of his society.

27. Those who have focused on the psychic suffering of the child have also addressed such issues as child abuse, child neglect, and the case of street children. See Sylla, Guèye, and Collignon 1995; Guèye et al. 1997; Agossou 2000; Barry 1998–99; Douville, 2003–2004. A series of training seminars in several countries of western Africa, initially organized by Marie-Cécile Ortigues and Thérèse Agossou and subsequently taken up by younger colleagues, has contributed to the development of child psychiatry, now in the hands of by the younger African generations. The continuing existence of living dialogue between the generations, despite the advanced age of Ortigues, is evinced by the comments she has recently made on the case studies published by her Burkina col-leagues (M. C. Ortigues 2005–2006).

28. Professor Thérèse Agossou joined the World Health Organization's Regional Of-fice for Africa (located in Brazzaville) in 2003 as regional advisor for mental health and substance abuse.

29. The issue includes an annotated bibliography of works produced in Mali, contain-ing nearly 200 items (Collignon and Koumaré 1992) and works by Koumaré, Coudray,

and Miquel-Garcia (1992); Koumaré, Diaoure, and Miquel-Garcia (1992); Corin et al. (1992a and 1992b); and Miquel-Garcia et al. (1992).

30. These researchers from the Université de Montréal include Gilles Bibeau, Ellen Corin, and Elizabeth Uchôa.

31. The works of the team have been published in several volumes (Coppo 1988, 1993, and 1998; Coppo and Keita 1990).

32. It is striking how frequently the titles of these meetings begin with "The First . . . ," as if inaugurating a series, although no sequels appear.

33. The journal's website is http://www.refer.sn/psychopathologieafricaine.

REFERENCES

Agossou, T., ed. 2000. *Regards d'Afrique sur la maltraitance.* Paris: Karthala.
Association des Chercheurs Sénégalais, ed. 1997. *La folie au Sénégal.* Dakar: Association des Chercheurs Sénégalais.
Ba, M. 1987a. "Actualité de la sémiologie en psychiatrie, à travers une tentative d'utilisation d'une échelle d'évaluation (BPRS)." Dakar: Mémoire de CES [Certificat d'études spéciales] de Psychiatrie. [Diss. For the speciality in Psychiatry, after M.D.]
———. 1987b. "Approche des schizophrénies dysthymiques, à propos de dix cas colligés au CHU de Fann." Dakar, med. thesis. [Université Cheikh Anta Diop de Dakar]
Ba, M., and M. Guèye. 1984. "Les états dépressifs en Afrique: Actualités cliniques." *Médecine d'Afrique noire* 31: 673–76.
Ba, M., O. Ndoye, and M. Guèye. 1998–1999. "Crise d'hystérie et thérapie traditionnelle, ou la quête initiatique d'une acculturée." *Psychopathologie africaine* 29 (3): 275–86.
Ba, M., and B. Samuel-Lajeunesse. 1984. "Sémiologie et pathologie transculturelle." *Psychopathologie africaine* 20 (2): 133–41.
Ba, M., and O. Sylla. 1997. "Éléments de réflexion sur les perspectives d'avenir de la psychiatrie au Sénégal." In *La folie au Sénégal,* edited by Association des Chercheurs Sénégalais: Dakar: Association des Chercheurs Sénégalais.
Badji, B. 1993. *La folie en Afrique: Une rivalité pathologique, le cas des psychoses puerpérales en milieu Sénégalais.* Paris: L'Harmattan.
Barry, A. 1998–1999. "Marginalité et errance juvénile en milieu Africain: La place de l'aide psychologique dans les dispositifs de prise en charge des enfants de la rue." *Psychopathologie africaine* 29 (2): 139–90.
Chirara, A. K. 1984. "Bouffée délirante au Sénégal: Approche statistique et clinique (à propos de 109 observations)." Dakar, med. thesis.(Université Cheikh Anta Diop de Dakar).
Collignon, R. 1978. "Vingt ans de travaux à la clinique psychiatrique de Fann-Dakar." *Psychopathologie africaine* 14 (2–3): 133–323.
———, ed. 1981. "Psychiatrie et culture: Symposium régional, WPA [World Psychiatric Association] et SPHMD [Société de Psychopathologie et d'Hygiène mentale de Dakar] (Dakar, 6–9 avril 1981)." *Psychopathologie africaine* 17 (1–3): 1–526.
———. 1982. "Social Psychiatry in French-Speaking Africa: The Case of Senegal." In *Mental Health in Africa,* edited by O. A. Bell and N. W. Bell, 8–27. Erinosho, Ibadan: Ibadan University Press

———. 1983. "À propos de psychiatrie communautaire en Afrique noire: Les dispositifs villageois d'assistance: Éléments pour un dossier." *Psychopathologie africaine* 19 (3): 287–328.

———. 1995–96. "Some Reflections on the History of Psychiatry in French-Speaking West Africa: The Example of Senegal." *Psychopathologie africaine* 27 (1): 37–51.

———. 2001. "Les pratiques institutionnelles dans le service de psychiatrie du l'Hôpital de Fann-Dakar: Leçons d'un réexamen critique." *Réseau anthropologique de la santé*, Bulletin no. 2, 11–25. [Unité de Recherche Socio-anthropologie de la santé SHADYC (EHESS-CNRS) Marseille]

———. 2002. "Pour une histoire de la psychiatrie coloniale française: À partir de l'exemple du Sénégal." *L'autre* 3 (3): 455–80.

Collignon, R., M. E. Gruénais, and L.Vidal, eds. 1994. "L'annonce de la Séropositivité au VIH en Afrique" *Psychopathologie africaine* 26 (2), 149–291.

Collignon, R., and M.Guèye. 1989. "Santé mentale et migration vers la ville." In *Urbanisation et santé dans le tiers monde: Transition épidémiologique, changement social et soins de santé primaires*, edited by G. Salem and E. Jannée, 297–303. Paris: Editions de l'ORSTOM. [Office de la Recherche Scientifique et Technique d'Outre-Mer].

———. 1995. "The Interface between Culture and Mental Illness in French-Speaking West Africa." In *Handbook of Culture and Mental Illness: An International Perspective*, edited by I. Al-Issa, 93–112. Madison, CT: International Universities Press.

———. 2003. *Psychiatrie, psychanalyse, culture/Psychiatry, Psychoanalysis, Culture*, First Pan-African Conference on Mental Health. (Dakar, 18–20 mars 2002). Proceedings edited by R. Collignon, and M.Guèye Dakar: SPHMD. [Société de Psychopathologie et d'Hygiène mentale de Dakar]

Collignon, R., and B. Koumaré. 1992. "La santé mentale au Mali: Éléments de bibliographie annotée." *Psychopathologie africaine* 24 (2): 243–87.

Collomb, Henri. 1965. "Les bouffées délirantes en psychiatrie africaine." *Psychopathologie africaine* 1 (2): 167–239.

———. 1973. "Rencontre de deux systèmes de soins: À propos de thérapeutiques des maladies mentales en Afrique." *Social Science and Medicine* 7: 623–633.

Coppo, P. 1988. *Médecine traditionnelle, psychiatrie et psychologie en Afrique*. Rome: Il Pensiero Scientifico Editore.

———, ed.. 1993. *Essai de psychopathologie Dogon*, Bandiagara, Mali/Perrugia, Italie: Editions CRMT [Centre de recherché sur la medicine traditionnelle]/PSMTM.

———. 1998. *Les guérisseurs de la folie: Histoires du plateau Dogon* (Ethnopsychiatrie). Paris: Collection les Empêcheurs de Penser en Rond.

Coppo, P., and A. Keita, eds. 1990. *Médecine traditionnelle: Acteurs, itinéraires et thérapeutiques*. Trieste, Italy: Edizionie.

Corin, E., E. Uchôa, G. Bibeau, and B. Koumaré. 1992a. "Articulation et variations des systèmes de signes, de sens et d'action." *Psychopathologie africaine* 24 (2): 183–204.

———. 1992b. "La place de la culture dans la psychiatrie africaine d'aujourd'hui: Paramètres pour un cadre de référence." *Psychopathologie africaine* 24 (2): 149–81.

Coulibaly, B., B. Koumaré, and J. P. Coudray. 1983. "La demande de soins psychiatriques au Mali: Données d'épidémiologie hospitalière." *Psychopathologie africaine* 19 (3): 261–86.

Dago-Akribi, H. A. 2001–2002. "Méthodes et conduite d'une consultation psychologique auprès des femmes enceintes infectées par le VIH à Abidjan (Côte-d'Ivoire)." *Psychopathologie africaine* 31 (2): 171–89.

D'Almeida, L., A. G. Diop, and C. Apovo. 1989. "Aspects neuro-psychiatriques du Sida." *Plurale* 1 (1): 57–67.

D'Almeida, L., and J.-G. Ouango. 1997. "À Propos des Villages Psychiatriques au Sénégal." *Afrique Médicale* 27e année (262), 199–202.

D'Almeida, L., P. Picard, O. Sylla, and A. M. Seck. 1986. "La thérapeutique psychiatrique dans l'œuvre écrite de Henri Collomb (1958–1978)." *Psychologie médicale* 18 (12): 1895–99.

Danfa, A. 1998. "Place de L'épilepsie dans Les Consultations Psychiatriques de La Division III de l'HP de Thiaroye." Dakar, Mémoire de Passage de 4e Année CES de Psychiatrie.

Diop, B. 1974. *Place de la santé mentale dans le développement des services de santé publique.* Brazzaville: OMS [Organisation mondiale de la Santé]: *Cahiers techniques* AFRO no. 8. [Bureau regional pour l'Afrique AFRO]

Diop, B., R. Collignon, and M. Guèye. 1976. "Présentation de l'étude concertée de l'OMS sur les stratégies pour l'extension des soins de santé mentale." *Psychopathologie africaine* 12 (2): 5–20.

Diop, B., R. Collignon, M. Guèye, and T. W. Harding. 1980. "Symptomatologie et diagnostiques dans une région rurale du Sénégal." *Psychopathologie africaine* 16 (1): 5–20.

———. 1982. "Diagnosis and Symptoms of Mental Disorders in a Rural Area of Senegal." *African Journal of Medical Science* 11 (3): 95–103.

Diop, M., A. Zempléni, P. Martino, and H. Collomb. 1964. "Signification et valeur de la persécution dans les cultures africaines." In *Comptes rendus du Congrès de Psychiatrie et de Neurologie de Langue Française,* (62e session, Marseille, 7–12 September 1964), 1: 333–43. Paris: Masson.

Douville, O. 2003–2004. "Enfants et adolescents en danger dans la rue à Bamako (Mali): questions cliniques et anthropologiques à partir d'une pratique." *Psychopathologie africaine* 32 (1): 55–89.

Dupont, G., and A. Ouedraogo. 1989. "À propos des psychoses puerpérales au Sénégal: Réflexion sur les psychoses aiguës africaines." *Information psychiatrique* 65 (10): 1011–16.

Ebin, V. 1990–1991. "'Laissez venir à moi vos peuples, vos émigrants exténués' . . . et je leur donnerai une boîte de gélatine en poudre: Étude d'un syndrome d'allure somatique parmi les émigrés sénégalais à New York." *Psychopathologie africaine* 23 (3): 365–85.

Fall, L., B. Seck, and D. Charlier. 2001–2002. "Pédopsychiatrie de liaison à Dakar." *Psychopathologie africaine* 31 (3): 345–64.

Faye, P. A., A. M. Seck, M. Kéré, and K. Karfo. 1994. "Traitement de la dépression." *Forum médical* 57–59.

Foucault, M. 1961. *Folie et déraison: Histoire de la folie à l'âge classique.* Paris: Plon.

Franklin, R. R., D. Sarr, M. Guèye, O. Sylla, and R. Collignon. 1996a. "Cultural Response to Mental Illness in Senegal: Reflections through Patient Companions—Part I. Methods and Descriptive Data." *Social Science and Medicine* 42 (3): 325–38.

———. 1996b. "Cultural Response to Mental Illness in Senegal: Reflections through Patient Companions—Part II. Statistical Correlates." *Social Science and Medicine*. 42 (3): 339–51.

Gbikpi, P. A. 1981. *"L'accompagnant en milieu psychiatrique africain: Bilan et synthèse"*. Dakar: Mémoire de CES de Psychiatrie, Dakar: med. thesis, Université Cheikh Anta Diop de Dakar.

Guèye, M. 1995. "Assistance psychiatrique au Sénégal: Bilan et perspective." *Information psychiatrique* 71 (6): 525–29.

———. 1998. "Résistance et chronicité en psychiatrie: L'expérience sénégalaise." *Nervure* 11 (4): 11–14.

———. 1998–1999. "Serigne Babakar Diop (1933–1998) ou L'art d'accomplir sa destinée." *Psychopathologie africaine* 29 (1): 3–6.

Guèye, M., R. Collignon, and M. M'Boussou. 1981. "Évolution du suicide et de la dépression au Sénégal et en Afrique." In *Dépression et suicide*, edited by J. P. Soubrier and J. Vedrinne, 38–48. Paris: Pergamon.

Guèye, M., K. Karfo, B. Seck, P. Lambert, and K. Sène. 1994. "Est-ce une dépression?" *Forum médical* 52–57.

Guèye, M., M. Loum, and O. Sylla. 1995. "La dépression de la personne âgée au Sénégal." *Information psychiatrique* 71 (6): 543–51.

Guèye, M., and M. M'Boussou. 1981. "Évolution des conceptions thérapeutiques des états dépressifs en 20 ans à Fann (1961–1980)." *Psychopathologie africaine* 17 (1–3): 197–208.

Guèye, M., and B. Seck. 1998. "L'humanitaire en santé mentale: L'exemple sénégalais du Centre Dalal Xel, de L'hôpital de Jour et du Dispositif Itinérant d'Assistance aux Malades Mentaux." *Synapse* 146:51–54.

Guèye, M., O. Sylla, B. Seck, P. Lambert, N. Huart, O Ly Kane, O Ndoye, eds. 1997. "La souffrance psychique chez l'enfant en Afrique noire." *Psychopathologie africaine* 28 (3): 293–356.

Harding, T. W., C. E. Climent, R. Collignon, B. Diop, R. Giel, M. Guèye, H. N. A. Ibrahim et al. 1979. "Santé mentale et soins de santé primaires. Premiers résultats d'une étude concertée de l'OMS." *Psychopathologie africaine* 15 (1): 5–28.

Kane, F. 1979. "Évaluation des Résultats Thérapeutiques du Centre Psychiatrique de Brousse de Kénia (Basse Casamance) Sénégal, Approche Sociologique," [Dakar, CRDI]. Centre de recherché pour le développement international [cooperation canadienne] Unpublished report.

Karfo, K. 1991. "Le vécu de l'épilepsie grand mal au Sénégal." Dakar: med. thesis. Université Cheikh Anta Diop de Dakar.

Karfo, K., M. Guèye, B. Seck, K. Sène, and I. P. Ndiaye. 1997. "L'épileptique et sa maladie en milieu dakarois: Enquête sur le vécu des patients." *Semaine des Hôpitaux* 73 (7–8): 218–22.

Karfo, K., M. Kéré, M. Guèye, and I. P. Ndiaye. 1993. "Aspects socio-culturels de l'épilepsie grand mal en milieu dakarois." *Dakar médical* 38 (2): 139–45.

Keita, B., E. Miquel-Garcia, and B. Koumaré. 1994. "Représentation et perception du *Sérébana*: malnutrition protéino-calorique du jeune enfant et grossesses rapprochées: Étude dans le cistrict de Bamako." *Psychopathologie africaine* 26 (3): 301–30.

Koumaré, B., ed. 1992. "Santé Mentale au Mali," *Psychopathologie africaine*, 24 (2), 133–287.

Koumaré, B., J.-P. Coudray,and E. Miquel-Garcia. 1992. "L'assistance psychiatrique au Mali: À propos du placement des patients psychiatriques auprès de tradipraticiens." *Psychopathologie africaine* 24 (2): 135–48.

Koumaré, B., R. Diaoure, and E. Miquel-Garcia. 1992. "Définition d'un instrument de dépistage des troubles psychiques." *Psychopathologie africaine* 24 (2): 229–43.

Ly, O. D. 1997. "Souffrance psychique, imaginaire et intervention dans la tradition: La valeur d'une interaction." *Psychopathologie africaine* 28 (3): 339–56.

———. 2003–2004. "Ibrahima: L'enfant mal nommé?" *Psychopathologie africaine* 32 (3): 273–89.

Mbassa Menick, D., and O. Sylla. 1995. "La conjugopathie au Sénégal: Une plainte ango-issée de la féminité." *Médecine tropicale* 56 (4): 423–29.

Mbodji, M. 1997a. "Indices de souffrance psychique de l'enfant dans l'imaginaire et le langage populaire en milieu Wolof et Lébou (Sénégal)." *Psychopathologie africaine* 28 (3): 295–311.

———. 1997b. "Réflexions sur l'individuation dans la pathologie mentale au Sénégal." In *La folie au Sénégal* edited by Association des Chercheurs Sénégalais [ACS], 283–304. Dakar: ACS [Association des chercheurs Sénégalais].

Miquel-Garcia, E., B. Keita, B. Koumaré, and G. Soula. 1992. "Malnutrition et troubles réactionnels mère-enfant en milieu urbain au Mali." *Psychopathologie africaine* 24 (2): 205–28.

Ndiaye, B. 1989. "L'hospitalisme à l'Hôpital Psychiatrique de Thiaroye." Dakar: med. thesis, Université Cheikh Anta Diop de Dakar.

Ndoye, O., ed. 2003. *Le sexe qui rend fou: Approche clinique et thérapeutique,* Paris: Présence Africaine.

Ndoye, O., A. Devos, and M. Guèye. 2000. "L'ethnopsychiatrie à Fann aujourd'hui." *Psychopathologie africaine* 30 (3): 265–82.

Ortigues, M. C. 2005–2006. "Commentaires sur l'observation clinique d'une jeune fille orpheline de père depuis l'âge d'un an, proposée par deux collègues Burkinabè," *Psychopathologie africaine* 33 (2): 249–56.

Ortigues, M.-C. and E. Ortigues 1966. *Œdipe africain,* Paris: Plon (2nd ed.: UGE "10/18," 1973; 3rd ed: L'Harmattan, 1984).

Ortigues, M. C., P. Martino, and H. Collomb. 1967. "L'utilisation des données culturelles dans un cas de bouffée délirante." *Psychopathologie africaine* 3 (1): 121–147.

Ouango, J.-G. 1984. "Contribution à l'étude des bouffées délirantes à Dakar: À propos de 373 cas relevés à la Clinique Moussa Diop de Fann," Dakar: med. thesis, Université Cheikh Anta Diop de Dakar.

———. 1987 "Les villages psychiatriques au Sénégal. Mythes et réalités: l'exemple de Botou." Dakar: 65 p. multigr. (Mém. CES psychiatrie, 32)

Ouedraogo, A., T. L. Ouedraogo, and P. T. Sanou. 2001–2002. "Dépression chez les personnes vivant avec le VIH en milieu africain à Ouagadougou." *Psychopathologie africaine* 31 (3): 333–44.

Ouedraogo, A., and S. Siranyian. 2003–2004. "Facteurs socioculturels et problématique du support identificatoire paternel à l'adolescence: À propos d'un cas clinique à Ouagadougou (Burkina Faso)." *Psychopathologie africaine* 32 (3): 261–71.

Picard, P. 1985. "Réflexion sur le phénomène de la double demande" Dakar: Mémoire de CES de psychiatrie. [Unpublished paper, Université Cheikh Anta Diop de Dakar].

Picard, P., and L. d'Almeida. 1985. "La double demande d'assistance psychiatrique et traditionnelle: Approche statistique à partir d'une population de consultants (clinique psychiatrique Moussa Diop, CHU de Fann)." *Afrique médicale* 24 (231): 305–14.

Réseau de Recherche en Santé de la Reproduction en Afrique. 1991. *Guide de counseling VIH/SIDA*. Dakar: Réseau de Recherche en Santé de la Reproduction en Afrique.

Sarr, D., and M. Guèye. 1994. "L'école ethnopsychiatrique de Dakar: mythe ou réalité?" *Synapse* 108: 33–40.

Seck, A. M., and D. Sarr. 1997."Approche thérapeutique de la folie au Sénégal." *Psychopathologie africaine* 28 (3): 257–82.

Seck, B., J. Stéphany, B. Koumaré, H. Stach, S. Dia, and P. Gbikpi. 1981. "Un modèle de désinstitutionalisation au Sénégal: le Dispositif itinérant d'assistance aux malades mentaux (DIAMM)." *Psychopathologie africaine* 17 (1–3): 271–78.

Selguetia J. 1997. *Évaluation d'une pratique thérapeutique: Le pënc de Fann*. Dakar: Diplôme d'initiation en psychopathologie.

Siranyian, S. 2003–2004. "Destin personnel, destinée familiale, ou le risque lié à la position d'aîné: Illustration clinique chez un adolescent à Ouagadougou (Burkina Faso)." *Psychopathologie africaine* 32 (2): 141–52.

Sow, I., L. d'Almeida, O. Sylla, P. Picard. 1986. "Le pënc de Fann ou la parole normative." *Psychologie médicale* 18 (12): 1855–59.

Sylla, A. 2002. "Malaise dans la famille africaine." In *Les repères dans la famille africaine,* edited by Claude Duprat and Roger Wartel, 51–59. Paris: L'Harmattan (*Cahiers du Grappaf,* No. 2).

Sylla, A, O. Ndoye, and M. Guèye. 2001. "Importance du contexte socioculturel dans la psychopathie en Afrique: Une observation clinique." *L'évolution psychiatrique* 66 (4): 647–54.

Sylla, O., M. Guèye, and R. Collignon, R., eds. 1995. *Les mauvais traitements de mineurs: Réalités, Caractéristiques, Enjeux, Réponses,* Séminaire international ISPCAN [International Society for Prevention of Child Abuse and Neglect], AFIREM [Association française d'information et de recherche sur l'enfance maltraitée] (Dakar, 8–23 avril 1994). Dakar: SPHMD [Société de Psychopathologie et d'Hygiène mentale de Dakar].

Sylla, O., and M. Mbaye. 1990–1991. "Psychopathologie et migration, un cas de 'wootal.'" *Psychopathologie africaine* 23 (3): 353–64.

Thiam, M. H., P. O. Ndiaye, and M. Guèye. 2001–2002. "Relation médecin/malade et observance thérapeutique en psychiatrie: À propos d'une étude chez des patients suivis en ambulatoire à Dakar." *Psychopathologie africaine* 31 (3): 379–392.

Uchôa, E. 1988. "Les femmes de Bamako (Mali) et la santé mentale: Une étude anthropopsychiatrique." PhD diss., University of Montreal.

Uchôa, E., E. Corin, G. Bibeau, and B. Koumaré. 1993. "Représentations culturelles et disqualification sociale: L'épilepsie dans trois groupes ethniques au Mali." *Psychopathologie africaine* 25 (1): 33–57.

Vaughan, M. 1983. "Idioms of Madness: Zomba Lunatic Asylum in the Colonial Period." *Journal of Southern African Studies* 9 (2): 218–38.

———. 1991. *Curing Their Ills: Colonial Power and African Illness*. Cambridge, UK: Polity.

Zempléni, A. 1968. "L'interprétation et la thérapie traditionnelle du désordre mentale chez les Wolof et les Lebou (Sénégal)." Paris: Faculté des lettres et sciences humaines, Doctoral Thèse de 3e cycle.

———. 1980. "Henri Collomb (1913–1979) and the Fann Team." *Social Science and Medicine* 14 (2): 85–90.

———. 1983. "Quelques problèmes de méthode en psychopathologie africaine." In *Une anthropologie médicale en France?,* edited by A. Retel-Laurentin, 23–28. Paris: Editions du CNRS [Centre national de la Recherche scientifique, France].

7 WOMEN'S SELF-REPORTED MENTAL HEALTH IN ACCRA, GHANA

ALLAN G. HILL AND VICTORIA DE MENIL

IN RECENT YEARS, interest in international comparisons of health across populations has grown considerably. So has interest in the concept of global health and the concern with measuring a country's progress towards set targets, especially the Millennium Development Goals. The key assumption in tracking international progress towards such targets is that information on health can be collected in similar ways and compared on similar scales across countries. This makes good sense when dealing with objective measures such as height, weight, and blood pressure, but it becomes more questionable when dealing with conditions that are subjective, socially shameful, difficult to assess with simple physical examinations, and possibly intermittent or recurring. Most mental health disorders fall into this last category.

Nonetheless, a substantial literature has grown up around how best to compare self-reported health states, both physical and mental (Üstün et al. 2010). This literature addresses the development of reliable instruments and the introduction of better measuring approaches. These approaches include the replacement of categorical variables with visual analog scales and applying standardization techniques, including the "anchoring vignettes" for standardization used in several studies supported by the World Health Organization (Salomon, Tandon, and Murray 2004). The comparisons of test and self-report data around the world have largely focused on physical measures, often with confusing findings on the links between the two (Ploubidis and Grundy 2011; Halabi et al. 1992; Lawlor et al. 2002; Louie and Ward 2010; Zurayk et al. 1995). Many studies have found major discrepancies and inconsistencies in both level and distribution of outcomes, even when comparing so-called objective measures with self-reports on the same family of conditions. The conclusion to be drawn is that health states have several dimensions, and although many of them are complementary, it is difficult to collapse them all into any single summary measure.

Notably, the more general and less symptom-specific the questions are, the better the answers predict health-related behavior. Broader questions about general health ("How would you describe your general health?") or questions about health transitions ("Compared to a year ago, would you describe your health as better, worse, or about the same?") are often preferred when the aim is to predict health-related behavior such as seeking professional care. Analysts have often resorted to histories of care-seeking as alternatives, but even with that approach, cultural factors can affect the tendency to seek care (Murray and Williams 1986). Further, the psychiatric state of the person can also affect health-seeking behavior significantly (Dowrick, Bellon, and Gomez 2000).

Recently, there have been several major attempts to improve the population-level reporting of mental health status and mental disorders (including depression and schizophrenia) through the development of standardized instruments with established psychometric properties. In 2002 and 2003, the World Health Survey conducted research at the population level into the health of a wide range of countries (Ghana among them), including some mental health measures. Only two conditions—depression and schizophrenia—were systematically investigated, and the results were cross-classified by sex, urban or rural residence, income quintile, and age. The prevalences found for diagnoses of depression and schizophrenia in Ghana were very low: 1.5 percent and 0.7 percent, respectively (World Health Organization 2005). Very little interpretation of these data is provided, but the prevalence is low in comparison to that in countries with good mental health surveillance. For example, in the United Kingdom and France, the World Health Survey reported that depression affected 16 percent and 17 percent of the population, respectively, and that of those affected, 39 percent and 41 percent respectively, had been treated (World Health Organization 2003). Even in comparison with the facility-based data for Accra discussed below, the Ghana figures on a few aspects of mental illness are plainly not credible.

Alternative sources of information have also been sought by attempting to improve the routinely reported facility-based data. Despite the scanty data currently available on mental health in Ghana (Osei 2003), the picture is changing and becoming increasingly balanced, thanks in part to the landmark introduction of a new national mental health surveillance system begun in 2009. The new information system was developed as part of the Mental Health and Poverty Project, an applied research study in Ghana, Zambia, Uganda, and South Africa led by a consortium of researchers with funding from the UK Department for International Development (2005). The system draws on diagnoses from the tenth edition of the World Health Organization's *International Statistical Classification of Diseases and Related Health Problems* (ICD-10) (World Health Organization 2010) and has increased the number of conditions surveyed from four to ten.

Although it is too early to evaluate them systematically, preliminary findings from the new system indicate that approximately equal numbers of women and men use the out-patient mental health departments of the government facilities, countering a local misperception that women more frequently develop mental illness and seek care for it than men do (Ofori-Atta et al. 2010). Epilepsy and related seizure disorders represent 10 percent of all neuropsychiatric disorders chronicled by the national health information system. Sixty percent of patients with mental illness were employed while receiving treatment, again dispelling a common misperception: in this case, that people with a mental illness are unable to work.

The main limitation of facility-based health information, however, is that rather than measuring the true prevalence of illness, it measures health-seeking behaviors. A better way to measure the burden of psychiatric disorders in a population is through community surveys. In 2003 researchers in Ghana launched the first large-scale community health study to include mental health, called the Women's Health Study of Accra. The study involved a sample of 3,200 women from Accra and combined self-reported health questions with a clinical examination (Hill et al. 2007). The study used instruments developed and tested elsewhere to allow for comparisons with other populations. It collected a rich array of contextual data, such as the household circumstances of people suffering from mental distress. Part of the importance of the study is that it provides some of the first information on the prevalence of mental distress in a large urban population in Africa, together with relevant contextual information. The investigators had the advantage of being able to compare the prevalence of mental distress in subpopulations drawn from very different backgrounds, such as various language groups, townspeople and rural immigrants, rich and poor, and educated and uneducated. This chapter also explains the process used to conduct the Women's Health Study in Accra, Ghana and examines some of the main mental health findings from that study, some of which are described more quantitatively elsewhere (de Menil et al. 2012). The chapter provides an empirical account of how the instruments were selected and how women reported their mental health, as well as providing the basis for the study of the several correlations of mental distress and health with common risk and protective factors.

CHOOSING A TOOL FOR ASSESSING MENTAL HEALTH IN AFRICA

Choosing a tool to measure population-level mental illnesses or disorders in communities in Ghana is challenging, as there is no general consensus on the most appropriate way to capture the prevalence and severity of mental disorders in African societies, as chapters 2 and 3 in this volume illustrate. A good tool needs to be reliable—in other words, measuring similarly the same phenomena in repeated studies in different cultures—and valid, so as to allow for generalization and comparison.

Some of the early community studies of mental health began as enquiries into the health of relatively small communities with a particular medical problem in mind (Coleman et al. 2006; Walraven et al. 2001; Zurayk and Harfouche 1970; Zurayk et al. 2007). Others, such as the Giza studies in Egypt, were accompanied by more in-depth anthropological work and interventions (Younis et al. 1993). More recently, studies assessing mental health have become larger, more complex, and hence much more representative of the general population . Gradually, the process of standardization of instruments has increased the utility of such studies for comparative purposes.

The first psychiatric epidemiological surveys of the 1980s used variations of the Diagnostic Interview Schedule (DIS) (Robins et al. 1981). This interview schedule bases its mental illness categories on the third edition of the American Psychiatric Association's *Diagnostic and Statistical Manual of Mental Disorders* (DSM-III) (American Psychiatric Association 1980). The US National Institute of Mental Health, which encouraged the development of the DIS, encouraged the researchers to make the connection with the ICD-10. The result was the World Health Organization's Composite International Diagnostic Interview (CIDI), which was first used in the United States in 1994.

In 1995 the World Health Organization sponsored a World Mental Health Survey Initiative (Kessler and Üstün 2004), which to date has applied the CIDI in twenty-eight countries, although only two of them—Nigeria and South Africa—are in Africa. The wide application of the CIDI, mostly in Europe and North America, revealed the pressing need to understand more about illness severity. Many mild or self-limiting disorders may not have needed treatment, but the studies were initially not refined enough to produce reliable gradations of severity (Kessler and Üstün 2008, 6). In response to this challenge, a new World Mental Health Survey was launched, using an updated version of the CIDI—CIDI 3.0 —with a much stronger emphasis on severity of illness. Embedded in the new questionnaire are diagnostic criteria from both the ICD-10 and the fourth edition of the *Diagnostic and Statistical Manual of Mental Disorders* (DSM-IV) (American Psychiatric Association 1994).

Another study to use the original CIDI was the World Health Organization's Multi-country Survey Study, conducted in 2000–2001. This survey drew on 300 research instruments, covering a wide range of health conditions and was implemented in more than fifty countries. The only questions related to mental health pertain to depression and alcohol use and are based on the relevant sections of the CIDI. The CIDI questions have now been extensively employed in many international studies (Haro et al. 2006; Kessler and Üstün 2004; Wittchen 1994).

In parallel with the development and upgrading of the CIDI, the 1990s saw the creation of new tools for assessing mental health at the population level, rather than at the level of the individual. One of these tools, which became standardized as the Short Form 36 (SF-36), was originally developed as part of the Medical Outcomes Study sponsored by the RAND Corporation to examine the link between physicians' practice styles and patients' outcomes across different health systems and to assess post-treatment improvements in health at the individual level. Nonetheless, it lends itself to population-based assessments by the addition of norm-based scoring and the establishment of standard values adjusted by age and gender. The SF-36 been used to measure both physical and mental disorders and to assess quality-adjusted life-years (QALYs) which are the basis for much cost-effectiveness analysis. In the SF-36 there are two sets of health domains, with four physical and four mental domains. Full details on the scales and the psychometrics of the SF-36 are provided by the developers (Ware et al. 1993). SF-36 measures have been calculated for a wide range of populations, mostly in Europe and North America, but increasingly in low-income countries. It has been used only rarely in Africa, except for surveys in specialized clinical studies.

Other population health studies have made an effort to include a mental health dimension, but often either the questions used have not been tested or the findings are not presented in a way that can be compared across studies. One such example is the World Health Survey launched in 2002 (World Health Organization 2003). This survey was designed to collect data on a wide range of health issues in nine main domains: socio-demographic characteristics, health state descriptions, health state valuations, risk factors, mortality, health system coverage, health system responsiveness, health goals, and social capital. The study's coverage of mental illness (even in the long form of the survey) is very brief. It mentions the general impact of illness on physical and mental health (questions 2000 and 2001 in the health state descriptions) and asks some additional questions in the twelve-month recall period about sadness and hallucinations, as well as about explicit diagnoses—namely, depression, schizophrenia, and psychosis. Summary results and micro data are available for eighteen African countries. Without the accompanying social and cultural background, however, the summary results are difficult to interpret for those countries, leaving the reader with considerable uncertainty about the reliability and consistency of the different prevalence of mental health findings across the countries.

Another example is the World Health Organization's Study on Global AGEing and Adult Health (SAGE) (World Health Organization n.d.). SAGE collects data on respondents aged eighteen or older, with an emphasis on populations aged fifty or older, from nationally representative samples in six countries, including Ghana and South Africa. The survey also contains a sub-study that has been applied in several longitudinal studies or demographic surveillance sites in Africa, including Navrongo, in Ghana; Agincourt, in South Africa; Nairobi, in Kenya; and Ifakara, in Tanzania. SAGE contains twenty-one questions on depression or anxiety and suicidal tendencies. There are some overlaps with standard instruments such as the SF-36, but it is difficult to make direct comparisons between data from SAGE and information from other sources. This is particularly true for comparing sets of questions, rather than individual questions.

As a whole, these mental health measures reveal several important assumptions about mental health. In general, their framework, which builds on the ICD-10 or DSM, is essentially biologically based, reflecting contemporary knowledge about disease agents. In addition, the perspective on illness adopted for the surveys is that of the individual patient, rather than that of the population and its broader patterns of illness prevalence and incidence. This perspective leads to the inclusion of individual-level risk factors in the questionnaires rather than to the collection of information on broader determinants of mental health such as a recent bereavement, unemployment, or an insecure social and economic environment.

These instruments adopt two main approaches to assessing mental suffering. Some of the instruments—for example, those used in the World Health Survey and SAGE—have preferred to ask direct diagnostic questions, such as "Have you been depressed?" and "Have you experienced psychosis or schizophrenia?" Other instruments, including the SF-36, ask about selected symptoms rather than about a diagnosis.

Taking into account the histories as well as the advantages and disadvantages of the different research instruments, the researchers in Accra ultimately chose to use the SF-36 to measure self-reported health status, including mental health, in the women they studied. They selected the SF-36 because it has proven psychometric properties, allows comparisons with other studies, is quick to administer, and provides information at a population level. Since the study in Accra focused on mental distress in the population, the researchers were more interested in an instrument that could provide information about the distribution of disorders at that level than they were in an instrument that focused on clinical diagnosis and treatment of individuals. The final questionnaire added to the SF-36 a few additional questions on mental health that were asked of a smaller group of participants. The respondents were first asked the questions at home and then asked them again in the very different environment of a hospital clinic.

USING THE TOOL

In Ghana, as in many other African countries, very little information is available on the epidemiology of mental illnesses. Generally, mental illnesses—especially the common mental disorders—are not well reported in data based on facilities, whether government-run or private. Until recently, for example, only four conditions associated with mental illness were recognized in the official data: acute psychosis, substance abuse, epilepsy, and neurosis.

In 2005, there were 2,668 cases in metropolitan Accra of the four mental disorders; 1,562 cases (59 percent) were men. For both men and women, the largest numbers of cases were in the 25–34 age group (Ghana Health Service 2005). Converting these numbers to rates by dividing by the population by age, the overall prevalence for men for the four conditions were 0.69 percent for psychosis, 0.55 percent for substance abuse, 0.43 percent for epilepsy, and 0.20 percent for neurosis. For women, the rates were 0.68 percent for psychosis, 0.54 percent for substance abuse, 0.42 percent for epilepsy, and 0.20 percent for neurosis. Although the rates of psychosis are consistent with those found in other countries (Van Os and Kapur 2009), the rates of substance abuse elsewhere are typically closer to 5 percent (ten times the reported rate in Ghana), and three to four times higher among men than among women. In addition, rates of neurosis (that is, depression and anxiety) would be expected to be considerably higher in populations with good mental health surveillance. Due to the low levels of diagnosis and reporting, all the rates in Ghana are severe underestimates of the true prevalence of these conditions.

Adapting research tools into the local language is a crucial step for any research on mental health, since the vocabulary and concepts describing many mental health conditions are not as readily shared across languages and cultures as the terms for the more common infectious diseases with well-known physical symptoms. For the study in Ghana, the research tools were translated into three local languages—Ga, Akan, and Ewe—in the course of a focus group with all of the interviewers, most of whom were young female college graduates, some from the nursing school. The translations were then typed up as a reference document for the interviewers, while the data were entered on the original English language form. No backward translation was conducted, since the original translation had been reviewed by all members of the group.

A sample of 3,200 women was chosen to represent the population of the Accra metropolitan area living in the community (that is, not living in a health or welfare institution). The population was stratified by age and social position to ensure representation across all types of people. A quarter of the women were fifty or older, to provide enough cases for an analysis of illness among the elderly. People from some outlying towns and the port city of Tema—which are not part of the Accra metropolitan area, the study region—were excluded from the sample. A subset of 1,316 women chosen for a medical examination and tests were asked additional questions on mental health, including their experience with selected symptoms such as anxiety, sadness, depression, and suicidal thoughts.

The study consisted of two parts: a self-reported interview at the home and a medical assessment at the clinic. Both clinical assessments and self-reported information collected at the women's homes were available for over one-third of the women. The home interview contained a suite of questions on the dwelling, household members, and the health of the woman, including the SF-36 instrument for assessing mental health. Below we draw out the salient general findings from this work, since many of the more technical and statistical issues have been addressed elsewhere (see list of references at the end of the chapter).

WHAT WOMEN IN ACCRA REPORT ABOUT THEIR MENTAL HEALTH

The first finding of general importance is that the results on the mental health domains were highly correlated with the answers to the set of questions on general health, providing the first evidence from Africa that this international scale remains internally consistent when used within the Ghanaian population. The study found a strong association between all eight domains of the SF-36 instrument, indicating that the respondents replied consistently to the standardized questions and with patterns similar to those of US and European respondents. The results were also consistent by age and social class across the diverse linguistic groups, suggesting that the questions were understood similarly by different linguistic and cultural groups, and the tabulations of the norm-based scores on all the SF-36 indicators showed no significant differences by ethnicity or language. With this reassurance about the reliability and internal consistency of the self-reported measures, we can now turn to examine the differences in self-reported mental health that might provide clues to the underlying risk factors.

Differences by Age

The analysis focuses on four domains of interest: vitality, social functioning, role limitations (social activities affected by physical or emotional problems) and mental health (feelings of nervousness and depression). First, we present the results of the analysis of the outcomes using norm-based scores tabulated by age, as shown in figure 7.1.

There is a very strong negative association with age on all four measures of mental health. All of the measures except mental health worsen at about the same rate with age; the mental health measure declines more slowly. The norm-based

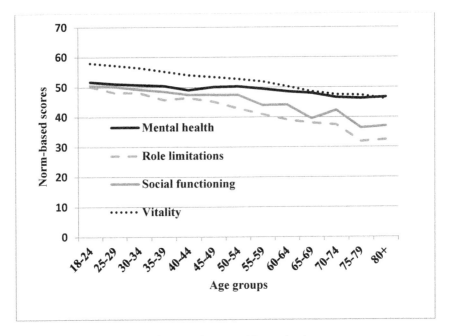

Figure 7.1. SF-36 Mental Health Scores for Accra Women by Age.
The vertical scale runs from 100 (very good) to 0 (very poor).

scoring system is designed to produce a population average score of 50; thus, on all four dimensions of mental health and well-being, the Accra women's scores are quite high. How do these results compare with other relevant populations?

Comparison with Nigeria

The Nigerian World Mental Health Survey was conducted in 2003 among 2,143 adults in different parts of the country, beginning with the Yoruba-speaking areas and extending to other language groups (for full results, see Gureje, Lasebikan, and Makanjuola 2006).Two features of this survey are worth noting here. First, the lifetime prevalence for any disorder (ibid., table 10.2) was 12 percent, peaking in the age range 35–64 rather than in an older population. For the twelve-month prevalence, overall 6 percent of the respondents reported any disorder. These were mostly anxiety disorders and only 13 percent of the respondents showed indication of a severe condition (reporting two or more symptoms). The authors of the study surmise that the conditions were probably underreported. They found very few systematic or significant differences by sex, age, income, marital status, or level of education (ibid. 227).

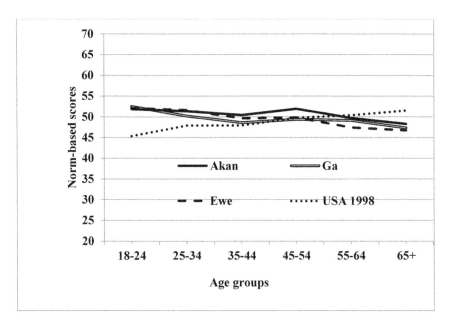

Figure 7.2. SF-36 Mental Health Scores for Accra and US Women by Age.
The vertical scale runs from 100 (very good) to 0 (very poor).

Comparison with the United States

The unusual nature of the Ghana age gradient results is further demonstrated in a comparison with norms for US women of the same ages. Figure 7.2 shows the trend by age in SF-36 mental health scores for the three main ethnic groups in Accra compared with the trend for US women, where mental health improves with age. The striking finding is that the gradient with age in Accra is in the opposite direction from that for the US women. This difference in scores by age is also found for the other three scales within the mental health measure, so it is not an aberrant finding for a single scale.

Differences by Socioeconomic Status

The same four measures were next examined by level of education, standard of living, and marital status—common indicators of social position.

Figure 7.3 shows that the average mental health scores are better for people with higher levels of education. The differentials are relatively narrow, although they widen with age. But overall, it seems that a greater amount of education is protective against mental distress.

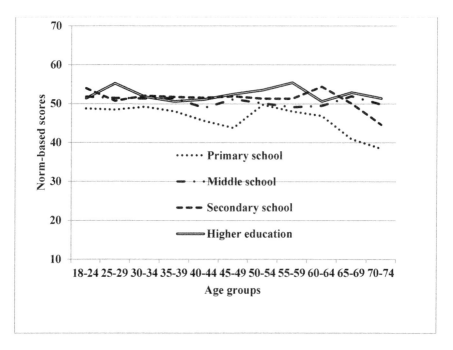

Figure 7.3. SF-36 Mental Health Scores for Accra Women by Age and Level of Education. The vertical scale runs from 100 (very good) to 0 (very poor).

For household wealth, the study used a wealth measure based on a selection of household possessions and facilities. Women living in relatively poor households had the worst mental health, across all ages (figure 7.4). The same differences are seen for individual socioeconomic characteristics in general, including work status (the formally employed had the best health, the unemployed the worst) and income. Material conditions in the household have some bearing on mental health, but crowding paradoxically appeared to be protective against mental illness.

Factors Related to Gender

The study found that marital status—particularly whether the respondent's husband had one or more additional wives—had very strong effects on mental health. Since almost all of the women in the study had at least one surviving child, it was not possible to assess the effects of childlessness on mental health.

Assessing Conditions' Severity

One of the more difficult aspects of mental health assessment is distinguishing between conditions that require treatment and could even be life-threatening

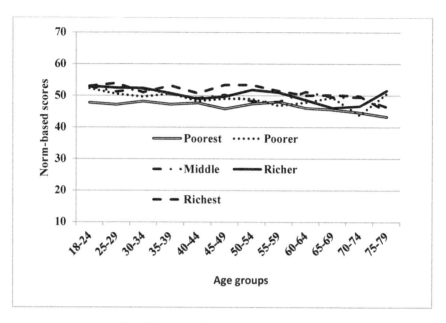

Figure 7.4. SF-36 Mental Health Scores for Accra Women by Age and Wealth
Note: The vertical scale runs from 100 (very good) to 0 (very poor).

and other conditions that may simply reflect common levels of stress in the population. Standardized scores such as those on the SF-36 scales are of little help in this regard, especially in the case of the Accra women, where the differences in scores were not very large. In the household interviews, women were asked about worry, anxiety, and feeling sad, low, or depressed. Very few women gave answers indicating that these feelings had reached the "severe" level (table 7.1). Taking the "moderate" and "severe" categories together however, we find that overall, 26 percent of women reported such problems, with a clear cut increase in the prevalence of sadness or depression with age. This increase in the prevalence of such mental health disorders with age is, however, much less steep than the increase in physical ill-health—a finding common to all of the populations surveyed with the SF-36 around the world.

Suicidality

Overall, just 1.5 percent of the women in the study reported having had suicidal thoughts in the last month. Interestingly, the pattern by age on this variable, as on other variables relating to severe mental health conditions, was U-shaped, being quite high among women younger than twenty-five, then falling slightly and

Table 7.1. Proportions of Women by Age Group Reporting Feeling Sad, Low, or Depressed in the Previous 30 Days

| SURVEY AGE GROUPS | | PROBLEM WITH FEELING SAD, LOW, OR DEPRESSED | | | | | |
		NONE	MILD	MODERATE	SEVERE	CANNOT DO ANYTHING	TOTAL
18–24	Number	507	222	93	21	0	843
	% of age group	60.1	26.3	11.0	2.5	0.0	100.0
25–34	Number	445	219	109	41	1	815
	% of age group	54.6	26.9	13.4	5.0	0.1	100.0
35–54	Number	416	221	108	41	0	786
	% of age group	52.9	28.1	13.7	5.2	0.0	100.0
55+	Number	299	237	138	51	0	725
	% of age group	41.2	32.7	19.0	7.0	0.0	100.0
Total	Number	1,667	899	448	154	1	3,169
	% all groups	52.6	28.4	14.1	4.9	0.0	100.0

rising again at higher ages. In the interviews, many more young women reported severe depression and occasionally suicidal thoughts. With high unemployment and under-employment in the younger age groups, it seems that graduating from school and not finding work or beginning a family has a depressing effect on young women in the city.

INTERPRETING THESE RESULTS

A significant portion of the women in the study exhibited symptoms of mental distress and of anxiety or depression. A salient finding is that mental distress is a heavier burden among older women in Accra than among younger women. The reason for this negative response to aging is not clear from the data. There are, however, indications that mental distress is correlated with polygynous marriage and a wife's status in such a marriage. This finding is corroborated by an earlier study of depression among 131 women in Accra who were seeking care for the first time at the University of Ghana Medical School psychiatric clinic (Turkson and Dua 1996). The earlier study noted an association between marriage and depression among these women, who typically sought treatment for the first time between the ages of thirty and forty. Although polygyny is less common in Accra than in rural areas of Ghana, its effects on the Accra women indicate that, as elsewhere, women's mental health is markedly affected by the threat of divorce or of relegation to a secondary role by the arrival of another wife.

A recent situational analysis of mental health in Ghana (Doku et al. 2008) further supports the explanation that women's inferior status in marital relationships causes considerable mental distress among women in Ghana. One of the study respondents quoted in the review, a district health worker from Kintampo District, noted,

> Our traditional way of marrying . . . sometimes, you marry about three women and then you may neglect the other one, then she will start thinking. . . . Or she is the only wife, but the husband may not pay good attention and may be moving with other women. And that may lead to mental illness, because a majority of the cases come from this point. (Doku et al. 2008, 147)

A police officer from Kintampo offered a similar explanation:

> For men, . . . you see, [the problem] is the marijuana. . . . But normal mental illness is the [problem for] women. They don't normally take drug, but many of them are in [with] the psychiatrist, immediately you fail them small [receive small set-backs], then they become dejected. (ibid., 148)

Another reason for poorer mental health among older women in Accra may be health problems related to aging. This is particularly clear in a comparison of Accra and US women. The life expectancy of a sixty-five-year-old woman in Ghana in 2011 was estimated to be 14.9 years, slightly higher for women in Accra, whereas the life expectancy of a sixty-five-year-old woman in the United States for the same years was estimated to be 24.2 years (World Health Organization 2013).

Equally important to the physical health and expectations of these women is the role they can occupy in society. In the course of the interviews, several older women remarked that they felt marginalized and no longer engaged in the family's daily affairs. One woman even reported that she was "just waiting to die." We speculate that the dramatic drop in fertility to near replacement levels in Accra may have decreased the importance of grandmothering (Douptcheva and Hill 2011, 60).

The younger women who reported mental distress explained, during unstructured portions of the interview, that unemployment and lack of job prospects—despite good levels of education—made them feel unwanted and discouraged about their prospects. In addition, symptoms of depression and anxiety in younger women may also relate to the fertility transition. Since the age at marriage and at first birth is now quite high in Ghana, 23 years for women in Accra in 2000, there is a much longer gap between the end of schooling and the beginning of family life (Ghana Statistical Service [GSS], Ghana Health Service [GHS], and ICF Macro 2009). In the past, marital life probably established a women's role in society at an earlier age than today, thus potentially increasing some younger women's feelings of not having a place in society.

Although it is possible to analyze with some accuracy the differences in mental distress across subsets of the study population, it is more challenging to compare the overall burden of mental distress between populations in Ghana and those in other countries. One reason for this is that the Ghanaian women may be generally underreporting their symptoms, possibly because of stigma associated with emotional complaints or limited awareness of mental conditions other than psychosis. In general, increased awareness of a condition translates into higher reported prevalence of it. A good example comes from The Gambia, where asking about cases of epilepsy in the context of a survey about non-communicable diseases led to the uncovering of a range of other mental health conditions (Coleman, Loppy, and Walraven 2002; Van der Sande et al. 1997).

CONCLUSIONS

This study demonstrates that community-based enquiries about mental health in Africa are feasible and worthwhile, with respondents able to provide consistent and interpretable answers to questions developed in very different contexts. This is important for future comparative work as well as for intervention studies, in which it is important to be able to measure changes between rounds. In Accra, repeat interviews with the majority of the women interviewed in 2003 have already been completed and future analyses will report on the reliability of the reports across the rounds.

The study also shows that mental distress constituted a considerable health burden among a community sample of women in urban Ghana. Levels of mental distress were found to be markedly higher among older women, suggesting the possible marginalization of these women in their various social roles, including as wives and grandmothers. In addition, it should be noted that many of the socioeconomic gradients seen elsewhere are present in Accra. Thus, people who are less wealthy or less well educated, as well as those who are unemployed or in difficult domestic circumstances, display higher levels of psychological stress and mental health problems than their more fortunate peers. To address this burden, these morbidities have to attract the attention of both the community and the government. There are new opportunities to deal with such issues, since mental health care in the community has been promoted by a Mental Health Act passed in 2012 (Doku, Wusu-Takyi, and Awakame 2012).

Finally, this study shows that standard instruments developed elsewhere—in particular, SF-36—can be used to detect patterns and differences in mental illness across various groups in Ghana. This was demonstrated by the consistency of responses across different indicators, languages, and ethnic groups. Thus, health researchers should not dismiss inquiries into mental health for fear that symptoms will differ too much across cultures. It is possible to meaningfully translate these concepts into the local idiom and thereby shed light onto emotional questions that would otherwise remain in the dark.

NOTE

The Women's Health Study of Accra 2003 was directed by Allan G. Hill and Rosemary B. Duda, both from Harvard University, with co-directors John K. Anarfi, Richard Adanu, Rudolph Darko, and Joseph Seffah, all from the University of Ghana. Funding was provided by WHO/Geneva, USAID/Ghana, the Fulbright New Century Scholars Program, and the Harvard School of Public Health. All tables are derived from the Women's Health Study of Accra, Wave I, 2003.

REFERENCES

American Psychiatric Association. 1980. *Diagnostic and Statistical Manual of Mental Disorders.* Third edition. Arlington, VA: American Psychiatric Association.

———. 1994. *Diagnostic and Statistical Manual of Mental Disorders.* Fourth edition. Arlington, VA: American Psychiatric Association.

Coleman, R., L. Loppy, and G. Walraven. 2002. "The Treatment Gap and Primary Health Care for People with Epilepsy in Rural Gambia." *Bulletin of the World Health Organization* 80 (5): 378–83.

Coleman, R., L. Morison, K. Paine, R. A. Powell, and G. Walraven. 2006. "Women's Reproductive Health and Depression: A Community Survey in the Gambia, West Africa." *Social Psychiatry and Psychiatric Epidemiology* 41 (9): 720–27.

de Menil, V., A. Osei, N. Douptcheva, A. G. Hill, P. Yaro, and A. de-Graft Aikins. 2012. "Symptoms of Common Mental Disorders and Their Correlates among Women in Accra, Ghana: A Population-Based Survey." *Ghana Medical Journal* 46 (2): 95–103.

Doku V., A. Ofori-Atta, B. Akpalu, U. Read, A. Osei, K. Ae-Ngibise, et al. 2008. *Phase 1. Country Report: A Situational Analysis of the Mental Health System in Ghana.* Cape Town, South Africa: Mental Health and Poverty Project 2008.

Doku, V., A. Wusu-Takyi, and J. Awakame. 2012. "Implementing the Mental Health Act in Ghana: Any Challenges Ahead?" *Ghana Medical Journal* 46 (4): 241–50.

Douptcheva, N., and A. G. Hill. 2011. "Final Report on the Women's Health Study of Accra, Wave II conducted in 2008–2009." In *Technical Publication No. 91.* Accra, Ghana: The Institute of Statistics, Social and Economic Research (ISSER) of University of Ghana.

Dowrick, C. F., J. A. Bellon, and M. J. Gomez. 2000. "GP Frequent Attendance in Liverpool and Granada: The Impact of Depressive Symptoms." *British Journal of General Practice* 50 (454): 361–65.

Ghana Health Service. 2005. *The Health Sector in Ghana: Facts and Figures.* Accra, Ghana.

Ghana Statistical Service (GSS), Ghana Health Service (GHS), and ICF Macro. 2009. *Ghana Demographic and Health Survey 2008.* Accra, Ghana: GSS, GHS, and ICF Macro.

Gureje, O., V. O. Lasebikan, L. Kola, and V. A. Makanjuola. 2006. "Lifetime and 12-Month Prevalence of Mental Disorders in the Nigerian Survey of Mental Health and Well-Being." *The British Journal of Psychiatry* 188 (5): 465–71.

Halabi, S., H. Zurayk, R. Awaida, M. Darwish, and B. Saab. 1992. "Reliability and Validity of Self and Proxy Reporting of Morbidity Data: A Case Study from Beirut, Lebanon." *International Journal of Epidemiology* 21 (3): 607–12.

Haro, J. M., S. Arbabzadeh-Bouchez, T. S. Brugha, G. De Girolamo, M. E. Guyer, R. Jin, J. P. Lepine, F. Mazzi, B. Reneses, and G. Vilagut. 2006. "Concordance of the Composite International Diagnostic Interview Version 3.0 (CIDI 3.0) with standardized clinical assessments in the WHO World Mental Health surveys." *International Journal of Methods in Psychiatric Research* 15 (4):167–80.

Hill, A., R. Darko, J. Seffah, R. Adanu, J. Anarfi, and R. Duda. 2007. "Health of Urban Ghanaian Women as Identified by the Women's Health Study of Accra." *International Journal of Gynecology & Obstetrics* 99 (2): 150–56.

Kessler, R. C., and T. B. Üstün. 2004. "The World Mental Health (WMH) Survey Initiative Version of the World Health Organization (WHO) Composite International Diagnostic Interview (CIDI)." *International Journal of Methods in Psychiatric Research* 13 (2): 93–121.

Kessler R. C. and T. B. Üstün (eds.). 2008. *The WHO Mental Health Survey: Global Perspectives on the Epidemiology of Mental Disorders.* Cambridge University Press in collaboration with the World Health Organization, Geneva.

Lawlor, D. A., C. Bedford, M. Taylor, and S. Ebrahim. 2002. "Agreement between Measured and Self-Reported Weight in Older Women. Results from the British Women's Heart and Health Study." *Age and Ageing* 31 (3): 169–74.

Louie, G. H., and M. M. Ward. 2010. "Association of Measured Physical Performance and Demographic and Health Characteristics with Self-Reported Physical Function: Implications for the Interpretation of Self-Reported Limitations." *Health and Quality of Life Outcomes* 8 (84): 1–13.

Murray, J., and P. Williams. 1986. "Self-Reported Illness and General Practice Consultations in Asian-Born and British-Born Residents of West London." *Social Psychiatry* 21 (3): 139–45.

Ofori-Atta, A., S. Cooper, B. Akpalu, A. Osei, V. Doku, C. Lund, A. Flisher, and the Mhapp Research Programme Consortium. 2010. "Common understandings of women's mental illness in Ghana: results from a qualitative study. "*International Review of Psychiatry* 22 (6): 589–98.

Osei, A. 2003. "Prevalence of Psychiatric Illness in an Urban Community in Ghana." *Ghana Medical Journal* 37 (2): 62–67.

Ploubidis, G. B., and E. Grundy. 2011. "Health Measurement in Population Surveys: Combining Information from Self-Reported and Observer-Measured Health Indicators." *Demography* 48 (2): 699–724.

Robins, L. N., J. E. Helzer, J. Croughan, and K. S. Ratcliff. 1981. "National Institute of Mental Health Diagnostic Interview Schedule: Its History, Characteristics, and Validity." *Archives of General Psychiatry* 38 (4): 381–89.

Salomon, J. A., A. Tandon, and C. J. L. Murray. 2004. "Comparability of Self Rated Health: Cross Sectional Multi-Country Survey Using Anchoring Vignettes." *British Medical Journal* 328 (7434): 258–64.

Turkson, S., and A. Dua. 1996. "A Study of the Social and Clinical Characteristics of Depressive Illness among Ghanaian Women (1988–1992)." *West African Journal of Medicine* 15 (2): 85.

UK Department for International Development. 2005. "The Mental Health and Poverty Project: Mental Health Policy Development and Implementation in Four African Countries." See http://r4d.dfid.gov.uk/Project/50165/.

Üstün, T. B., S. Chatterji, N. Kostanjsek, J. Rehm, C. Kennedy, J. Epping-Jordan, S. Saxena, M. von Korff, and C. Pull. 2010. "Developing the World Health Organization Disability Assessment Schedule 2.0." *Bulletin of the World Health Organization* 88 (11): 815–23.

Van der Sande, M. A., R. Bailey, H. Faal, W. A. S. Banya, P. Dolin, O. A. Nyan, S. M. Ceesay, et al. 1997. "Nationwide Prevalence Study of Hypertension and Related Non-Communicable Diseases in the Gambia." *Tropical Medicine and International Health* 2 (11): 1039–48.

Van Os, J., and S. Kapur. 2009. "Schizophrenia." *Lancet* 374 (9690): 635–45.

Walraven, G., C. Scherf, B. West, G. Ekpo, K. Paine, R. Coleman, R. Bailey, and L. Morison. 2001. "The Burden of Reproductive-Organ Disease in Rural Women in the Gambia, West Africa." *Lancet* 357 (9263): 1161–67.

Ware, J. E., K. K. Snow, M. Kosinski, B. Gandek, and New England Medical Center Hospital Health Institute. 1993. *SF-36 Health Survey: Manual and Interpretation Guide.* Boston: The Health Institute New England Medical Center.

Wittchen, Hans-Ulrich. "Screening for Serious Mental Illness: Methodological Studies of the K6 Screening Scale." *International Journal of Methods in Psychiatric Research* 19, no. S1 (2010): 1–3.

World Health Organization. 2003. World Health Survey 2003 Country Reports. http://apps.who.int/healthinfo/systems/surveydata/index.php/catalog/whs.

———. 2005. "Report of Ghana. World Health Survey—Sage Wave 0—2003." In *World Health Survey Country Reports.* Geneva: WHO.

———. 2010. International Classification of Diseases (ICD): ICD-10. http://www.who.int/classifications/icd/ICD10Volume2_en_2010.pdf?ua=1.

———. 2013. WHO Global Health Observatory Data Repository http://apps.who.int/gho/data/node.main.688?lang=en.

——— n. d. SAGE Longitudinal Multi-Country Study. http://www.who.int/healthinfo/sage/cohorts/en/. Accessed on August 21, 2013.

Younis, N., H. Khattab, H. Zurayk, M. el-Mouelhy, M. F. Amin, and A. M. Farag. 1993. "A Community Study of Gynecological and Related Morbidities in Rural Egypt." *Studies in Family Planning* 24 (3): 175–86.

Zurayk, H., H. Khattab, N. Younis, O. Kamal, and M. El-Helw. 1995. "Comparing Women's Reports with Medical Diagnoses of Reproductive Morbidity Conditions in Rural Egypt." *Studies in Family Planning* 26 (1): 14–21.

Zurayk, H. C., and J. K. Harfouche. 1970. "Family Health and Population Profile in a Peri-Urban Setting." [In English]. *Le Journal médical libanais.* 23 (3): 287–304.

Zurayk, H., C. Myntti, M. T. Salem, A. Kaddour, F. El-Kak, and S. Jabbour. 2007. "Beyond Reproductive Health: Listening to Women about Their Health in Disadvantaged Beirut Neighborhoods." *Health Care for Women International* 28 (7): 614–37.

8 ONE THING LEADS TO ANOTHER

Sex, AIDS, and Mental Health Reform
in South Africa

PAMELA Y. COLLINS

SOUTH AFRICA, LIKE many other African countries, struggled with the reality of limited mental health resources as it entered the era of democracy. Under these circumstances, how did the mental health system address the specter of a growing AIDS epidemic? The development of public mental health policy and interventions is not always a linear process. Often, a chance collision of epidemiology (a devastating AIDS epidemic), politics (a society in transition to democracy), policies (changing health priorities), and people with overlapping interests catalyzes events and spurs systemic change. This chapter describes a series of HIV and mental health service research and policy activities that helped make the needs of people with mental illness more visible in the South African AIDS epidemic.

DEINSTITUTIONALIZATION

In 1998 in a small town in the Eastern Cape that was surrounded by rolling green hills dotted with thatch-roofed *rondavels,* a middle-aged black woman, her face made up with *umcako* (a white paste made from lime), captured the attention of a group of European and North and South American mental health service providers. The woman, a traditional healer, explained to the group how she had instituted a training program for healers, many of whom were young people with symptoms of mental illness. Of particular interest to the group was her explanation of how she distinguished between people with serious, persistent psychotic disorders (who needed to be evaluated and treated in the local hospital) and those whose symptoms could qualify them for apprenticeship as a traditional healer. She described an integrated approach to care: treatment in the formal mental health system accompanied by the rehabilitation and purification services she provided. A number of her students stood by, features obscured beneath their white make-up, listening to her and gazing at the group of foreigners. The leader of the group of Western mental health professionals, Melvyn Freeman, then head of South Africa's National Directorate of Mental Health and Substance Abuse, explained the mission of his project: to explore how people might be discharged from the psychiatric hospital and cared for in the local community. The project marked another step on the path to mental health reform.

SOUTH AFRICA'S MENTAL HEALTH SYSTEM

More than a century before these events, mental health reformers in the Cape Colony (by then a semiautonomous British colony) began to shape the structure and values of South African mental health services (Swartz 1999). Psychiatric services replicated the British system, and although reforms improved the general conditions in the asylum, differential treatment based on race and social class was normative. From 1891 to 1910, the number of people treated in psychiatric asylums grew dramatically. By 1910, when the Union of South Africa was established, eight mental institutions were providing care for more than 3,000 patients (Emsley 2001). The number of institutions tripled during the twentieth century, but racial disparities in quality of care and access to varied forms of care persisted for decades. The majority of black South Africans in need of services received custodial care in state institutions and care provided by indigenous or traditional healers (Foster and Swartz 1997).

With the election of Nelson Mandela as president in 1994 and the transition to democracy, reform of the mental health system began in earnest. Reformers and policymakers sought to provide for all South Africans comprehensive services that included community-based care, mental health promotion, and mental illness prevention. Traditionally, public mental health services had focused on people with psychotic disorders, developmental disabilities, and epilepsy (Emsley 2001). A comprehensive mental health policy, developed in 1995, promoted a new, broader approach to services and included integrating mental health services into primary care.

Several factors affected the impact of the reforms. First, with the arrival of the democratic government, administrative restructuring led to an increase in the number of official provinces from four to nine. An uneven distribution of clinical sites (hospitals and clinics) and mental health funding across the provinces resulted. In some settings, public and private mental health services created an array of treatment options that included residential facilities for people with severe mental illness; psychoanalysis; clubhouses and day programs sponsored by nongovernmental organizations; and access to social workers, psychologists, and psychiatric nurses in public clinics. In other sites, mental health services consisted of the monthly provision of psychiatric medication by a nurse.

Psychiatric nurses in some primary care settings managed the maintenance care of people with severe mental illness—a result of efforts to integrate mental health care into primary care (Emsley 2001). Observers of the initiative pointed out its weaknesses (Petersen 2000). Nurses were not equipped to manage the trauma, violence, learning problems, or intellectual disabilities with which some community members and their families struggled, and thus—when patients arrived with relatively less severe symptoms—nurses often avoided the patients' psychosocial problems (Petersen 2004). Nurses complained of their lack of technical and emotional support, lack of time to attend to psychosocial needs, and lack of knowledge about psychological problems. Similar issues would arise when nurses and other mental health providers were confronted with the need to add HIV prevention and attention to patients' sexuality to their other tasks.

Insufficient numbers of mental health care providers further limited the impact of mental health service reforms, and the problem of inadequate staffing persists (Emsley 2001; World Health Organization 2005). Data from 2005 suggest that as many as 20 percent of psychiatrists trained in South Africa soon emigrate to work abroad (Lund et al. 2010). According the World Health Organization (2007), there were 0.28 psychiatrists, 0.32 psychologists, 7.45 psychiatric nurses, and 0.4 social workers per 100,000 people working in mental health facilities of South Africa's Department of Health in 2005. At the time of that study, 56 percent of psychiatrists in South Africa were working in private practice and providing services to 20 percent of the population. Only 11 percent were able to communicate fluently in one or more African languages. Perhaps as a result, psychopharmacology remains the predominant form of treatment in the public sector, and psychiatric hospitals remain the point of entry into care for many (Emsley 2001; Lund et al. 2010).

AIDS AND THE NEW SOUTH AFRICA

The encounter with the traditional healer described above occurred during the national mental health program's pilot project of deinstitutionalization. As the National Directorate of Mental Health and Substance Abuse and its consultants considered alternatives to hospital-based care, they discussed the implications of discharging patients from long-term hospitalizations into a vastly changed society. Some of the patients had been in institutions for a decade or more, and many had no relatives living in the surrounding community. Although deinstitutionalized men and women with severe mental illness would reap the benefits of the new South African democracy, they would also face the threat of HIV infection.

Studies in North America and Europe had shown for many years that in settings of low HIV prevalence among the general population, the prevalence of HIV infection among people with psychiatric disorders was disproportionately high (Kalichman et al. 1994; McKinnon et al. 1996; Meade and Sikkema 2005; Otto-Salaj et al. 1998; Rosenberg et al. 2001). Investigators linked this to factors such as having multiple sexual partners, not using condoms consistently, substance abuse, exchanging sex for money or other goods, and having impaired judgment as a secondary psychiatric symptom. People with severe mental illness in the United States also wrestled with poverty, the effects of gender inequality, and social marginalization, all of which were known to contribute to HIV risk (Farmer 1996).

The North American experience raised questions for the South African setting. In 1998 South Africa faced one of the fastest growing HIV epidemics in the world. The HIV prevalence among women attending antenatal clinics was 23 percent, a 34 percent increase over 1997 figures (Republic of South Africa Department of Health 2000). By 2005 the prevalence among women attending antenatal clinics had risen to 30 percent (Republic of South Africa Department of Health 2006). An estimated 5.6 million South Africans were living with HIV in 2009, and the epidemic in the country remains the largest in the world (Republic of South Africa 2010). Did the prevalence among people with mental illness reflect the epidemic in the general population? Mental health care providers held differing views. Some believed that the most severely ill patients were too withdrawn to engage in sexual activity (Collins 2001). Others suspected that the stigma of mental illness might lead to persistent rejection, thereby protecting them from infection (Collins 2006). Still other providers suspected that uncontrolled psychiatric symptoms and a high rate of rape and coerced sex placed women with mental illness, in particular, at great risk of infection. Did existing policies affect how HIV could be dealt with in psychiatric settings? How should HIV prevention and care be incorporated into the movement toward greater community-based mental health services?

The attitudes and knowledge of mental health care providers would play an important role in the success of HIV prevention activities for people with mental illness. North American studies showed that lack of knowledge, stigmatizing ideas, and institutional barriers limited providers' ability to respond to HIV prevention needs in psychiatric settings (Herman et al. 1994; Wright and Martin 2003). Providers often struggled with ethical and moral questions related to the sexual activity that occurred in hospitals. Should sexual activity be permitted in a hospital? Were clinical staff members responsible for protecting inpatients from HIV infection (Thom 2003)? These questions catalyzed a series of research and policy activities in South Africa that sought to reduce HIV risk among people with severe mental illness and address the mental health needs of people living with HIV.

SEX AND MENTAL HEALTH SERVICES

AIDS prevention requires frank discussion of sexuality. A South African clinician once said to me: "Mental health and sexuality are two things that you don't talk about. We've come from a society where those are taboos. Things have been so controlled." Historically, mental health policy facilitated avoidance of this discussion, but it did attempt to address certain aspects of sexual behavior in institutional settings. The Cape Colony mental health acts of 1891 and 1897 made it an offense for a male person to have custody of female patients (Swartz 1999). The Mental Health Act 1973—which remained effect into the late 1990s—was reminiscent of these earlier laws, declaring that "any person who has carnal intercourse with a female who is detained under the provision of this Act or who is under care of control as a mentally ill person shall be guilty of an offence." The act also stated that "the consent of the female shall not be a defence to any such charge."

Under this act, therefore, a female patient could not give consent to sexual activity. This sole reference to sexual behavior in the act criminalized sexual activity, ignored sex between men, and emphasized the protection of women (Collins 2001). Because sex was treated as a punishable offense, clinicians believed that they could be implicated in any actions that acknowledged, or could be construed as condoning, sex in their institution. Of relevance to the AIDS epidemic, an attempt to make condoms available to patients could be interpreted as a violation of the act.

In 1996 a national forum on mental health policy in South Africa specifically considered policies related to the management of HIV infection in psychiatric hospitals (Lindegger and Crewe 1997). Participants in the forum discussed the dilemma of protecting HIV-positive people from segregation in the institutions and protecting HIV-negative patients from infection. Implicit in these discussions was the recognition that sexual activity occurred in hospitals. These issues presented important challenges to the management of HIV infection in psychiatric hospitals, but they remained unresolved.

The passsage of a new act—the Mental Health Care Act (Act 17 of 2002)—helped remove barriers to HIV prevention. The new act minimizes the language of restriction and recognizes that sexuality is part of the lives of people in the mental health care system. It grants people in institutions the right to consensual intimate relationships: "Subject to conditions applicable to providing care, treatment and *rehabilitation* services in *health establishments,* the *head of the health establishment* may limit intimate adult relationships of adult mental health care users only if due to mental illness, the ability of the user to consent is diminished." The new language on sexuality emerged from meetings with some of the foreign consultants on the deinstitutionalization pilot project in 1998. The rapid acceptance and inclusion of the language into the new act reflected the progressive attitudes of the National Directorate of Mental Health and Substance Abuse and policymakers in the new democracy. It also revealed the influences of international mental health consultants, who had witnessed the devastation of the AIDS epidemic in the 1980s and early 1990s in urban U.S. settings.

DARING TO TALK ABOUT SEX IN PSYCHIATRIC HOSPITALS

A series of studies in South African psychiatric treatment settings systematically explored the influence of state and hospital policies and provider attitudes on institutional HIV prevention practices. Esther Moors (2000) assessed HIV prevention policies and practices at six psychiatric hospitals in the Western Cape. Through group discussions and individual interviews with 152 nurses, she identified practices that impeded HIV prevention among staff and patients: many nurses did not adhere to universal precautions; condoms were not consistently available in the institutions; and nurses often lacked adequate training on HIV transmission and how to address patients' sexual activity. More than one-third of participants believed that developmentally disabled people were sexually active; however, facilities that served this population offered the least HIV-related information of the institutions studied.

My colleagues and I conducted two studies that helped underscore the need for HIV prevention activities in psychiatric settings (Collins 2001 and 2006; Collins et al. 2006). In the first study, qualitative interviews identified providers' perceived barriers to HIV prevention among people with mental illness (Collins 2001 and 2006). The second study developed and tested the efficacy of an HIV education intervention for providers at two psychiatric institutions. Providers participating in the first study almost unanimously agreed that health care professionals outside of the mental health system were not likely to address the needs of people with psychiatric illness. They attributed this to the social stigma associated with mental illness. In the mental health system, psychiatric symptoms, transitions in the health care system, and cultural ideas about sex formed interlocking barriers to prevention activities (Collins 2006).

Barriers to HIV Prevention

Many providers expressed doubt about the possibility of communicating HIV prevention messages to psychiatric patients in a manner that they could understand and act on. They noted that their patients' poor levels of education, combined with symptoms like delusional beliefs, presented a barrier to comprehension. One nurse explained: "The person had misconceptions before mental illness. It gets worse. He will attach delusions to the whole concept, which makes it worse. They do pass their ideas to each other, so it spreads."[1]

Experiences with this population led a small number of providers to believe that the repetition of prevention messages along with focused skills building could reduce risky sexual behavior. But most feared patients would simply misuse condoms if they were distributed widely. As a result, many clinicians gave condoms or HIV-related information only to specific patients known to have a sexually transmitted infection or known to be sexually active.

Providers' skepticism probably reflected the dynamics of the mental health system. Clinicians in most public psychiatric hospitals tended to treat very ill patients, since alternatives to hospitalization were often scarce, except in provinces with more resources. Some of these providers found it difficult to envision interventions that could successfully alter the behavior of people with chronic mental illness. Furthermore, shortages in staff and the demands of patient care overwhelmed and stretched the resources of these institutions, leading providers to question whether HIV should really be a priority in mental health service settings.

The disorder inherent in the reorganization of health services after 1994 left many providers feeling skeptical about the integration of HIV prevention activities into mental health services. Efforts at HIV education followed the more urgent tasks of managing psychiatric symptoms, discharge planning, meeting with families to educate and support them, and assisting patients in getting a disability grant, a monthly income benefit provided by the South African government for people with disabilities who meet income and health qualifications. These concerns required providers' full-time attention. "We're all so busy trying to keep them in balance and trying to solve relationship problems in the family," commented one nurse.

The legislation of sexual inclusiveness and tolerance in the country's new constitution and mental health act forced a reorganization of ideas about sex, and some providers struggled with the implications. They emphasized that South Africans typically had conservative attitudes toward sex and that secrecy about sexuality was normative. Although the majority of providers said that they were comfortable talking about sex with patients, some felt ill-equipped to initiate these conversations. Cultural taboos in various ethnic groups challenged providers. A black nurse said of one ethnic group: "According to Shangaan culture, they won't talk much about sex. They don't feel comfortable. Vocabulary is restricted. They don't use these words." Having such a conversation with a person of a different gender or race added another layer of complexity. One white provider spoke of her anxieties about discussing sex with black patients: "I think [there is] suspicion in the sense that some of the black patients who are less educated think, 'now this white doctor is trying to tell me to stop sleeping around.' Suspicion in terms of, 'should I buy what they're telling me?' They might think you're trying to impose your culture on them."

Providers were faced with caring for people whom they often believed to be at risk for HIV infection, managing the stresses of demanding patient loads with few resources, and learning to work in a system with increasingly liberal ideas about sexuality. The HIV/AIDS epidemic demanded that they confront these issues, and the new, liberal legislation removed policy barriers that could inhibit action—yet the legislation outpaced the readiness of many providers to institute change.

How did these cultural barriers to addressing HIV prevention operate in practice? The following two examples, experiences of a primary care nurse in a community clinic and HIV training activities in a general hospital's psychiatric unit, illustrate these challenges.

Tackling HIV and Mental Health in a Community Clinic

Two psychiatric nurses worked in this public clinic, which served a large urban area that included a number of poor Afrikaans and colored communities. Some of the patients were residents of black communities who preferred to travel to this clinic where they could receive psychiatric care without being observed by friends and neighbors.

One nurse, Alice (not her real name), a young Indian woman, described her attraction to the mental health field.[2] She explained: "The treatment is individual. Patients are very individual. You can be you. What you see is what you get. They're easy to communicate with. You can be yourself."

Alice reported that the clinic had received more patients since the 1994 democratic elections. She attributed this to adjustments that people were having to make to the new South Africa: "I think there's a lot of stress. Taking back what they have . . . I think a lot of people have problems coming to grips. They're used to having everything done for them. They can't cope. Not just the whites." She believed this stress had been worse for people with mental illness and was compounded by stigma and related joblessness.

Ethnic differences between the nurses and the patients complicated the interactions at the clinic. Alice explained: "We work with an Afrikaans community. It's an adjustment for them to have us here. You know the thoughts are still very ancient. It's something people have grown up with. I have a lady who refuses to come to clinic because she doesn't want to see the 'coolie' doctor. I hope she doesn't mind the 'coolie' nurse." The clinic experienced frequent staff turnover that also limited the depth of relationships between providers and patients.

These tensions, as well as other societal constraints around discussion of sex, affected Alice's ability to provide information about HIV. She believed that most of her patients had troubled interpersonal relationships, although she rarely discussed these issues since she opted not to initiate such conversations:

> Many come from relationships that aren't very happy—short standing, on and off. They are sexually active. I think it's also the community we're involved with—you don't talk about these things unless there's abuse. . . . Perhaps it's too painful to talk about. Also, they have a problem meeting people and the little they have they want to hold on to. We do get condoms occasionally, but the box stayed full. It's not possible for us to dish them out on a one-to-one basis.

Alice was acutely aware of how the patients might respond if she were to distribute condoms: "They would think, 'What is this one thinking about?'" She believed that the clinic attendees were ashamed to pick up condoms, and that a discussion of safer sex would place a strain on her relationship with them. She described how people from various ethnic groups would respond, noting that reticence about sex was the norm: "With the Indian community it's even worse. Whites reserve who they want to tell. With blacks—you have to earn their trust. We have a lot of issues."

Yet Alice was also aware that, with respect to HIV, most of the clinic attendees have "just a superficial knowledge because they hear [about] it on TV." She added that the attendees were not "clued in to the consequences." She suspected that the patients' exposure to HIV- related information most frequently occurred in health care settings, but the information was not available at her clinic: "We do have pamphlets we give to people we think may be susceptible. But many can't read. The video machines [that could provide the information] got stolen."

In addition to the lack of information, larger problems in the lives of the men and women who attended the clinic made protecting them from HIV difficult. Alice believed the biggest barrier to HIV prevention was "social circumstances." She explained: "We can give wonderful talks, but they go home where there's nothing. You know, their basic biological needs are not met. You can't talk to them about fancy stuff. They're hungry when they come to the clinic. Their self-esteem is in their shoes. They feel worthless. They can't worry about infection. They have nothing to lose."

Staff Concerns in a General Hospital's Psychiatric Unit

Team A served a large public general hospital.[3] The psychiatric section was divided into admission, short-term rehabilitation, long-term rehabilitation, security, and geriatric wards. The team admitted patients with acute and chronic mental illness. The length of hospitalizations ranged from one month to several years.

During a five-day needs-assessment and training workshop on HIV prevention and care, a multidisciplinary group of seventeen providers practiced role-playing activities, engaged in debate, and—at the end of the workshop—practiced teaching men and women on the wards about HIV. The members of Team A spoke openly about their reservations and their hopes of providing HIV prevention activities in the hospital. Four issues in particular prompted lively discussion among the participants that increased providers' levels of confidence and commitment to addressing HIV: beliefs about sexual morality, beliefs about the use of traditional medicines in managing AIDS, concerns about confidentiality, and the personal burden of the AIDS epidemic.

Despite the shared perception that some men and women were at risk of being infected with HIV in the hospital (due to unprotected sex), the prospect of making condoms available conflicted with the religious beliefs of several group participants, and many feared that making condoms available would make it seem that they condoned sexual relationships on the wards. The group debated this issue intensely. Team members with conservative religious views insisted that adherence to biblical moral law was the best way to prevent HIV infection. Other providers wrestled with their moral responsibility to the spouses of patients, and they wondered how these relatives would respond if they knew that condoms had been made available in the hospital. Others asserted that the duty to provide a means of protection from HIV infection should take precedence over religious beliefs that might not be shared by all. The diversity of viewpoints on this single issue made consensus around action difficult.

Another contentious issue—providers' mixed views about the efficacy of traditional African remedies for AIDS—affected their ability to provide clear information about HIV prevention and treatment to patients. A number of providers felt strongly that traditional African medicines and herbs, which were more readily available than Western medicines, might be able to treat—if not cure—AIDS. Many felt that the traditional healers who provided these interventions should be integrated into HIV prevention programs because of their popularity in the larger society and the frequency with which many people sought their help. Providers' uncertainties about these issues were apparent as they listened to patients on the wards say they had used African potatoes and other local remedies to treat HIV infection. Mental health care providers who expressed their beliefs in the efficacy of traditional medicines sometimes seemed unsure of how to use biomedical information to respond to patients' questions about HIV and AIDS. These beliefs probably affected both providers' and patients' perceptions of the risk of HIV infection and its long-term consequences.

The confusion about treatment options was understandable in one sense. The community around the hospital had little if any access to antiretroviral drugs in 2000, when the training occurred. By the end of 2005, although the rate of highly active antiretroviral therapy treatment had risen dramatically, it was still being given to only a minority of people who needed treatment (Nattrass 2006). And only an estimated 55 percent of those who needed antiretroviral therapy in South Africa were receiving it in 2010 (World Health Organization 2011). All of the providers were familiar with the outcome of failed prevention and care: HIV infection, AIDS, and death. The burden of HIV on the families of patients worried providers. Moreover, they needed to manage their own anxieties about ill friends and relatives. Members of Team A expressed frustration about the absence of treatment for HIV-infected people. The workshop presenters provided information on the use of medications for prophylaxis of opportunistic infections and emphasized the role that these could play in keeping people with HIV-related disease or AIDS healthy in the absence of antiretroviral therapy.

Throughout the workshop, the discussion consistently returned to the issue of patients' needs for (or rights to) protection from HIV while in the hospital and the duty of the providers to ensure patients' safety. What were the boundaries of the provider's duties? Some providers felt that disclosing to family members that a psychiatric patient was HIV positive would help ensure the patient's well-being. Others wanted to disclose the information to the patient's known sexual partners in the hospital. They interpreted confidentiality requirements as a hindrance to the proper care of HIV-infected patients and to prevention activities. Team A members wondered how to protect themselves from lawsuits by families who might suspect that a relative had become infected with HIV in the hospital.

FOCUSING ON PSYCHIATRIC HOSPITALS

These exploratory studies demonstrated that attitudinal, cultural, and systemic barriers to introducing HIV prevention into psychiatric services were similar across a variety of treatment settings. Both providers and trainers had to tackle the complexities of sociocultural ideas about sexuality and HIV/AIDS. As clinicians grappled with the challenges of HIV infection that faced patients, families, and other relatives—and sometimes with the challenges involved in their own infection—they needed the opportunity to voice their anxieties, reservations, and personal beliefs. They needed information about HIV transmission and care that would take into account local views of the illness and locally available resources for treatment. Staff members in some settings, like hospital inpatient units, could be responsible for preventing behaviors that increased HIV risk from occurring in their sites and for equipping people with mental illness to live safely after being discharged. Preliminary findings from these studies and training experiences were presented to the provincial mental health directors and the National Directorate of Mental Health and Substance Abuse. The directorate mobilized support for HIV-related training and research activities in hospital settings.

As a consequence of the expansion of community mental health services, psychiatric hospitals faced an important dynamic that had implications for their role in the AIDS epidemic. The growth in community treatment coincided with a reduction in the duration of hospitalizations. The average length of admissions fell from more than one month to four or fewer weeks. In theory, this rapid turnover of patients increasingly exposed them to HIV infection through sexual transmission in the institutions. It was well known that sexual activity occurred in psychiatric institutions. The staff members of the directorate reasoned that if psychiatric patients could be exposed to HIV prevention interventions before being discharged from an institution, they would receive crucial information that they were unlikely to receive in other health care settings (personal communication from Melvyn Freeman, mental health consultant, August 2007).

TRAINING MENTAL HEALTH CARE PROVIDERS

Armed with substantial data on the challenges facing providers, my colleagues and I formed a collaboration with staff members of the National Directorate of Mental Health and Substance Abuse, a South African research team, and a group of administrators and clinicians from three psychiatric hospitals. The group aimed to develop and test training materials for mental health care providers working in three public mental health facilities in one province (Collins et al. 2006). The research team studied a setting in which HIV infection was prevalent among staff members, deaths were increasing, and funerals were frequent. The risk of shame and social exclusion associated with HIV infection prevented open discussion of AIDS and its impact on the hospitals.

The team worked with small core groups of providers at each facility. These providers identified a range of issues that required attention: integrating HIV prevention into their daily work routine, developing policies on sexual behavior, managing violent patients and their HIV risk, addressing the hospital's liability for HIV infections among patients, managing sex in the institution, addressing the stigma of mental illness and HIV, and addressing staff needs for HIV support and treatment.

A nine-session curriculum, designed to impart relevant information about HIV and to introduce skills for communicating with patients, emerged (Collins et al. 2006). The first session, "What is the situation?," presented local HIV prevalence data and reviewed the basics of HIV infection and transmission, defined terms such as "opportunistic infection" and "CD-4 cells," and explained concepts such as "viral load." Session 2, "Am I at risk?," personalized the epidemic by inviting participants to complete a personal risk assessment. That exercise was followed by a guided discussion of stigma related to HIV. Providers were encouraged to brainstorm about the reasons for stigma as well as solutions.

Session 3, "What can we do?," began to offer solutions. Two physicians from the communicable disease clinic at a local public hospital shared with providers the treatments available in the community for opportunistic infections and described what antiretroviral therapies were available. They reviewed costs of medication, eligibility for antiretroviral therapy, medical insurance plans and their coverage of antiretroviral therapy, and nutrition and diet, and showed how to refer patients to the clinic.

Session 4, "What more can we do?," addressed the need to talk about sex with inpatients to explain the institution's policy on sexual activity and to teach patients how to reduce risky sexual behavior. The session's exercises accustomed providers to using sexual terms and taught them to understand the terms used by most of their patients. In Session 5, "Talking about sex," providers demonstrated their approaches to discussing HIV with patients. Next, trainers modeled empathic interactions with patients. The group identified key messages to convey about sex and HIV and practiced delivering these messages in role-playing activities.

In Sessions 6 and 7, "Legalities 1 and 2," local human rights lawyers answered questions about confidentiality, the disclosure of psychiatric patients' HIV status, and rights to privacy and protection for staff and patients. They explained the institution's liability with respect to HIV testing and prevention and provided guidelines for developing policies for sexual activity in the institution.

Session 8, "Our daily routine," focused on integrating HIV prevention messages into the ward routine. Providers identified which wards were amenable to integrating HIV prevention activities and the kinds of activities that would be appropriate. And the final session, "Supporting our community," facilitated a discussion of staff support needs, strategies for sustaining the core group, and service provision to staff members affected by or infected with HIV.

Training workshops lasted one and a half days. An evaluation of the workshops showed that this contextually relevant HIV education curriculum significantly changed providers' attitudes and knowledge, demonstrated the feasibility of administering the training program, and provided a foundation for further prevention activities (Collins et al. 2006).

ADAPTING MANUALS

The workshops prepared providers to administer interventions, but prevention efforts at psychiatric institutions in South Africa focused primarily on education and awareness. Providers needed access to risk reduction interventions developed and tested in a South African context that could change behavior, taking into account the individual and contextual factors that mediate risk. In the next step of the project, the research team worked with the core groups to adapt for use in South Africa HIV prevention manuals that had been developed for people with severe mental illness in the United States.

The adaptation process began with a review of three U.S. manuals designed for people with severe mental illness. *Sex, Games, and Videotapes* is a sixteen-session curriculum for HIV risk reduction among homeless mentally ill men that was tested in a randomized clinical trial by Ezra Susser and colleagues (1998) and found to be effective in reducing risky sexual behaviors in that population. The curriculum emphasized rehearsal and repetition of safe sex methods and condom application, using practice condoms and plastic models, among men troubled by mental illness and substance use disorders. A second manual, *HIV Prevention for People with Severe Mental Illness,* had been used extensively by Francine Cournos and colleagues for men and women with psychiatric illness in clinical settings. The third manual, *Our Selves, Our Bodies, Our Realities,* was developed and pilot-tested by my colleagues and me for use with women with severe mental illness (Collins et al. 2001; Collins et al. 2011). These manuals addressed, explicitly or implicitly, the context of HIV risk for people with severe mental illness in the United States and used skills-building approaches appropriate for audiences with cognitive deficits. *Our Selves, Our Bodies, Our Realities* introduced the female condom, a female-initiated HIV prevention method, to women with severe mental illness and emphasized providing women with options for protection. *HIV Prevention for People with Severe Mental Illness* included sessions focused on substance abuse and HIV risk. To make HIV prevention relevant to homeless men with severe mental illness, *Sex, Games, and Videotapes* used real-life situations in which such men traded sex for money or drugs.

The research team introduced the manuals to the group, role-played the sessions with the providers, and encouraged the providers to review the sessions independently. In the three months following the training, the providers field-tested sessions from the manuals in selected wards in their hospitals. In core group meetings, providers and research team members discussed modifications for the South African setting. These changes were incorporated into a new manual. The team eliminated presentation styles or exercises deemed inappropriate for a South African audience. For example, the use of a talk-show format was a successful way to engage U.S. women with severe mental illness, but that format was unfamiliar to South African patients. South African sexual conservatism led the team to modify some of the exercises, such as those that focused explicitly on specific language for sexual acts, to suit local norms. Conversely, many of the scenarios used in role-playing exercises in the United States—such as negotiating condom use with an unwilling partner, discussing violence in relationships, and the use of illicit drugs—were quite relevant for the institutionalized population in South Africa.

The final adapted manual *Shosholoza for Health,* contained selections from each of the three original manuals and exercises developed specifically for the South African setting. Specifically, exercises guiding male participants to examine the role of violence in relationships were added. The manual ultimately targeted the patient populations served at two of the hospitals. The team provided alternate resources for use at the third hospital that were more suited to the needs of people with developmental disorders.

As noted above, the project provided an opportunity for my colleagues and me to form a collaboration with the National Directorate of Mental Health and Substance Abuse, a South African research team, and a core group of clinical care providers and administrators from each site. All of us learned several lessons.

The collaboration with the directorate, a government agency, eased the research team's entry into the psychiatric institutions and facilitated their working with staff at all levels—from ward staff members to administrators.

Building rapport and establishing trust with institution staff members required time. Some participants initially feared being "studied" and suspected they would not reap any benefits from the project. Others assumed that intervention ideas from the United States would be irrelevant and too expensive in South Africa. Delays in the release of funding ultimately worked to the researchers' advantage, because they allowed time for the development of trusting relationships with the core teams.

The investigators sought to understand and support existing AIDS programs in the institutions, and these efforts proved essential. The project built on these programs rather than discounting progress that had already been made.

The research team facilitated access to other resources in the community that could provide additional services to patients, such as the communicable disease clinic at a local hospital. Psychiatric institutions tend to be marginalized in the health care system. Establishing contact with provincial and national AIDS departments and connecting the mental health care providers to community-based AIDS organizations can help reduce the isolation of mental health services while increasing their access to resources. The team helped make the initial contacts in some cases, but strengthening the relationships between community institutions should play a larger role in HIV care and prevention in resource-constrained settings. Outsiders often have more time and energy to organize these kinds of introductions.

Continual communication among the local research team, international team, core groups, and hospital administrators stimulated changes at all levels of the institution and broadened the impact of the intervention. Senior managers established an HIV/AIDS committee. Core group leaders introduced the adapted HIV prevention manual to the wards and trained other providers in its use. The creation of sustainable structures should be an explicit outcome of the process.

Although the core groups were established to participate in the research, the groups became a valuable forum in which members could air frustrations and receive support. The members began to feel empowered as they discussed solutions to problems related to HIV and sexuality with the support of the research team. Hierarchical barriers were broken in the core groups, facilitating communication and support. Even within the group, however, barriers due to race remained. Issues related to affirmative action, racism, and political party support filtered into the dynamics of the groups. Some providers felt that their opinions and roles were not duly acknowledged, and this hampered their motivation to participate in the study and reduced their contributions. And what providers perceived as mixed messages regarding HIV/AIDS from the administration of President Thabo Mbeki also limited the motivation of some participants.

Ambivalence about sexuality in the psychiatric institutions in South Africa constituted a powerful force that stalled widespread attention to HIV/AIDS in these settings. The difficulties of dealing with sexuality in psychiatric hospitals for providers and managers will probably continue to influence implementation of HIV interventions. The presence of the research team in this case served as a stimulus for change. Situating the project as part of a process of change rather than as a single, time-limited intervention was an important approach.

SUSTAINING CHANGE AND PROGRESS

During the course of these research activities, the National Directorate of Mental Health and Substance Abuse established a task force on HIV/AIDS that developed guidelines for the management of HIV/AIDS in psychiatric institutions. The guidelines provided a resource for addressing issues of HIV testing, confidentiality, and management of HIV in psychiatric settings. Groups of providers in specific provinces carried this process further (Thom 2003; Joska, Kaliski, and Benatar 2008). During this period, pilot studies in two institutions demonstrated HIV prevalence rates of 9 percent in one state psychiatric hospital and 29 percent on the acute psychiatric admission ward at a large tertiary care hospital (Zingela et al. 2002; Singh, Berkman, and Bresnahan 2009). Since that time data from one of the study sites described above has been published, showing a 26.5 percent prevalence of HIV infection among men and women in a predischarge unit in a public psychiatric hospital (Collins et al. 2009). These findings affirmed the importance of focusing on prevention activities in the severely mentally ill population.

These studies demonstrate the importance of political, socioeconomic, cultural, and health system contexts in the development and implementation of interventions. In particular, policy, attitudinal, and structural barriers arising from any of these contexts can hinder initial development of HIV prevention interventions and limit the ability of hospital administrators and clinical staff members to sustain educational and prevention activities for people under their care. The research team's experiences suggest, first, that the close collaboration of researchers, clinicians and policymakers can accelerate institutional and policy change; and, second, that the maintenance of change, as well as the implementation of interventions, requires a sustained flow of resources and continuous advocacy.

Advocacy must be a key component of ongoing activities (Collins and Freeman 2009). One goal of such activities should be to enable the health system to sustain adequate numbers of mental health service providers. These providers require ongoing training and effective systems of supervision to implement and maintain HIV prevention and treatment activities in mental health settings across the country.

A critical missing voice in these studies is that of people using the mental health services, who are a potential resource in advocacy, mental health reform, and HIV prevention. A new network of collaboration needs to grow from these experiences—one that includes the support of the National Directorate of Mental Health and Substance Abuse, the South African National AIDS Council, mental health researchers, clinicians and administrators in clinical settings, and the people who use these services.

NOTES

Alan Berkman, Melvyn Freeman, and Kezziah Mestry provided thoughtful feedback during the preparation of this chapter. I am grateful to Sifiso Phakathi, head of the South African National Directorate of Mental Health and Substance Abuse, for his reflections. I would like to thank Emmanuel Akyeampong and the African Psychiatry Workshop at Harvard University for their support of this work. The views expressed in this chapter do not necessarily reflect the viewpoints of the National Institute of Mental Health or the US government.

1. The data in this section are presented in their entirety in Collins (2006).

2. This interview was conducted, though not previously reported in its entirety, as part of the 1998 study whose findings are published in Collins (2001 and 2006).

3. The training activities described here were conducted by the author and colleagues in collaboration with the National Directorate of Mental Health and Substance Abuse in 2000.

REFERENCES

Collins P. Y. 2001. "Dual Taboos: Sexuality and Women with Severe Mental Illness in South Africa. Perceptions of Mental Health Care Providers." AIDS and Behavior 5 (2): 151–61.
———. 2006. "Challenges to HIV Prevention in Psychiatric Settings: Perceptions of South African Mental Health Care Providers." Social Science in Medicine 63 (4): 979–90.

Collins, P. Y., A. Berkman, K. Mestry, and A. Pillai. 2009. "HIV Prevalence among Men and Women Admitted to a South African Public Psychiatric Hospital." *AIDS Care* 21 (7): 863–67.

Collins, P. Y., and M. Freeman. 2009. "Bridging the Gap between HIV and Mental Health Services in South Africa." In *HIV/AIDS in South Africa 25 Years On: Psychosocial Perspectives,* edited by P. Rohleder, L. Swartz, S. C. Kalichman, and L. C. Simbayi, 353–371. New York: Springer.

Collins, P. Y., P. A. Geller, S. Miller, P. Toro, E. Susser. 2001. "Ourselves, Our Bodies, Our Realities: An HIV Prevention Intervention for Women with Severe Mental Illness." *Journal of Urban Health* 78 (1): 162–75.

Collins, P. Y., K. Mestry, M. Wainberg, T. Nzama, G. Lindegger, et al. 2006. "Training South African mental health providers to talk about sex in the era of AIDS," *Psychiatric Services* 57 (11): 1644–47.

Collins, P. Y., H. von Unger, S. Putnins, N. Crawford, R. Dutt, and M. Hoffer. 2011. "Adding the Female Condom to HIV Prevention Interventions for Women with Severe Mental Illness: A Pilot Test." *Community Mental Health Journal* 47 (2): 143–55.

Emsley, R. 2001. "Focus on Psychiatry in South Africa." *British Journal of Psychiatry* 178: 382–86.

Farmer, P. 1996. "Women, Poverty and AIDS." In *Women, Poverty, and AIDS: Sex, Drugs, and Structural Violence,* edited by P. Farmer, M. Connors, and J. Simmons, 3–38. Monroe, ME: Common Courage.

Foster, D., and S. Swartz. 1997. "Introduction: Policy Considerations in Mental Health Policy Issues for South Africa." In *Mental Health Policy Issues for South Africa,* edited by D. Foster, M. Freeman, and Y. Pillay, 1–22. Pinelands, South Africa: Medical Association of South Africa Multimedia.

Herman, R., M. Kaplan, J. Satriano, F. Cournos, and K. McKinnon. 1994. "HIV Prevention with Persons with Serious Mental Illness: Staff Training and Institutional Attitudes." *Psychosocial Rehabilitation Journal* 17 (4): 97–104.

Joska, J. A., S. Z. Kaliski, and S. R. Benatar. 2008. "Patients with Severe Mental Illness: A New Approach to Testing for HIV." *South African Medical Journal* 98 (3): 213–17.

Kalichman, S. C., J. A. Kelly, J. R. Johnson, and M. Bulto. 1994. "Factors Associated with Risk for HIV Infection among Chronically Mentally Ill Adults." *American Journal of Psychiatry* 151 (2): 221–27.

Lindegger, G. and M. Crewe. 1997. "HIV/AIDS: Managing the Madness." In *Mental Health Policy Issues for South Africa,* edited by D. Foster, M. Freeman, and Y. Pillay. Pinelands, South Africa: Medical Association of South Africa Multimedia.

Lund, C., S. Kleintjes, R. Kakuma, A. J. Flisher, and MHaPP Research Programme Consortium. 2010. "Public Sector Mental Health Systems in South Africa: Inter-Provincial Comparisons and Policy Implications." *Social Psychiatry and Psychiatric Epidemiology* 45 (3): 393–404.

McKinnon, K., F. Cournos, R. Sugden, J. R. Guido, and R. Herman.. 1996. "The Relative Contribution of Psychiatric Symptoms and AIDS Knowledge to HIV Risk Behaviors among People with Severe Mental Illness." *Journal of Clinical Psychiatry,* 57 (11): 506–13.

Meade, C. S., and K. J. Sikkema. 2005. "HIV Risk Behavior among Adults with Severe Mental Illness: A Systematic Review." *Clinical Psychology Review* 25 (4): 433–57.

Moors, E. 2000. "An Assessment of Measures to Contain HIV/AIDS within Mental Health Facilities in the Western Cape." Unpublished report to the English National Health Service.

Nattrass, N. 2006. "South Africa's 'Rollout' of Antiretroviral Therapy: A Critical Assessment." *Journal of Acquired Immune Deficiency Syndromes* 43 (5): 618–23.

Otto-Salaj, L. L., T. G. Heckman, L. Y. Stevenson, and J. A. Kelly. 1998. "Patterns, Predictors, and Gender Differences in HIV Risk among Severely Mentally Ill Men and Women." *Community Mental Health Journal* 34 (2): 175–90.

Petersen, I. 2000. "Comprehensive Integrated Primary Mental Health Care for South Africa: Pipedream or Possibility?" *Social Science and Medicine* 51 (3): 321–34.

———. 2004. "Primary Level Psychological Services in South Africa: Can a New Psychological Professional Fill the Gap?" *Health Policy and Planning* 19 (1): 33–40.

Republic of South Africa. 2010. *Country Progress Report on the Declaration of Commitment on HIV/AIDS: 2010 Report,* Pretoria: National Department of Health.

Republic of South Africa Department of Health. 2000. *National HIV and Syphilis Sero-Prevalence Survey of Women Attending Public Antenatal Clinics in South Africa,* Pretoria: National Department of Health.

———. 2006. *National HIV and Syphilis Antenatal Sero-Prevalence Survey in South Africa, 2005,* Pretoria: National Department of Health.

Rosenberg, S. D., S. L. Trumbetta, K. T. Mueser, L. A. Goodman, F. C. Osher, R. M. Vidaver, and D. S. Metzger. 2001. "Determinants of Risk Behavior for Human Immunodeficiency Virus/Acquired Immunodeficiency Syndrome in People with Severe Mental Illness." *Comprehensive Psychiatry* 42 (4): 263–71.

Singh, D., A. Berkman, and M. Bresnahan. 2009. "Seroprevalence and HIV-Associated Factors among Adults with Severe Mental Illness—A Vulnerable Population," *South African Medical Journal* 99 (7): 523–27.

Susser, E., E. Valencia, A. Berkman, N. Sohler, S. Conover, J. Torres, P. Betne, et al. 1998. "Human Immunodeficiency Virus Sexual Risk Reduction in Homeless Men with Mental Illness." *Archives of General Psychiatry* 55 (3): 266–72.

Swartz, S. 1999. "Work of Mercy and Necessity: British Rule and Psychiatric Practice in the Cape Colony, 1891–1910." *International Journal of Mental Health* 28 (2): 72–90.

Thom, R. 2003."HIV/AIDS and Mental Illness: Ethical and Medico-Legal Issues for Psychiatric Services." *South African Psychiatry Review* 6 (3): 18–21.

World Health Organization and University of Cape Town Department of Psychiatry and Mental Health. 2007. *WHO-AIMS Report on Mental Health System in South Africa.* Geneva: World Health Organization.

———. 2011. *Global HIV/AIDS Response: Epidemic Update and Health Sector Progress towards Universal Access: Progress Report 2011.* Geneva: World Health Organization.

Wright, E. R., and T. N. Martin. 2003. "The Social Organization of HIV/AIDS Care in Treatment Programmes for Adults with Serious Mental Illness." *AIDS Care* 15 (6): 763–73.

Zingela, Z., F. Esterhuizen, C. Kruger, and L.M. Webber. 2002. "Prevalence of HIV Infection in a Group of Adult Psychiatric Inpatients in Two Wards in Weskoppies Hospital." Paper presented at 12th National Psychiatry Congress of the South African Society of Psychiatrists, Cape Town 2002.

9 HEALTH CARE PROFESSIONALS' MENTAL HEALTH AND WELL-BEING IN THE ERA OF HIV/AIDS

Perspectives from Sub-Saharan Africa

GIUSEPPE RAVIOLA

THE PHENOMENON OF the demoralization and burnout of health care professionals practicing in environments characterized by significant lack of resources and high numbers of patients with HIV/AIDS constitutes a major crisis for African medicine, its practitioners, and the patients they treat. This chapter presents a biosocial perspective on issues of medical professionalism and health care professionals' distress and demoralization, both globally and in sub-Saharan Africa. That is, it seeks to examine such issues beyond the biological and clinical spheres, taking into consideration the social, political, and economic aspects of medicine as it is practiced in global and local contexts (Walton, Farmer, and Dillingham 2011). A stream of ethnographic research spanning the past decade, supplemented by research from other African medical milieus, has examined the moral and ethical dilemmas of public medical practice in East African teaching hospitals, illustrating the complexity of factors affecting health care workers' well-being in African contexts (Good et al. 1999; Iliffe 1998 and 2006; Raviola et al. 2002).

Although significant progress has been made in delivering antiretroviral medications (ARVs) to those for whom life-saving treatment had not previously been available, it has become clear over the past decade that, for a number of reasons, formal health care infrastructures and human resources in sub-Saharan Africa have been limited in their capacity to facilitate the expansion of this effort. This tragedy has unfolded in the context of what has been described as a global crisis in medical professionalism, due in large part to the nature of health care system reform and its impact on the practice of medicine (Working Party of the Royal College of Physicians 2005). Multiple factors—including technological advances, managed care, and the corporatization of doctoring (which does not occur only in the developed world), globalization, computerization, growing access to information for patients, rising health care costs, and increasing competition across health care workers in different fields—have dramatically altered the nature of medical practice for health care professionals (McKinlay and Marceau 2002). Larger social, institutional, and disease-related forces as well as clinical challenges are also affecting health care workers' well-being and mental health. This is not only shaping how future generations of physicians will practice, but also how they will view their professional lives. For example, the effects of privatization on the practice of medicine have created challenges in instilling and maintaining in physicians an ethic of professionalism that is essential to both protecting the interests of patients and providing health care systems of reasonable quality (Blumenthal and Hsiao 2005). A growing literature from the United States and Europe has described not only a widespread erosion of patients' trust in providers but also the adverse impacts of changing working conditions on providers themselves, including trainees and nurses as well as physicians. In the West much of this analysis has focused on outcomes relating to increasing management of health care by corporate entities and increasing pressures on providers for greater efficiency and reduced costs. Following the implementation of "structural adjustment" policies, privatization has also taken hold in certain regions of Africa, with managed care also emerging there. Studies examining the situation of providers in sub-Saharan Africa have begun to appear, not only exploring the significant impact of HIV/AIDS on providers' health and morale, but also describing other factors related to resource shortages, working conditions, and local professional medical cultures.

A mental health perspective has been largely absent from discourse at the global policy level on the "brain drain" of health care providers in the region. Given the general paucity of research and intervention concerning this major crisis within a crisis, there exists an opportunity for African psychiatry to take a lead role in research and in the composition of a formal response that is not only clinical but also political and systemic, paying comprehensive attention to the multiplicity of causative factors. The aims of this chapter will be to encourage African mental health professionals to educate policymakers about the psychological impact of overwhelming everyday practice, to demonstrate the relationship of this impact to broader structural problems, and to advocate for the basic mental health and well-being of colleagues working on the front lines of the HIV/AIDS pandemic. The chapter will conclude with a call for African mental health professionals to also work toward the development of formal support services for clinicians. Together with other important policy measures, these services could be instrumental in mitigating demoralization, professional crises, and emotional and physical exhaustion among African health care providers.

GLOBAL PERSPECTIVES ON HEALTH CARE PROVIDERS' DISTRESS AND WELL-BEING

Historical Perspectives

The terms "health care professional," "health care provider," "health care worker," and "formal caregiver" will be used interchangeably in this chapter. They all include health professionals, behavioral health specialists, and social workers who are trained and compensated for their caregiving activities (O'Neill and McKinney 2003). Informal caregivers—including relatives, spouses, partners, and friends who provide in-home care, usually on an unpaid basis—will not be discussed here.

An increased focus on the distress and well-being of health care providers globally can be traced to what has become known as the impaired physician movement. The movement started in the United States in 1972 following a report by the American Medical Association's Council on Mental Health titled "The Sick Physician"(1973). The increased awareness of the need for physician self care promoted the mandatory reporting, evaluation, and treatment of impaired practitioners and led to increased attention to the mental health of physicians. The more recent attention given to the stresses that the changing political economy of the medical professions has imposed on physicians and other health care workers is reflected in the acknowledgment by some national medical associations that the reorganization of health care systems is having a profound and adverse effect on physicians' health and well-being (Canadian Medical Association 1998). Approaches from organizational and clinical psychology have increasingly been applied to the problem of stress in health professionals (Firth-Cozens and Payne 1999). Investigations into doctors' diseases, despair, substance abuse, burnout, and dysfunctional relationships—as well as positive influences on their mental health such as the effective treatment of patients—have been characterized by a preponderance of emphasis on psychopathology and disease models rather than sources of positive functioning (Yamey and Wilkes 2001).

Burnout, Compassion Fatigue, and Demoralization

Methods employed to measure stress in physicians have included measures of burnout, utilizing the Maslach Burnout Inventory, developed by Christina Maslach (1982) to assess aspects of emotional exhaustion, depersonalization, and personal accomplishment; measures of compassion fatigue, or secondary traumatic stress, utilizing the Compassion Fatigue Self Test, developed by Charles Figley and Beth Stamm (1996); clinical interviews based on the American Psychiatric Association's *Diagnostic and Statistical Manual of Mental Disorders* (2000); general surveys of practitioners; and collections of practitioners' narrative. Burnout has been described as a "health care professional's occupational disease" (Felton 1998, 248). Demoralization—arguably the main reason people seek psychiatric treatment—is another term used in literature that reviews health care workers' well-being, although it does not appear in the psychiatric nomenclature (Clarke and Kissane 2002). There are controversies about the conceptualization and construct validity of terms such as burnout, and compassion fatigue, and other terms applied to health care providers such as vicarious traumatization (Jenkins and Baird 2002; Sabin-Farrell and Turpin 2003; R. Thomas and Wilson 2004). Despite recent advances in knowledge, there continues to be a need for prospective, longitudinal studies that further explore the causes and ramifications of physicians' distress, as well as a need for new instruments to specifically measure physicians' well-being (Gundersen 2001; Shanafelt, Sloan, and Haberman 2003; Yamey and Wilkes 2001).

Distress and well-being have been increasingly evaluated in nurses (Edward and Herselinskyj 2007; Maytum, Bielski-Heiman, and Garwick 2004; Radziewicz 2001; Sabo 2006; Wright 2004) and mental health professionals (Pross 2006) as well as in physicians. Collectively, these studies have been international in scope, with a range of methodologies and emphases used across medical specialties and professions. A random sample of such studies, not including examples from sub-Saharan Africa, includes the investigation of: physician burnout in the United States and Holland, the first application of this model across cultures (Linzer et al. 2001); burnout among intensive care physicians and nurses in Croatia (Cubrilo-Turek, Urek, and Turek 2006); occupational stressors and coping as determinants of burnout in female hospice nurses in the United Kingdom (Payne 2003); burnout and psychiatric morbidity in new medical graduates in Australia (Willcock et al. 2004); burnout, stress, and styles of coping among hospital nurses in Poland (Jaracz, Gorna, and Konieczna 2005); burnout, role conflict, job satisfaction, and psychosocial health among health care staff in Hungary (Piko 2006); predictors of burnout and job satisfaction among physicians in Turkey (Ozyurt, Hayran, and Sur 2006); and burnout among critical care nursing staff in France (Poncet et al. 2007). A twelve-year longitudinal study of UK medical graduates reported that personality and learning styles on entering medical school served as predictors of future stress and burnout, suggesting that how doctors perceive and respond to stressors plays an important role in the development of burnout (McManus, Keeling, and Paice 2004).

Medical training, particularly the experience of medical students, has also been increasingly scrutinized in the context of a rapidly shifting professional landscape. As an example, recent U.S. studies have evaluated decreasing empathy over the course of training (Bellini, Baime, and Shea 2002; Bellini and Shea 2005), the effects of lack of sleep and fatigue on the mood of trainees (Kiernan et al. 2006), the impact of work hours on burnout of trainees (Barack et al. 2006), the impact of burnout on patient care by trainees (Shanafelt et al. 2002), and burnout among trainees in different medical specialties (Martini et al. 2004). A review of resident burnout by Niku Thomas (2004) reported that literature on the subject is still in the preliminary stages. Most studies so far have probed for associations in small samples, and larger, more carefully planned prospective studies are needed. Thomas postulated that preventive structural reform may prove more effective than time-intensive stress management training and noted that more research is also needed to guide training directors in preventing, recognizing, and managing burnout in trainees.

The Stresses of Coping with HIV/AIDS

With regard to HIV/AIDS, health care professionals' distress, and how they cope with it, a more substantive literature has begun to emerge over the past decade, with attention to the causes of distress and interventions to address it (Bennett, Miller, and Ross 1995; Miller 2000). Most of the research conducted on coping by health workers has been descriptive in nature, highlighting various ways in which workers are influenced by HIV/AIDS at the workplace and identifying root causes that often include lack of knowledge, protective measures, and emotional and technical support to deal with HIV/AIDS at work (Dieleman et al. 2007). Marjolein Dieleman and coauthors, reporting on health care professionals' distress in Zambia, noted that existing studies are difficult to compare because they have used a variety of designs, most with self-developed instruments, and have no common theoretical framework. The authors also noted that most research in this area has been conducted in resource-rich countries, with a focus on burnout and individual coping strategies and with specific attention given to staff fears, issues of association with patients, professional and role issues, stigma, discrimination, and ethical issues.

A comparison of burnout in nurse samples working in HIV, oncology, medicine, and intensive care in the United States has found comparable levels of job tension across these fields. However, nurses in the HIV intensive care unit show more evidence of feeling emotionally exhausted and drained (Van Servellen and Leake 1993). M. L. Bellani and coauthors have studied burnout and related factors among HIV/AIDS health care workers in Italy, and their result suggest important correlations among burnout, sense of personal accomplishment, anxiety, and depression. Burnout correlates negatively with advancing age. Anxiety, depression, emotional reactions, attitudes, ego strength, and aptitude for interpersonal relationships and teamwork are significant factors in outlining a profile of highly burned out versus "personally accomplished" HIV/AIDS health care providers (Bellani et al. 1996, 207). These results suggest the need to develop strategies of prevention, intervention, and treatment of burnout in the context of HIV/AIDS that consider the importance not only of occupational and institutional characteristics but also of individual ones. Over the past decade Lydia Bennett and colleagues have investigated the importance of internal versus external coping styles and the positive psychological and sociological dimensions of providing AIDS care on the well-being of providers in Australia (Bennett and Kelaher 1994; Bennett, Ross, and Sunderland 1996). Violaine Gueritault-Chalvin and coauthors, seeking to replicate their findings with a sample of nurses specializing in AIDS care in the United States, concluded that both external and internal coping styles predict burnout significantly better than age and workload. The authors found that the use of external coping strategies was positively correlated with levels of burnout, while internal coping strategies had a protective effect: People using more internal coping strategies reported experiencing lower levels of burnout. In addition, the authors concluded that age was a significant factor in burnout in nurses, and perceived workload was positively correlated with burnout and significantly predicted it (Gueritault-Chalvin et al. 2000). F. Lert, J. F. Chastang, and I. Castano (2001) examined psychological stress among hospital doctors caring for patients with AIDS in the late 1990s, reporting that in a French sample of 670 physicians, stress was not related to time spent in clinical work, to HIV work, or to patients' suffering. Rather, work overload and stress derived from social relationships at work were the main predictors of psychological distress, emotional exhaustion, and depersonalization. Carrying out in-depth interviews with physicians in San Francisco, B. Gerbert and coauthors (2004) related not only burnout but also personal and systemic stresses to HIV stigma among providers, as well as to systemic challenges such as restrictive insurance policies and the influence of the pharmaceutical industry. More recently, Lydia Bennett and Margaret Kelaher (2006) have reported that in a sample of 134 Australian health care professionals, grief is associated with higher levels of identification with patients and anxiety; higher levels of grief are associated with burnout due to lack of personal accomplishment; and lower levels of grief are associated with burnout related to depersonalization, reliance on internal coping strategies, and social support or belonging. The authors' results suggest that staff members should be taught ways of separating their work from their private lives to reduce the risks of overidentification with patients and that teaching techniques for reducing anxiety, providing support groups for staff, and encouraging the use of coping strategies that emphasize personal agency could reduce the intense feelings of grief experienced by many health care providers.

Research examining the experience of health care workers in settings where resources are more limited has tended to focus on occupational safety concerns with regard to the risk of needle sticks and contact with bodily fluids of infected patients; knowledge, attitudes, and practices of health workers with respect to HIV/AIDS; and the specific parameters of stress and burnout, working conditions, and organizational support (Dieleman et al. 2007). A. M. Benevides-Pereira and R. Das Neves Alves (2007) have noted that very few studies have investigated the emotional and affective conditions of health care providers, in spite of the importance of the quality of their services, or the way in which their services are offered and, consequently, their influence on the management of HIV disease in patients. Investigating the occurrence of burnout in health care providers caring for HIV-positive patients in the state of Paraná, Brazil, the authors described considerable stress and burnout among providers, also noting a "contagion" effect, whereby providers' burnout contributes to burnout in those around them (Benevides-Pereira and Das Neves Alves 2007, 570). Recommendations by the authors included the need for caregivers to take better care of themselves, more studies on burnout that are national in scope, the identification of social and institutional factors that may contribute to the development of burnout, raising of awareness about possible stressing agents and about the drawbacks of stress and burnout, and improved training and the formation of support groups for people who work directly with HIV-positive patients.

The research available to date on health care professionals' mental health, well-being, and burnout in the context of treating patients with HIV is limited in both scope and volume. It does, however, provide an indication of the complex variables, both individual and systemic, that must be considered in larger, prospective studies in the future and in the development of interventions for formal caregivers. The first steps have been taken toward the development of effective and rational interventions for health care professionals working in diverse contexts.

MEDICAL PROFESSIONALS IN THE ERA OF HIV/AIDS

Defining Medical Professionalism in African Contexts

Fredric Hafferty and John McKinlay (1993) have described meaningful differences and variations that exist in the condition and status of medicine across different countries, shaped by political, cultural, and economic forces and reflected in the way medical work is structured, carried out, and valued. Rather than there being one profession of medicine that is undergoing some universal change, there are as many professions and cultures of medicine as there are nations, societies, and cultures that have created them. Just as physicians have their own universal and local professional cultures, so do nurses, trainees (in medicine and nursing), and health care providers in other professions, with each of these provider groups' cultures deserving attention. Physicians also work within subspecialty cultures—such as those of internal medicine, surgery, obstetrics and gynecology, psychiatry, and pediatrics—that further define their professional identities, activities, and experience.

Mary-Jo Good and colleagues (1999), comparing medical practice in East Africa and the United States, have noted that tensions exist between universal and local standards of practice, and between expectations of professional development and competence and distinctive social and cultural settings. These tensions shape the moral discourses of medicine's multiple voices and produce multiple realities of practice. If medical professionalism is defined as a set of values, behaviors, and relationships that underpin the public's trust in doctors (Working Party of the Royal College of Physicians 2005), then the exercise of medical professionalism in sub-Saharan Africa and other parts of the world has been hampered by the shifting political and cultural environments of health. The conditions of medical practice are critical determinants for the future of professionalism, with a number of complex factors—including, but not limited to, HIV/ AIDS—collectively presenting tremendous challenges for medical professionalism and professionals in African contexts. The dilemmas presented by HIV/AIDS for African practitioners have compounded—but not created—a number of professional concerns, with HIV/AIDS representing only one of a number of stressors that adversely affect the professional and personal self-perceptions of practitioners and their ability to effectively work with and treat the sick.

Focusing his analysis on East African medicine, the historian John Iliffe (1998) has noted that very little is known about the power, prestige, culture, and practice of the profession today. His analysis suggests an impressive diversity and complexity of the profession of medicine across Africa. Describing the essence of medical professionalism in East Africa as ambiguous, embracing "specialized knowledge, altruistic service, thirst for power and blatant self-interest," Iliffe has shown how medical professionalism evolved in local contexts of disintegrating state power, capitalism, and socialism (in Uganda, Kenya, and Tanzania, respectively) (1998, 3). He reports that an ability to meet great challenges has been a consistent thread throughout the histories of medicine in East Africa, citing the remarkable lives and careers of James Ainsworth and Adrien Atiman in the early twentieth century and Elly Katabira in the late twentieth century as examples (Iliffe 1998 and 2006). His call for a program, conducted by East Africans, to collect the life histories and papers of modern doctors is relevant here, given the continuing scarcity of research on the culture of biomedicine in Africa relating to the experiences of health care professionals.

Iliffe (1998) has also reported that the impact of HIV/AIDS on the practice of physicians in East Africa has been complex and is intelligible only in the context of the profession's historical evolution. Given the entrepreneurial strand of

the profession in Kenya, for example, it is likely that in the 1990s many doctors—especially private practitioners—spent less time with HIV/AIDS patients
than might have been expected. With the emergence of HIV/AIDS, the public
perception of physicians as impersonal figures from whom patients sought treatment for serious illness rather than assistance in distress may have contributed
to the finding that some 30 percent of patients in Kenya in the mid-1990s were
dying without ever contacting the health system (Iliffe 1998). Increasingly, however, HIV-related illness became the most common presenting problem in hospitals and clinics, with psychiatrists, for example, seeing organic complications
of AIDS more frequently than other conditions. Over time, given the increasing
burdens on physicians, many aspects of the education, counseling, and care of
the infected were passed on to nurses, auxiliary staff members, counselors, vol-
unteers, or the patients' family and friends. Iliffe (1998) has cited the incurability
of patients, poor and unsafe working conditions, the effects of stigma, challenges
regarding diagnosis and issues of confidentiality, physicians' infection with HIV,
and their general demoralization—accompanied by an erosion of confidence
and ability to cope with the situation—as features complicating the practice of
medicine in East Africa since the emergence of HIV/AIDS. Iliffe (1998 and 2006)
has noted that despite these challenges, East African physicians performed an
important service in maintaining the objective rationality that lies at the heart
of their professional tradition: displaying their continuing faith in modern medicine and exhibiting devotion to their patients in the midst of a widespread collapse of morale.

Moral and Ethical Dilemmas of Practice

An overview of emerging narratives and perspectives of health care providers'
well-being and mental health in sub-Saharan benefits from an examination of the
moral and ethical dimensions of the profession of medicine—that is, bioethics—
and its practice in Africa. In the East African context, ethnographic research by
Good and coauthors with physicians between 1997 and 1999 at Kenyatta National
Hospital, East Africa's largest public hospital, suggests that many physicians in
specialty residencies and many attending faculty clinicians were experiencing
profound professional and emotional distress (Good et al. 1999; Machoki 1998;
Machoki et al. 1999; Mwaikambo 2000). The researchers initiated discussions
with senior physicians on how the brute fact of the HIV/AIDS pandemic—compounded by poverty, scarcity of resources, and deep inequalities of wealth within
and between societies—has been stripping medicine of its instrumental efficacy
as well as its cultural power over the past two decades (Good et al. 1999). Unsettling physician experiences were attributed to the pandemic, scarce medical and
economic resources, structural adjustment, and the clinical realities and intense

personal dilemmas clinicians face in treating patients dying of AIDS. The authors noted that in practice environments where the ability to cure was becoming increasingly limited by the growing number of people contracting the illness, not only were physicians facing very specific moral dilemmas—for example, how to ration scarce resources and acquire costly medications, or how to inform families that a loved one was HIV-positive—but the very moral foundations of medicine as a scientific and caring profession were themselves starting to be called into question (Good et al. 1999). With the loss of the variety of disease patterns due to the scope of the pandemic, HIV/AIDS was perceived to be contributing to an erosion of fundamental intellectual assumptions about medicine as a system of knowledge. As the ability of physicians and trainees to effectively respond to human suffering with medical interventions was being compromised, so too was their sense of professional competence and empowerment. Some physicians expressed concern that discussing and researching HIV/AIDS and related infections were receiving so much attention that there was not much time left for other disease conditions, which adversely affected both the training of medical students and the care of patients suffering from other conditions. One senior physician noted that the "overcrowding of death" was disempowering physicians, threatening the most basic goals of medical education: the reproduction of a sense of competence in a new generation of physicians and an embodied ability to respond to human suffering in an effective manner (Good et al. 1999, 173).

Based on their preliminary explorations, Good and coauthors identified four kinds of concerns. The first was, how to preserve medicine as an intellectual enterprise and ensure the training of competent physicians and the upholding of "universal" standards of biomedicine in the face of HIV/AIDS, with the ideal of medical professionalism being perceived as grounded in the challenge of diagnosis, the excitement of curing diseases, and the potential to stem the consequences of disease and to manage illness (Good et al., 1999, 178). The second type of concern was that HIV was threatening the ideals of "doing good," "good doctoring," quality patient care, and the modeling of good caretaking behavior for trainee physicians (ibid., 178–80). The third was that the political economy of medical care in East Africa and the international global market—specifically, the local and global inequities, the scarcity of resources, and the implicit and explicit rationing of therapeutic treatments in terms of time and pharmaceuticals that have been part of daily practice since the emergence of HIV/AIDS—have limited the instrumental effectiveness of physicians and trainees. And the fourth was how to redefine the care of HIV/AIDS patients from curative medicine to palliative care with the management of associated diseases. This preliminary work indicated that the demoralization of medical professionals in urban East Africa was more complex and historically shaped than had previously been realized. Not only clinical but also economic, social, and even political stresses appeared to be having serious negative effects on the professional and emotional experiences of physicians.

During the mid- to late 1990s, anecdotal evidence emerged from a number of other African medical sources that reinforced the notion that the burden of HIV/AIDS was creating significant professional dilemmas for physicians and other health care providers. A 1994 investigation of stress and burnout, measured through questionnaires sent to South African physicians, found that 78 percent of doctors reported experiencing symptoms consistent with burnout since graduation from an English medical school (Schweitzer 1994). This study showed that when a doctor was suffering from burnout, he or she tended to endure the symptoms rather than seek help. Many doctors viewed joining a support group as reflecting an inability to cope. Nevertheless, 63 percent of doctors in this study thought that such a group would be helpful. The low incidence of burnout in doctors who were in their own practices, as opposed to working in clinics and hospitals, gave some indication of the importance of an internal locus of control as protection against burnout. B. Schweitzer reported being impressed by how many doctors had indicated that they were burned out and had encouraged him to do the study, and he recommended the recognition of early signs of burnout, the teaching of concepts of stress and burnout in medical schools, the development of strategies for prevention and management of burnout, and the increased availability of nonjudgmental counseling.

Some subsequent reports and investigations have sought to describe and clarify the relationships among the knowledge, attitudes, and practices of health workers in caring for people with HIV/AIDS (Dieleman et al. 2007), including issues such as risk and fear of infection, lack of resources, and stigma and discrimination (Adebajo, Bamgbala, and Oyediran 2003; Awusabo-Asare and Marfo 1997; Ezedinachi et al. 2002; Grinstead et al. 2000; Mungherera et al. 1997; Ogunbodede, Folayan, and Adedigba 2005; Oyeyemi, Oyeyemi, and Bello 2006; Rahlenbeck 2004; Walusimbi and Okonsky 2004). Other reports have increasingly focused specifically on the stresses experienced by both formal and informal caregivers. A UNAIDS report that focused on nongovernmental organizations working in AIDS care in Uganda and South Africa concluded that "caring for the carers of people with AIDS is not only a humanitarian imperative, it is a social and economic necessity" (2000, 54). Identifying a number of factors that cause stress and burnout, including lack of preparation, lack of training for new tasks, and inadequate support and lack of supervision and recognition, this report made several general observations about the requirements of managing stress and burnout among caregivers. It recommended in general terms strengthening the capacity of the individual caregiver to cope with the duties and responsibilities of the role; ensuring that the working conditions, practices, and policies of care programs offer a supportive environment to caregivers and are not causes of stress in themselves; and advocating for national policies and laws that are sensitive to the needs of caregivers (UNAIDS 2000). The report also suggested several specific prevention strategies, including peer counseling, personal mentors, supervision, appropriate training, and better distribution of tasks (UNAIDS 2000; Dieleman et al. 2007). Among other important conclusions, the report called for more systematic studies of stress among caregivers at all levels and in all settings, with more formal documentation of findings. Despite these recommendations, few studies since have focused on specifically relating formal caregivers' concerns to their mental health.

EMERGING NARRATIVES OF THE DISTRESS OF AFRICAN HEALTH CARE PROVIDERS

East Africa

Building on questions previously generated in East Africa by Iliffe (1998) and Good and coauthors (1999), my colleagues and I (Raviola et al. 2002) sought to further investigate the complex relationships between burnout, demoralization, and depression, on the one hand, to larger social, institutional, and disease-related forces, on the other hand. Using qualitative methods to better understand the perspectives of physicians in training on social supports, medical training, patients with HIV/AIDS, limited resources, working relationships in the hospital, and burnout, we used a standardized clinical assessment of major depression and post-traumatic stress disorder. We found that of fifty physicians in training who were interviewed at Kenyatta National Hospital, 82 percent reported being at least moderately affected by burnout, 48 percent met the criteria for major depression, and 32 percent met the criteria for post-traumatic stress disorder (Raviola et al. 2002). Sixty-two percent of the trainees reported that they were at least moderately affected physically by their anxiety.

With regard to the perceptions of trainees regarding their professional development and implications for future practice, 80 percent reported that, when they chose the medical profession, their main motivations, expectations, and aspirations had been to help alleviate pain and suffering or to fight disease. Ninety percent reported that their main motivations, expectations, and aspirations changed after they entered medical school. Inadequate hospital facilities and congested, crowded wards were cited by trainees as the largest contributors to such changes, closely followed by the poverty of patients and the overwhelming HIV/AIDS pandemic. Sixty-eight percent reported doubting their choice to practice medicine, and 58 percent reported thinking of leaving medicine altogether. Eighty percent reported that they would discourage their children or close family members from pursuing medicine as a career. Extensive statements by interviewees provided worrisome signs of how the pandemic, inside and outside the hospital; the lack of resources, including drugs and equipment; and an unmanageable patient load were having a significant effect on how trainees perceived themselves and their patients. Most notable with regard to sources of stress was the role that hospital relationships played in contributing to trainees' dissatisfaction and hopelessness, particularly with regard to meeting the expectations of, and even experiencing ridicule from, senior physicians. Themes relating to lack of support from senior physicians and hospital administrators, as well as nurses, were consistently expressed by trainees both in questionnaires and interviews. It was notable that after the interviews, many respondents reported that the interviews had helped them better understand the professional issues that were central to their lives. Given this receptivity to the interview experience, my colleagues and I wished that we had attempted to measure the interviews themselves as a supportive intervention. The findings also support previous data suggesting that as the ability of physicians and trainees to respond to human suffering with medical interventions has been compromised by HIV/AIDS, so too has their emotional well-being and their sense of competence and empowerment as practitioners (Raviola et al. 2002). An important conclusion is that although poor pay and financial incentives have been identified as significant reasons why physicians leave the public sector, another overriding incentive to move to the private sector has been the basic psychological necessity to reduce stress. The study findings support prior work by one of the authors suggesting the importance of examining issues of mentorship; role modeling; good doctoring in care of all patients, including those who are HIV-positive; communication flows through the training hierarchy; and faculty members' commitment, accountability; and obligations. In the hope of bolstering physician resilience, my colleagues and I noted that future research might try to find ways to help overwhelmed physicians in Africa remain intellectually engaged in medicine and teaching, maintain a sense of empathy for patients without becoming emotionally numb, and retain a sense of hope and idealism under difficult circumstances (Raviola et al. 2002). Following the publication of this study, we reported the findings to the Kenyan Ministry of Health. As a result, there was an apparent increase in the willingness to consider policy reforms to address health care professionals' stress and burnout. More recently, a group of Kenyan psychiatrists has sought to build on previous findings, measuring burnout and compassion fatigue at Kenyatta National Hospital in 2003 with a sample of 345 physicians and nurses (Kokonya 2007).

West Africa

Noting that there have been few studies examining burnout in health care workers in Nigeria, Benjamin Olley (2003) carried out a comparative study of burnout syndrome among health professionals in a teaching hospital in Ibadan. He sampled 260 health professionals across disciplines using the Maslach Burnout Inventory, the thirty-item General Health Questionnaire, and the State Trait Anxiety Inventory. Nurses had greater psychological distress, with consistently higher scores on all measures of burnout when compared with other health care providers, including physicians, pharmacists, medical social workers, and nursing assistants. Olley attributed nurses' problems to long work hours, additional professional activities, institutional disregard for the needs of patients in favor of administrative and bureaucratic needs, gender-biased leadership and supervisory style, obsolete and fractionalized training, and unnecessary class consciousness. Increased years of education and increased job experience appeared to decrease the risk for burnout among physicians, and Olley suggested that the tendency among new doctors and nurses to strive for excellence early in their careers makes them more vulnerable to burnout. This is in contrast to findings in South Africa by L. S. Thomas and A. Valli (2006), who found that junior physicians experienced more job satisfaction.

I. Agyepong and colleagues (2004) sought to identify factors affecting health workers' motivation and satisfaction in the public sector in Accra, Ghana. An interviewer administered a structured questionnaire, with respondents identifying workplace obstacles that caused dissatisfaction and reduced their motivation. The most frequently mentioned obstacles, in the following order, were: salaries so low that obtaining the basic necessities of life was a problem; lack of essential equipment, tools, and supplies to work with; delayed promotions; difficulties and inconveniences with transportation to work; staff shortages; housing; additional allowances for overtime; and the quality of in-service training. More recently, Amy Hagopian and coauthors examined the flight of physicians from West Africa, reporting that in Ghana there exists a "culture of emigration" for physicians in training (2005, 9).

Southern Africa

Since 2000 numerous reports have emerged from South Africa regarding widespread dissatisfaction, distress, and demoralization of nurses and physicians working in the public sector. A 2003 report, responding to new statistics that 16 percent of public health workers were HIV-positive and nearly half were found exhausted and stressed from a fourfold increase in AIDS patients over the previous five years, indicated a growing health-sector crisis (Bateman 2003). The report noted that the main reasons for exhaustion and stress among the workers were the lack of knowledge about AIDS among caregivers or patients, volume of patients, lack of equipment, lack of patient support from relatives, and drop in the quality of care, with heavy workload cited as the most debilitating factor. A study of perceptions of nurses working in a public hospital in Gauteng Province found that the majority of nurses working with HIV/AIDS patients were experiencing feelings of significant helplessness, emotional stress, and fatigue (Smit 2004). Nurses reported significant apprehension, fear, anxiety, anger, and frustration, related both to work with patients and to the government's slow response to the HIV/AIDS crisis. They expressed concerns about the deterioration of the hospital's infrastructure, inadequate availability of medical equipment, shortage of nurses, and increasing workload. The study's recommendations included improved biomedical education regarding HIV/AIDS, sufficient medical supplies, increased emphasis on the emotional and psychological needs of patients, and increased recognition of the importance of more proactive institutional initiatives to support nurses in coping with occupational stress and addressing their emotional concerns. Specific recommended strategies were stress management courses, nurses' support groups, and increased recognition—both formal and informal of people for valuable occupational contributions. Another recommendation was that, because of the lack of research focusing on nurses' experiences in HIV-related nursing care in South Africa, similar studies should be conducted at other hospitals in both rural and urban areas in the country to ascertain whether the findings could be replicated. E. J. Hall (2004) reports that, given the stressful and unsupportive work environment for nurses in the public sector and nurses' perception that they are no longer able to provide adequate health care for reasons perceived to be out of their control, increased nursing attrition could be expected. Hall recommends stress-management programs and counseling services that are free and available to all staff members to help them cope, observing that employers need to reject the old-fashioned but persistent belief that nurses who find it hard to cope do not belong in the profession. Subsequent investigations at hospitals in South Africa have identified poor morale and similar problems related to factors in the health care system—including workload, staff shortages, occupational safety concerns, physical and psychosocial stress, autocratic and dehumanizing management structures, distrust of hospital administration, lack of career advancement, poor pay and benefits—and factors outside the system, such as poverty, poor nutrition, home stresses, and HIV/AIDS (Gaede et al. 2006; King and Mcinerney, 2006; Lephokoet al., 2006; Thomas and Valli, 2006; Zelnick and O'Donnell 2005). Reporting on the public sector in rural areas, B. Gaede and coauthors (2006) conclude that limitations to practicing holistically in the public sector in South Africa go beyond mere issues of resource allocation, which are often claimed to be the only problem. The resource limitations, in terms of both numbers of health care workers and their skills, are real. However, there are also problems in organizational reorientation and the management of a paradigmatic change. Practices could be made more holistic practice with relatively modest increases in resource allocation if they were accompanied by better management, such as improved collaboration among the sectors.

L. S. Thomas and A. Valli (2006) have reported that evidence is increasing to support the view that stress in the workplace can have national implications for health policy initiatives and developments. Noting that occupational stress in the public health sector in South Africa is still a new concept, the authors conclude that, although it is important to teach doctors how to manage stress, it is just as important to change the hospital environment, both from provincial and national perspectives.

A more recent study examined perceptions of the impact of HIV/AIDS on health workers in two districts in Zambia through a qualitative study, complemented by a survey using self-administered questionnaires at four selected health facilities in two rural districts (Dieleman et al. 2007). The authors note that it is one of the few studies to have explored the impact of HIV/AIDS from the perspective of health workers in the region. In this study, despite the fact that health workers were still relatively motivated, emotional exhaustion occurred among 62 percent of the forty-two respondents. HIV/AIDS was found to have had a negative impact on workload and to have considerably changed or added tasks to already overburdened health workers. Approximately 77 percent of respondents reported fear of infection at the workplace, and HIV-positive health workers remained "in hiding," not talking about their illness and suffering in silence (Dieleman et al. 2007, 139). The authors found that organizational support for health workers to deal with HIV/AIDS was either haphazard or not available at all. HIV/AIDS was felt to complicate the already difficult work environment. Managers, like health workers, were found to need support in dealing with AIDS at the workplace. The authors also reported that "emotional coping with HIV/AIDS at the workplace was considered difficult, and health workers confirmed that there were no official structures in place to help them to cope better. . . . Management support was considered important by health workers, but they confirmed that this was almost absent. Respondents suggested several types of support in order to better deal with HIV/AIDS, such as sharing experiences with each other, receiving professional advice on dealing with certain cases and training for new tasks" (ibid., 145).

The two professional groups found to be most at risk for emotional exhaustion were counselors and nurses on the wards. The authors reported that counselors had established professional meetings and support systems at their own initiative, although not systematically. Nurses on the wards, often not trained in emotionally and technically supporting AIDS patients, did not have a support system in place. This study highlighted the pressing need to provide organizational support to health workers and to managers: "HIV/AIDS requires health policy makers and planners to implement multi-faceted workplace policies and programs in order to support valuable health workers who are at their limits. Urgent action is necessary" (Dieleman et al. 2007, 146).

A larger-scale, longitudinal study, begun in 2004 by the Population Council and still continuing, has followed more than 1,400 hospital employees in Zambia, with a similar investigation in Kenya, and has provided additional information about the needs of formal caregivers (Kiragu et al. 2005). The study's findings have included: significant occupational risk of HIV infection, with approximately half of the respondents reporting work-related incidents where they could have been infected; significant psychosocial stress at home and at work, with 70 percent of respondents reporting that HIV had increased stress at work and 40 percent either having had an immediate family member die of AIDS or having one living with HIV; substantial risk of sexual transmission of HIV, with a quarter reporting multiple sexual partners in a twelve-month period, and nearly a third reporting having never used a condom during that time; and high risk from intimate partner violence, with 40 percent of men and 34 percent of women reporting feeling that it is acceptable for a man to hit a woman under certain circumstances, and about 45 percent of women who had ever been abused reporting violence during the past year. Recommendations from the study included urgent implementation of HIV/AIDS programs for hospital employees that would address occupational and sexual risks, differential risks by gender, and psychosocial support (Kiragu et al. 2005).

Incorporating the Well-Being of Formal Caregivers into Organizational Structures

The complex phenomenon of the brain drain of health care providers from sub-Saharan Africa has received increasing attention recently (Ahmad 2004; Chen and Hanvoravongchai 2005; Friedman 2004; Hagopian et al. 2004; Kirigia et al. 2006; Kober and Van Damme 2006; "Migration of Health Workers" 2005; Mullan 2005; Muula 2005; Schrecker and Labonte 2004). The devastating effects of the combination of HIV/AIDS and the brain drain on systems of care and patients are clear. The discourse about the brain drain has correctly emphasized a number of important issues, including the pull from resource-rich nations that are themselves experiencing shortages of health care worker shortages and the push from poorer nations, where caregivers face not only low financial remuneration but also fear of infection and mortality. The issues of personal and professional crises and ensuing psychological distress have implicitly permeated this discourse. Despite the changing nature of HIV/AIDS in sub-Saharan Africa, with infection rates slowing in some areas and increased availability of ARVs in others, some recent reports have suggested that conditions in many African hospitals are worsening, with an increased brain drain both within and between countries (Integrated Regional Information Networks, UN Office for the Coordination of Humanitarian Affairs 2003; "Brain Drain Now a Gush" 2004). Nevertheless, there is increasing promise for those who are HIV-positive, with African governments increasing their political and economic commitment to the production and distribution of ARVs to patients in both hospital and community settings. An adequate response to the brain drain is increasingly being understood to require national, regional, and global efforts of organization and cooperation (Chen et al. 2004).

A comprehensive action plan to address the brain drain presented by the Physicians for Human Rights (Friedman 2004) included important recommendations regarding the implementation of psychosocial support for health workers—which could take various forms—in the context of HIV/AIDS prevention and treatment services. It has been noted, however, that despite the urgent need for creative and caring responses to support health care workers in the delivery of services so that they, in turn, can provide sensitive, compassionate care for the individuals, families, and communities affected by HIV/AIDS, caring for carers is often spoken of yet seldom operationalized (Mayers 2005). Reframing our understanding of tropical infectious diseases with a biosocial analysis, David Walton, Paul Farmer, and Rebecca Dillingham (2005) have noted that health personnel flight is not simply a question of desire for more equitable remuneration. We still lack adequate data on the brain drain, which makes it difficult to determine the real extent of health care professionals' migration from and within Africa. This, in turn, makes the development of effective remedial policies harder (Connell et al. 2007). A biosocial analysis of this complex phenomenon, including attention to both broad structural and policy issues as well as to the immediate concerns of individual mental health and well-being in local contexts, would provide a better understanding of why caregivers leave the practice of medicine. This would lead to increased momentum toward political and structural solutions that included dedicated interventions for caregivers in distress and that incorporated HIV prevention strategies and concerns for caregivers' mental health and well-being.

Despite using a variety of methodologies as well as being limited in number and scope, existing studies of the effects of working conditions on health care workers in sub-Saharan Africa have provided a strong indication that there exists not only a human resource crisis, but also individual personal and professional crises, all of which significantly affect the well-being and mental health of health care providers, particularly in the public sector. HIV/AIDS is a critical factor. However, both global and local factors related to the changing cultures of medicine, their institutions, and the political economy of the professions of medicine are also profoundly affecting the health and well-being of health care providers. Studies in the United States and the United Kingdom have provided evidence that burnout among health care workers is not only an organizationally induced phenomenon but is also caregiver-dependent, and that education, training, and the fostering of workers' sense of mastery and self-esteem can be preventive (Egan 1993; McManus, Keeling, and Paice 2004). From a number of perspectives, therefore, evidence indicates that a mental health perspective can inform and enrich the discourse on the current crisis of African medical professionalism and human resources and inform a more organized response that also incorporates the mental health professions. In addition to the use of standardized measures of burnout, compassion fatigue, depression, and anxiety, qualitative narrative and ethnographic techniques remain critical for obtaining the most complete understanding of the reasons for health care professionals' distress and dysfunction in local contexts and their relationship to broader social maladies, such as the brain drain. African mental health professionals can play a critical role in articulating the place of mental health concerns in current debates, in the design of interventions for health care workers, and in educating policymakers about the psychological and mental health aspects of the current crisis. This would illuminate the relationship of this crisis to the political economy of medical practice in local contexts, and highlight the need for an increased commitment of financial and human resources to support formal caregivers.

Health Care Worker Support Programs

Dieleman and colleagues (2007) have noted that few intervention studies exist of efforts to improve the knowledge and practice of health workers in Africa, and none have focused on interventions addressing stress and mental health (Vos et al. 1998; Ezedinachi et al. 2002). Anecdotal evidence suggests that some attending physicians have resisted the notion that, in addition to HIV/AIDS, established systems of training and education may contribute to stress and difficulties in coping among trainees, junior physicians, and nurses. Formal statements acknowledging the reality and the multicausality of the stresses of medical practice by ministries of health and other government agencies may lead to a wider acceptance of the problem, greater openness to research, and the development of solutions. To be lasting, interventions will have to be tailored to contextual realities, and creative thinking about what would be most effective in particular clinical, professional, and cultural contexts will be needed. Given the shortage of psychiatrists in Africa, if psychiatry is to play the leadership role there, its efforts would have to be focused and circumscribed, with collaboration and sharing of information among allied mental health and health care professionals who are involved in interventional organization and training. With a movement toward increasing the number of community health workers as part of the effort to scale up the use of ARVs, interventions for caregivers will also need to be flexible in defining who would be eligible for such services. Because health care professionals tend to feel stigma regarding disorders among themselves, a focus on wellness and positive functioning—rather than on disorders—may make initiatives more likely to be accepted by practitioners (Yamey and Wilkes 2001).

Further investigation is needed regarding optimal ways to deliver comprehensive support services for clinicians in Africa that will bolster caregivers' resilience and well-being, thus increasing the quality and amount of care that they can provide. The Balint group model has been a powerful concept for some trainees in Australia and the United States, with mixed evidence in the literature suggesting its potential to mitigate compassion fatigue and burnout and to enhance professionalism (Adams et al. 2006; Benson and Magraith 2005; Lustig 2006; Smith and Anandarajah 2007). Potentially replicable models exist of more comprehensive support services for clinicians based in general hospital settings. Employee assistance programs have been established in U.S. hospitals that deliver counseling services to clinicians. More recently, offices of clinician support have been implemented, with the goal of giving clinicians a place to discuss and resolve both work-related and personal issues. These offices combine elements of the employee assistance program with those of an ombudsman's office in providing a safe, alternative, and confidential environment for voicing concerns and organizing thoughts and priorities (DeMaso et al. 2007; DeMaso and Skitt 2005). In Boston, the Children's Hospital's Office of Clinician Support, created in 2004, has reported increasing use by clinicians and very high satisfaction ratings from them (DeMaso et al. 2007).

Whether in developing educational presentations or programs, short-term and ongoing support groups, or various other possible interventions, those responding to clinicians' mental health needs will have to be sensitive to local medical culture and organizations and to integrate their interventions into existing and developing systems of care. Programs that implement rational interventions for health care providers by seeking to address the multiple direct and indirect causes and consequences of demoralization, fatigue, and burnout and that help individuals manage the significant emotional distress and difficulties of practice in local African contexts are urgently needed. Psychiatry and the allied mental health professions in Africa can begin to serve in a key leadership role in this regard.

NOTE

The author would like to thank colleagues in Kenya, Tanzania, and the United States for their significant contributions to the stream of East African ethnographic research cited in this chapter. M'Imunya Machoki, of the University of Nairobi, in Kenya, and Esther Mwaikambo, of the Hubert Kairuki Memorial University, in Tanzania, were Carnegie Fellows at the Department of Social Medicine at Harvard Medical School. Mary-Jo Good, a professor of social medicine at Harvard Medical School, has generously nurtured this international collaboration over the past decade.

REFERENCES

Adams, K., M. O'Reilly, J. Romm, K. James 2006. "Effect of Balint Training on Resident Professionalism." *American Journal of Obstetrics and Gynecology* 195 (5): 1431–37.
Adebajo, S. B., A. O. Bamgbala, and M. A. Oyediran. 2003. "Attitudes of Health Workers to Persons Living with HIV/AIDS in Lagos State, Nigeria." *African Journal for Reproductive Health* 7 (1): 103–12.
Agyepong, I., P. Anafi, E. Asiamah, E. Ansah, D. Ashon, and C. Nahr-Dometey. 2004. "Health Worker (Internal Customer) Satisfaction and Motivation in the Public Sector in Ghana." *International Journal of Health Planning and Management* 19 (4): 319–36.
Ahmad, O. 2004. "Brain Drain: The Flight of Human Capital." *Bulletin of the World Health Organization* 82 (10): 797–98.
American Medical Association, Council on Mental Health. 1973. "The Sick Physician: Impairment by Psychiatric Disorders, Including Alcoholism and Drug Dependence." *Journal of the American Medical Association* 223 (6): 684–87.
American Psychiatric Association. 2000. *Diagnostic and Statistical Manual of Mental Disorders.* 4th ed. Arlington, VA: American Psychiatric Association.
Awusabo-Asare, K., and C. Marfo. 1997. "Attitudes to and Management of HIV/AIDS among Health Workers in Ghana: The Care of Cape Coast Municipality." *Health Transition Review* 7 (Suppl.): 271–80.
Barack, R., L. Miller, W. Sotile, M. Sotile, and H. Rubash. 2006. "Effect of Duty Hour Standards on Burnout among Orthopedic Surgery Residents"; *Clinical Orthopedics and Related Research* 449 (August): 134–37.
Bateman, C. 2003. "Healthcare Workers Cracking under HIV/AIDS Workload." *South African Medical Journal* 93 (10): 734–36.
Bellani, M., F. Furlani, M. Gnecchi, P. Pezzotta, E. Trotti, and G. Bellotti. 1996. "Burnout and Related Factors among HIV/AIDS Health care Workers." *AIDS Care* 8 (2): 207–21.
Bellini, L., M. Baime, J. Shea. 2002. "Variation of Mood and Empathy during Internship." *Journal of the American Medical Association* 287 (23): 3143–46.
Bellini, L., and J. Shea. 2005. "Mood Change and Empathy Decline Persist during Three Years of Internal Medicine Training." *Academic Medicine* 80 (2): 164–67.
Benevides-Pereira, A. M. T., and R. Das Neves Alves. 2007. "A Study on Burnout Syndrome in Healthcare Providers to People Living with HIV." *AIDS Care* 19 (4): 565–71.
Bennett, L., and M. Kelaher. 1994. "Longitudinal Predictors of Burnout in HIV/AIDS Health Professionals." *Australian Journal of Public Health* 18 (3): 334–36.

———. 2006. "Variables Contributing to Experiences of Grief in HIV/AIDS Healthcare Professionals." *Journal of Community Psychology* 21 (3): 210–17.

Bennett, L., D. Miller, and M. Ross, eds. 1995. *Health Workers and AIDS: Research, Intervention and Current Issues in Burnout and Response.* Chur, Switzerland: Harwood Academic.

Bennett, L., R. W. Ross, and R. Sunderland. 1996. "The Relationship between Recognition, Rewards and Burnout in AIDS Caring." *AIDS Care* 8 (2): 145–54.

Benson, J., and K. Magraith. 2005. "Compassion Fatigue and Burnout: The Role of Balint Groups." *Australian Family Physician* 34 (6): 497–98.

Blumenthal, D., and W. Hsiao. 2005. "Privatization and Its Discontents: The Evolving Chinese Health Care System." *New England Journal of Medicine* 353 (11): 1165–70.

"Brain Drain Now a Gush." 2004. Accessed November 27, 2007. http://news.hst.org.za/view.php3?id=20040118 on 11/27/07.

Canadian Medical Association. 1998. "CMA Policy: Physician Health and Well-Being." Accessed October 6, 2013. http://policybase.cma.ca/dbtw-wpd/PolicyPDF/PD 98-04.pdf.

Chen, L., and P. Hanvoravongchai. 2005. "HIV/AIDS and Human Resources." *Bulletin of the World Health Organization* 83 (4): 243–44.

Chen, L., T. Evans, S. Anand, J. I. Boufford, H. Brown, M. Chowdhury, and M. Cueto, M., et al. 2004. "Human Resources for Health: Overcoming the Crisis." *Lancet* 364 (9449): 1984–90.

Clarke, D., and D. Kissane. 2002. "Demoralization: Its Phenomenology and Importance." *Australian and New Zealand Journal of Psychiatry* 36 (6): 733–42.

Connell, J., P. Zurn, B. Stilwell, M. Awases, and J. Braichet 2007. "Sub-Saharan Africa: Beyond the Health Worker Migration Crisis." *Social Science and Medicine* 64 (9): 1876–91.

Cubrilo-Turek, M., R. Urek, and S. Turek. 2006. "Burnout Syndrome: Assessment of a Stressful Job among Intensive Care Staff." *Collegium Antropologicum* 30 (1): 131–35.

DeMaso, D. R., L. Baptista, J. Andrus, L. Coyne, and A. Mowatt. 2007. *The Office of Clinician Support: Caring for Hospital Clinicians.* Boston: American Academy of Child and Adolescent Psychiatry.

DeMaso, D. R., and K. S. Skitt. 2005. "Clinician Support: Caring for Caregivers." *Children's Hospital Today,* 34–35.

Dieleman, M., G. Biemba, S. Mphuka, K. Sichinga-Sichali, D. Sissolak, A. van der Kwaak, and G. J. van der Wilt. 2007. "'We Are Also Dying Like Any Other People, We Are Also People': Perceptions of the Impact of HIV/AIDS on Health Workers in Two Districts in Zambia." *Health Policy and Planning* 22 (3): 139–48.

Edward, K., and G. Herselinskyj. 2007. "Burnout in the Caring Nurse: Learning Resilient Behaviors." *British Journal of Nursing* 16 (4): 240–42.

Egan, M. 1993. "Resilience at the Front Lines: Hospital Social Work with AIDS Patients and Burnout." *Social Work in Health Care* 18 (2): 109–25.

Ezedinachi, E. N., M. W. Ross, M. Meremiku, E. J. Essian, C. B. Edem, E. Ekure, and O. Ita. 2002. "The Impact of an Intervention to Change Health Workers' HIV/AIDS Attitudes and Knowledge in Nigeria: A Controlled Trial." *Public Health* 116 (2): 106–12.

Felton, J. S. 1998. "Burnout as a Clinical Entity: Its Importance in Health Care Workers." *Occupational Medicine* 48 (4): 237–50.

Figley, C. R., and B. H. Stamm. 1996. "Psychometric Review of Compassion Fatigue Self Test." In *Measurement of Stress, Trauma and Adaptation,* edited by B. H. Stamm, 127–30. Lutherville, MD: Sidan.

Firth-Cozens, J., and R. Payne, eds. 1999. *Stress in Health Professionals: Psychological and Organizational Causes and Interventions.* Chichester, UK: John Wiley and Sons.

Friedman, Eric A. 2004. *An Action Plan to Prevent Brain Drain: Building Equitable Systems in Africa.* Boston, MA: Physicians for Human Rights.

Gaede, B., S. Mahlobo, K. Shabalala, M. Moloi, and C. van Deventer. 2006. "Limitations to Practicing Holistically in the Public Sector in a Rural Sub-District in South Africa." *Rural and Remote Health* 6 (4): 1–8.

Gerbert, B., N. Casper, J. J. Moe, K. Clanon, P. Abercrombie, and K. Herzig. 2004. "The Mysteries and Demands of HIV Care: Qualitative Analyses of HIV Specialists' Views on Their Expertise." *AIDS Care* 16 (3): 363–76.

Good, M., M. Machoki, E. Mwaikambo, E. Amayo. 1999. "Clinical Realities and Moral Dilemmas: Contrasting Perspectives from Academic Medicine in Kenya, Tanzania and America." *Daedalus* 128 (4): 167–96.

Grinstead, O. A., A. van der Straten, and the Voluntary HIV-1 Counselling and Testing Efficacy Study Group. 2000. "Counsellors' Perspectives on the Experience of Providing HIV Counselling in Kenya and Tanzania: The Voluntary HIV-1 Counselling and Testing Efficacy Study." *AIDS Care* 12 (5): 625–42.

Gueritault-Chalvin, V., S. C. Kalichman, A. Demi, and J. L. Peterson. 2000. "Work-Related Stress and Occupational Burnout in AIDS Caregivers: Test of a Coping Model with Nurses Providing AIDS Care." *AIDS Care* 12 (2): 149–61.

Gundersen, L. 2001. "Physician Burnout." *Annals of Internal Medicine* 135 (2): 145–48.

Hafferty, F., and J. McKinlay, eds. 1993. *The Changing Medical Profession: An International Perspective.* New York: Oxford University Press.

Hagopian, A., A. Ofosu, A. Fatusi, R. Biritwum, A. Essele, L. G. Hart, and C. Wattse. 2005. "The Flight of Physicians from West Africa: Views of African Physicians and Implications for Policy." *Social Science and Medicine* 61 (8): 1750–60.

Hagopian, A., M. J. Thompson, M. Fordyce, K. Johnson, and L. G. Hart 2004. "The Migration of Physicians from Sub-Saharan Africa to the United States of America: Measures of the African Brain Drain." *Human Resources for Health* 2 (7): 1–10.

Hall, E. J. 2004. "Nursing Attrition and the Working Environment in South African Health Facilities." *Curationis* 27 (4): 28–36.

Iliffe, J. 1998. *East African Doctors: A History of the Modern Profession.* Cambridge: Cambridge University Press.

———. 2006. *The African AIDS Epidemic: A History.* Athens: Ohio University Press.

Integrated Regional Information Networks, UN Office for the Coordination of Humanitarian Affairs. 2003. "Africa: Hospitals Are Getting Worse—WHO." Accessed October 24, 2013. http://www.irinnews.org/report/35985/africa-hospitals -are-getting-worse-who.

Jaracz, K., K. Gorna, and J. Konieczna. 2005. "Burnout, Stress and Styles of Coping among Hospital Nurses." *Annales Academiae Medicae Bialostocensis* 50 (Suppl. 1): 216–19.

Jenkins, S. R., and S. Baird. 2002. "Secondary Traumatic Stress and Vicarious Trauma: A Validational Study." *Journal of Traumatic Stress* 15 (5): 423–32.

Kiernan, M., J. Civetta, C. Bartus, and S. Walsh. 2006. "24 Hours On-Call and Acute
Fatigue No Longer Worsen Resident Mood under the 80-Hour Work Week Regulations." *Current Surgery* 63 (3): 237–40.

King, L. A. and P. A. Mcinerney. 2006. "Hospital Workplace Experiences of Registered
Nurses That Have Contributed to Their Resignation in the Durban Metropolitan
Area." *Curationis* 29 (4): 70–81.

Kiragu, K., T. Ngulube, T. Nyumbu, P. Njobvu, P. Eerens, C. Mwaba, and A. Kalimbwe.
2005. "Caring for Caregivers: The HIV/AIDS Needs of Hospital Workers in Zambia."
Horizons Research Summary. Washington: Population Council.

Kirigia, J. M., A. R. Gbary, L. K. Muthuri, J. Nyoni, and A. Seddoh. 2006. "The Cost of
Health Professionals' Brain Drain in Kenya." *BMC Health Services Research* 6 (89):
1–10.

Kober, K., and W. Van Damme. 2006. "Public Sector Nurses in Swaziland: Can the
Downturn Be Reversed?" *Human Resources for Health* 4 (13): 1–11.

Kokonya, D. 2007. Untitled invited presentation at a regional meeting of the World
Psychiatric Association, Nairobi.

Lephoko, C. S. P., M. C. Bezuidenhaut, and J. H. Roos. 2006. "Organisational Climate as
a Cause of Job Dissatisfaction among Nursing Staff in Selected Hospitals within the
Mpumalanga Province." *Curationis* 29 (4): 28–36.

Lert, F., J. F. Chastang, and I. Castanol. 2001. "Psychological Stress among Hospital
Doctors Caring for HIV Patients in the Late Nineties." *AIDS Care* 13 (6): 763–78.

Linzer, M., M. R. Visser, F. J. Oort, E. M. Smets, J. E. McMurray, H. C. de Haes, and
Society of General Internal Medicine Career Satisfaction Study Group. 2001. "Pre-
dicting and Preventing Physician Burnout: Results from the United States and the
Netherlands." *American Journal of Medicine* 111 (2): 170–75.

Lustig, M. 2006. "Balint Groups: An Australian Perspective." *Australian Family Physician* 35 (8): 639–41.

Machoki, M. 1998. "Doing Good: Is It Possible in the HIV/AIDS Pandemic? The Impact of
HIV/AIDS and Depravity on Physician Practice in Kenya." Unpublished manuscript.

Machoki, M., M. Good, E. Mwaikambo, E. Amayo, and L. Muchiri. 1999. "Dilemmas in
Medical Education and Practice." Unpublished manuscript.

Martini, S., C. Arfken, A. Churchill, and R. Balon. 2004. "Burnout Comparison among
Residents in Different Medical Specialties." *Academic Psychiatry* 28 (3): 240–42.

Maslach, C. 1982. *Burnout: The Cost of Coping*. Englewood Cliffs, NJ: Prentice Hall.

Mayers, P. 2005. "HIV/AIDS and the ARV Roll-Out: What Support Do Health Care Providers Need?" *AIDS Bulletin* 14 (1): 37–42.

Maytum, J., M. Bielski-Heiman, and A. Garwick. 2004. "Compassion Fatigue and Burnout in Nurses Who Work with Children with Chronic Diseases and Their Families."
Journal of Pediatric Healthcare 18 (4): 171–78.

McKinlay, J. B., and L. D. Marceau. 2002. "The End of the Golden Age of Doctoring."
International Journal of Health Services 32 (2): 379–416.

McManus, I. C., A. Keeling, and E. Paice. 2004. "Stress, Burnout and Doctors' Attitudes
to Work Are Determined by Personality and Learning Style: A Twelve Year Longitudinal Study of UK Medical Graduates." *BMC Medicine* 2:29.

"Migration of Health Workers: An Unmanaged Crisis." 2005. *Lancet* 365 (9474): 1825.

Miller, D. 2000. *Dying to Care? Work Stress and Burnout in HIV/AIDS*. London: Routledge.

Mullan, F. 2005. "The Metrics of the Physician Brain Drain." *New England Journal of Medicine* 353 (17): 1810–18.

Mungherera, M., A. van der Straten, T. L. Hall, B. Faigeles, G. Fowler, and J. S. Mandel. 1997. "HIV/AIDS-Related Attitudes and Practices of Hospital-Based Health Workers in Kampala, Uganda." *AIDS* 11 (Suppl. 1): S79–85.

Muula, A. 2005. "Is There Any Solution to the 'Brain Drain' of Health Professionals and Knowledge from Africa?" *Croatian Medical Journal* 46 (1): 21–29.

Mwaikambo, E. 2000. "Medical Culture and Training—Ethical Issues and the Physician's Dilemmas of Disclosure in Tanzania." Unpublished manuscript.

Ogunbodede, E. O., M. O. Folayan, and M. A. Adedigba. 2005. "Oral Health-Care Workers and HIV Infection Control Practices in Nigeria." *Tropical Doctor* 35 (3): 147–50.

Olley, B. O. 2003. "A Comparative Study of Burnout Syndrome among Health Professionals in a Nigerian Teaching Hospital." *African Journal of Medicine and Medical Sciences* 32 (3): 297–302.

O'Neill, J., and M. McKinney 2003. "Care for the Caregivers: A Clinical Guide to Supportive and Palliative Care for People with HIV/AIDS." In *A Clinical Guide to Supportive and Palliative Care for HIV/AIDS,* edited by J. F. O'Neill, P. A. Selwyn, and H. Schietinger, chap. 20, Rockville, MD: Health Resources and Services Adminstration.

Oyeyemi, A., B. Oyeyemi, and I. Bello. 2006. "Caring for Patients Living with AIDS: Knowledge, Attitude and Global Level of Comfort." *Journal of Advanced Nursing,* 53 (2): 196–204.

Ozyurt, A., O. Hayran, and H. Sur. 2006. "Predictors of Burnout and Job Satisfaction among Turkish Physicians." *QJM* 99 (3): 161–69.

Payne, N. 2003. "Occupational Stressors and Coping as Determinants of Burnout in Female Hospital Nurses." *Journal of Advanced Nursing* 33 (3): 396–405.

Piko, B. 2006. "Burnout, Role Conflict, Job Satisfaction and Psychosocial Health among Hungarian Health Care Staff: A Questionnaire Survey." *International Journal of Nursing Studies* 43 (3): 311–18.

Poncet, M., P. Toullic, L. Papazian, N. Kentish-Barnes, J. Timsit, F. Pochard, S. Chevret, B. Schlemmer, and E. Azoulay. 2007. "Burnout Syndrome in Critical Care Nursing Staff." *American Journal of Respiratory Critical Care Medicine* 175 (7): 698–704.

Pross, C. 2006. "Burnout, Vicarious Traumatization and Its Prevention: What Is Burnout, What Is Vicarious Traumatization?" *Torture* 16 (1): 1–9.

Radziewicz, R. 2001. "Self-Care for the Caregiver." *Nursing Clinics of North America* 36 (4): 855–69.

Rahlenbeck, S. I. 2004. "Knowledge, Attitude and Practice about AIDS and Condom Utilisation among Health Workers in Rwanda." *Journal of the Association of Nurses in AIDS Care* 15 (3): 56–61.

Raviola, G., M. Machoki, E. Mwaikambo, and M. Good. 2002. "HIV, Disease Plague, Demoralisation and 'Burnout': Resident Experience of the Medical Profession in Nairobi, Kenya," *Culture, Medicine and Psychiatry* 26 (1): 55–86.

Sabin-Farrell, R., and G. Turpin. 2003. "Vicarious Traumatization: Implications for the Mental Health of Health Workers?" *Clinical Psychology Review* 23 (3): 449–80.

Sabo, B. 2006. "Compassion Fatigue and Nursing Work: Can We Accurately Capture the Consequences of Caring Work?" *International Journal of Nursing Practice* 12 (3): 136–42.

Schrecker, T., and R. Labonte. 2004. "Taming the Brain Drain: A Challenge for Public Health Systems in Southern Africa." *International Journal of Occupational and Environmental Health* 10 (4): 409–15.

Schweitzer, B. 1994. "Stress and Burnout in Junior Doctors." *South African Medical Journal* 84 (6): 352–54.

Shanafelt, T., J. Sloan, and T. Haberman. 2003. "The Well-Being of Physicians." *American Journal of Medicine* 114 (6): 513–17.

Shanafelt, T. D., K. A. Bradley, J. E. Wipf, and A. L. Back. 2002. "Burnout and Self-Reported Patient Care in an Internal Medicine Residency Program." *Annals of Internal Medicine* 136 (5): 358–67.

Smit, R. 2004. "HIV/AIDS and the Workplace: Perceptions of Nurses in a Public Hospital in South Africa." *Journal of Advanced Nursing* 51 (1): 22–29.

Smith, M., and G. Anandarajah. 2007. "Mutiny on the Balint: Balancing Resident Developmental Needs with the Balint Process." *Family Medicine* 39 (7): 495–97.

Thomas, L. S., and A. Valli. 2006. "Levels of Occupational Stress in Doctors Working in a South African Public-Sector Hospital." *South African Medical Journal* 96 (11): 1162–68.

Thomas, N. 2004. "Resident Burnout." *Journal of the American Medical Association* 292 (23): 2880–89.

Thomas, R. B., and J. P. Wilson. 2004. "Issues and Controversies in the Understanding and Diagnosis of Compassion Fatigue, Vicarious Traumatization, and Secondary Traumatic Stress Disorder." *International Journal of Emergency Mental Health* 6 (2): 81–92.

UNAIDS. 2000. *Caring for Carers: Managing Stress in Those Who Care for People with HIV and AIDS*. Geneva: UNAIDS.

Van Servellen, G., and Leake. 1993. "Burn-Out in Hospital Nurses: A Comparison of Acquired Immunodeficiency Syndrome, Oncology, General Medicine, and Intensive Care Unit Nurse Samples." *Journal of Professional Nursing* 9 (3): 169–77.

Vos, J., B.Gumudoka, H. A. van Asten, Z. A. Berege, W. M. Dolmans, M. W. Borgdorff, and M. W. Borgdorff. 1998. "Improved Injection Practices after the Introduction of Treatment and Sterility Guidelines in Tanzania." *Tropical Medicine and International Health* 3 (4): 291–6.

Walton, D., P. Farmer, and R. Dillingham. 2005. "Social and Cultural Factors in Tropical Medicine: Reframing Our Understanding of Disease." In *Tropical Infectious Diseases: Principles, Pathogens, and Practice,* edited by R. L. Guerrant, D. H. Walker, and P. F. Weller, 17–22. New York: Elsevier.

Walusimbi, M., and J. C. Okonsky. 2004. "Knowledge and Attitude of Nurses Caring for Patients with HIV/AIDS in Uganda." *Applied Nursing Research* 17 (2): 92–99.

Willcock, S., M. Daly, C. Tennant, and B. Allard. 2004. "Burnout and Psychiatric Morbidity in New Medical Graduates." *Medical Journal of Australia* 181 (7): 357–60.

Working Party of the Royal College of Physicians. 2005. "Doctors in Society: Medical Professionalism in a Changing World." *Clinical Medicine* 5 (6 Suppl 1): S5–40.

Wright, B. 2004. "Compassion Fatigue: How to Avoid It." *Palliative Medicine* 18 (1): 3–4.

Yamey, G., and M. Wilkes. 2001. "Promoting Well-Being among Doctors." *British Medical Journal* 322 (7281): 252–53.

Zelnick, J., and M. O'Donnell. 2005. "The Impact of HIV/AIDS Epidemic on Hospital Nurses in KwaZulu-Natal, South Africa: Nurses' Perspectives and Implications for Health Policy." *Journal of Public Health Policy* 26 (2): 163–85.

10 THE ROLE OF TRADITIONAL HEALERS IN MENTAL HEALTH CARE IN AFRICA

ELIALILIA OKELLO AND SEGGANE MUSISI

AFRICA HAS EXPERIENCED much strife in its recent history, especially south of the Sahara. Most of the continent's countries are characterized by low incomes, high prevalence of communicable diseases, malnutrition, low life expectancy, and poorly staffed services (World Bank 1998). Mental health issues are often last on the list of priorities for policy makers. Health care in general is still poorly funded in most African countries, and mental health services are the least developed and most poorly funded of all health services. Indeed, the majority of African countries do not have a mental health policy, nor do they have mental health programs or action plans (Okasha and Karam 1998).

Traditional healers perform a valuable role in the lives of people in Africa, especially in rural settings. A traditional healer often serves as the primary health care provider for people living in low-income, rural communities. Approximately 80 percent of Africans use traditional healers, and traditional medicine provides a major source of health care for more than 66 percent of the world's population (Kale 1995; Pillay 2002).

The purpose of this chapter is to review the literature on the role of traditional healers in mental illness in Africa. The chapter focuses on the following areas: traditional healers in Africa; traditional definitions and causes of mental illness and traditional healing practices in Africa; the reasons for use of traditional healers in the treatment of mental illness; integrating Western and traditional medicine; evidence on the role of traditional healers in health care; challenges and opportunities for traditional healing systems in Africa; and the legal environment.

TRADITIONAL HEALERS IN AFRICA

The World Health Organization (1978) defines a "traditional healer" as someone who is recognized in his or her community and other communities as competent to provide health services, using plant, animal, and mineral substances as well as other methods based on his or her social, cultural, and religious background. Traditional healers use the prevailing knowledge, attitudes, and beliefs in the community about physical, mental, and social well-being and the causes of disease and disability. Traditional healers share the history, culture, and environment of those who consult them. Because healers are so widely dispersed throughout the African continent, they are well positioned to provide primary health care in the African health care delivery system (Ndulo, Faxelid, and Krantz 2001). Unlike their Western-oriented counterparts, traditional healers do not receive formal training in medical procedures or dispensing medicines. Rather, they acquire their healing knowledge, methods, and skills from the spirits of deceased family healers. In some cases they are chosen by an ancestral spirit (*muzimu,* in Uganda). A study cited by Ann Beck (1985) noted that 74 percent of the sample of traditional healers claimed to have been possessed by a spirit, while 13 percent claimed to have learned the profession through being apprenticed to other healers. Traditional healing is a well-guarded family possession, with its knowledge and skills handed down through the generations. Diviners often look for "signs" in their children to distinguish those to whom they might eventually pass on the traditional healing art. Charles Good (1980) identified the signs of a predestined child, called to the profession of traditional healing. For example, such a child might hold onto some ritualistic object like a twig or an animal skin at a very early age. If the calling is manifested in adulthood, its signs include a prolonged illness characterized by symptoms such as dreams, visions, hallucinations, socially unusual or nonconformist behavior, and the inability to concentrate or stick to one subject. Other signs might manifest themselves through a series of misfortunes affecting the individual's entire family. In particular, women may experience a history of perceived barrenness or the death of their children. Depending on what type of healing is practiced in the community, the treatment of the person called to become a healer may include a calling to acquire traditional powers.

Good (1980) found twelve distinct categories of traditional medico-religious skills in use. Examples include a diviner who also treats patients, a midwife who can "rotate" a fetus, and someone who "opens" a bewitched person. During his study in the Kilungu Hills of Kenya, Good identified several specialties within traditional healing, including diviners, herbalists, midwives, and circumcisers. Other scholars found similar specialties as well as faith healers and traditional birth attendants in Zambia, for example (Ndulo, Faxelid, and Krantz 2001). One detailed investigation narrowed the categories to primarily two basic types, herbalists and the diviners or medium healers (Green 1999).

DEFINITIONS AND CAUSES OF MENTAL ILLNESS IN AFRICAN TRADITIONAL HEALING

In traditional African medicine, mental ill health is defined as a situation in which the victim tends to interpret reality in unusual ways (Ozekhome 1990). In extreme cases of mental illness, the patient may be unable to differentiate between reality and fantasy, may not pay attention to impending danger, and may be unable to recognize people previously known to him or her. Such a person's senses are obviously not functioning properly. Therefore, the traditional healer may need to redirect the patient's consciousness by the use of therapeutic devices. Francis Ozekhome, who practiced traditional medicine for several decades, opined that the mentally ill may be strangely protected by some auratic radiance against evil forces such as spells. According to Ozekhome, this is because there are spiritual aspects to the illness.

In this regard, there is a difference between Western and traditional African medicine, which is reflected in the treatments. Ozekhome writes: "Also, malevolent forces such as witches, wizards, sorcerers, demons and the sorts can cause brain disorder. The causes are usually aimed at punishing a parent through such evil visitations on the offspring, perhaps because attempts to undo such a parent directly or indirectly have proved utterly abortive. On another note, brain disorder could result from contact with a spiritual being whose coded rules might have been transgressed by the weary and at times restless young person" (1990, 113). Mental health care in traditional medicine tends to rely on spiritualism and divination, which often makes it difficult to provide good epistemic explanations to the uninitiated.

Thus, we should expect the management of mental illness by traditional healers in Africa to be radically different from the therapies and procedures used in Western medicine. Traditional healers use divination to understand the mental and psychological problems of their patients. In his influential study of persuasion and healing, Jerome Frank observed: "Since at least part of the efficacy of psychotherapeutic methods lies in the shared belief of participants that these methods will work, the predominant method would be expected to differ in different societies and in different historical epochs" (1974, 3). Psychotherapy has always formed an essential and dynamic basis of African medicine. The traditional healer as a diagnostician must first of all look into the patient's social, cultural, and intellectual environment and background. The healer can then evaluate and interpret the cause of the disease and prescribe the necessary treatment (Abbo 2003).

Many traditional healers show particularly keen insight into the social and psychological causes of illness. For example, when tension arises from the struggles of family members to achieve social recognition and assert their inherent rights, Africans usually seek help from traditional healers, who may perform rituals to restore social harmony. Thus, the traditional healer occupies an important place in social systems in Africa. In a study of traditional healers in Kampala, Uganda, Catherine Abbo (2003) found that they often dealt with social problems, including family problems related to children, a spouse or cowives, or other relatives; problems related to school, work, or finances; problems with neighbors; spiritual or cultural problems; psychosexual problems, including those having to do with relationships, sexual potency, love, and infertility; chronic illnesses that were sometimes not well defined; and epilepsy and madness. The healers' effectiveness, however, was most evident in the first three categories of problems. Abbo also noted that traditional healers used a broad range of practices, including herbalism and spiritualism, and included individuals who called themselves diviners, priests, and faith healers.

REASONS FOR THE USE OF TRADITIONAL HEALERS IN MENTAL ILLNESS

People have various reasons for using traditional healers. These include explanatory models of mental illness that are accepted by the community; the healers' accessibility and patients' convenience; and problems with other available health care systems.

Community Explanatory Models of Mental Illness

African communities believe some conditions are cultural and traditional rather than medical, and therefore they are not amenable to treatment by Western medicine. The consumer consciously and rationally decides which particular health service to consult for a particular ailment, even if this requires shopping around for treatment or even taking long trips to consult healers. Sometimes patients or their significant others feel that spirits have caused the illness. There is little to gain from challenging such views, as doing so would only make the person feel uncomfortable. Instead, health care providers should try to understand and respect these beliefs and try to explain the biomedical explanatory model in simple language.

The findings of studies conducted in Uganda on explanatory models for various subtypes of depression (Okello and Ekblad 2006; Okello and Musisi 2006; Okello and Neema 2007) are summarized as follows.

Nonpsychotic depressive symptoms were conceptualized as a problem related to thoughts (thinking too much) rather than emotions (sadness) or behavior, and the resulting condition was referred to as "illness of thoughts." This was considered a nonchronic condition caused by worrisome thoughts about psychosocial problems, which was not perceived to require Western medication. Lay help from the patient's social groups—such as religious groups, close relatives, elders, friends, and traditional healers—was seen as the appropriate solution.

Depression with psychotic features or with mood-congruent delusions was seen as a clan illness (*eByekika*) and was believed to have its origins in a faulty relationship between the living and the dead. Its management, therefore, required dealing with this relationship problem. The illness belonged to what the Baganda referred to as a Kiganda illness (an illness that has its origin in the collective group customs and the relationships of the Baganda people to others in their clans). The healing process might involve a traditional healer, the patient, and the clan members performing group ancestor worship (*kusamira*), for example.

The explanatory models of depression used by lay people, Western-trained psychiatrists, and traditional healers differed. However, there were similarities in the views that lay people and traditional healers had of the definition, cause, and treatment for depression. These similarities influenced people's choice of healers.

Accessibility and Convenience of Traditional Healers

The services provided by traditional healers are accessible, affordable, flexible, and appropriate to cultural settings. Every African village has a traditional healer, and these healers share the community's concepts of disease and offer clients a more convenient mode of payment than Western health care providers do.

Accessibility

Traditional healers often outnumber Western doctors by at least a hundred to one in most African countries. The healers provide a large pool of accessible, available, and affordable trained health care providers. The World Health Organization (2002) estimates that in sub-Saharan Africa today, approximately 80 percent of the general population consults traditional healers for health and/or personal reasons, regardless of the patient's social, economic, or educational status. In Uganda, for example, it is estimated there is one traditional healer per 100 people, while the number of medical doctors ranges from one to 10,000 people in the cities to one to 50,000 people in rural communities (Green 1999).

As in many developing countries, traditional healers in Uganda are consulted as doctors, counselors, and diviners for a wide range of physical and emotional issues. HIV/AIDS has presented traditional healers with a new challenge, and they have responded in a number of ways. Traditional healers have remained an important source of health care in Africa for the following reasons:

- They possess many effective treatments and treatment methods, especially for emotional, spiritual, and social issues.
- They provide client-centered, personalized health care that is culturally appropriate, holistic, and tailored to meet the needs and expectations of the patient.
- They are culturally close to clients, which facilitates communication about disease and related social issues.
- They often see their patients in the presence of other family members, which can allow the healer to promote social cohesion and stability.
- They are plentiful, accessible, and user-friendly (not arrogant).
- They deal with cultural illness or life concepts not addressed by Western medicine, such as bad luck and issues having to do with success in business, studies, love, or politics.

Since traditional healers occupy a critical role in African societies, they are not likely to disappear soon. They survived even strict colonial legislation forbidding their practices. And traditional healers play a crucial role in addressing a variety of psychosocial problems that arise from conflicting expectations of societies undergoing rapid social and cultural changes.

Convenience

Money is a problem in poverty-ridden Africa. Maja Naur (2000) has reported that the payment for traditional healers' services can be in the form of livestock or other personal possessions instead of money. Furthermore, although traditional healers may command high fees for their services, sometimes exceeding those of Western doctors, healers are paid in full only if the patient is cured. Traditional healers require an initial payment, at which time a future payment is discussed. If the patient is not cured or his or her condition does not improve, the healer usually receives nothing beyond the initial payment. Sometimes, of course, there are disagreements about the criteria used to determine whether a patient's health has improved enough for the healer to receive another payment. However, the main reason clients choose traditional healers is their effectiveness in curing ill health. Referrals and consultations are part and parcel of the traditional healing procedures. For example, if a patient's illness does not respond to herbal treatment, the herbalist concludes that there is something else present in the sickness. The diviner is called, and the cause is sought in a wider context. George Ndege (2001) has discussed the African's holistic perception of health and disease as an integrated concept that considers not only the biological malfunctions of the body but also the religious, moral, political, and economic influences that affect the body.

In addition, Africans view health as transcending the mere absence of disease, recognizing that the body and the mind must be in a harmonious state of wellness that is recognized and accepted by both the individual and society. Ndege's framework of health and disease include the role of the traditional healer and the following three underlying principles that he or she brings to health care delivery. First, the healer ensures that the patient and his or her symptoms are taken seriously and fears are abated. Second, the healer considers the whole individual, dealing with the mind and body together instead of separately. Finally, the healer never considers the individual in isolation but as a member of the family and the community. Accordingly, "the etiology and symptomology of disease is rarely, if ever, characterized as simply the result of a malfunctioning organ or bodily lesion, whether spontaneous or initiated by some physical cause. Instead, disease is . . . a rupture of life's harmony" (Good 1980, 17).

Problems with Other Health Care Systems

Dissatisfaction with the Western health care system—including its inadequate supplies of drugs, arrogant health care workers, and the long distances to health facilities—all mitigate against its use in treating mental illness. Practitioners of Western medicine realize that the holistic approach of traditional healers can work to calm a patient and facilitate healing through the elimination of stress, which instead can be increased by unfamiliar treatment. A patient who has faith in the healing powers of traditional medicines can derive from them a psychological sense of wellness, belonging, and awareness of self, which in turn can help alleviate pain and suffering and facilitate healing.

INTEGRATING WESTERN AND TRADITIONAL MEDICINE

Due to the high costs of Western medicine and fierce competition by other high-priority areas for scarce resources from national governments in Africa, adequate Western health services will probably not be made available to all in the foreseeable future. Therefore, both practical and economic reasons exist to integrate traditional and Western health care systems. This is not a new idea. Various options for integrating the two systems have been suggested by several studies:

Option 1: The complete professionalization of traditional healing along Western lines (Nzima, Edwards, and Makunga 1992). Traditional healers would end up being registered or licensed to practice their profession.

Option 2: Cooperation and collaboration (Freeman and Motsei 1992; Okello et al. 2006). Both systems would essentially retain their autonomy, but cooperate, with each respecting the importance and value of the other. Today joint treatment of patients, whether for psychiatric or other ailments, is forbidden in modern hospitals in most African countries. However, Western-trained healers often tolerate traditional healers' involvement because patients and/or their relatives insist on it. This occurs with both inpatients and outpatients, and with patients who are highly educated and/or prominent in politics and business. A major challenge in Africa is that there are often clashes between traditional and Western ways of doing things. However, this duality is part of modern Africa.

Option 3: Incorporation (Freeman 1992). Traditional healers would only carry out functions that were approved by their Western counterparts. This option is unlikely to be accepted by traditional healers.

Option 4: Total integration, or a complete merger between the two systems (Freeman 1992). This would entail creating a completely new healing system in which both systems would be equally acceptable and respectable. This, too, is unlikely to happen.

Several attempts at the integration of traditional and Western healing systems using one or more of the strategies discussed above have been undertaken in African countries such as the Côte d'Ivoire, Lesotho, Mozambique, Nigeria, Senegal, South Africa, and Zimbabwe (Freeman 1992). To some extent, all these experiments have met with some, but not complete, success. The lesson from these experiences is that the different strategies used by these countries reflect the possibilities of and problems with different approaches. Contextualized research is thus needed to investigate what will be suitable for each local situation.

The challenge of making mental health care in sub-Saharan Africa available to millions of poor people in remote rural areas, where few if any formal quality health services are available today, is a large one. Policy makers in resource-constrained situations have been unable to answer the question of who can deliver these essential services. Comprehensive mental health care would allow the use of available local resources, including traditional healers. Studies and experiences from other countries, such as China and Korea, have shown that an empowered network of traditional health practitioners, linked to adequate referral facilities, could effectively create an expanded health care system with minimal costs or delays. Traditional healers, traditional birth attendants, and faith healers are ubiquitous throughout Africa, where they represent the first line of care for the population. Traditional practitioners provide at least 80 percent of the health care of rural inhabitants in developing countries. In Africa, traditional healers and traditional birth attendants could thus fulfill the triple role of complementary care providers, treatment adherence counselors, and referral advisors. However, it is important to note that traditional healers will need to be supported if they are to maintain acceptable standards of care and if the effectiveness of their herbal treatments is to be assessed.

EVIDENCE ON THE ROLE OF TRADITIONAL HEALERS

Studies in Africa and Asia and among Native Americans (in both South and North America) have repeatedly shown traditional healing to be effective in treating many common forms of mental illness. Arthur Kleinman and Lilias Sung investigated the traditional healing practices of shamans in Taiwan and concluded that 90 percent of the shamans' patients presented with "chronic self-limited illnesses and masked minor psychological disorders," with 50 percent of patients with the latter conditions presenting as people with somatization (1979, 7). Most of these patients reported improvement after the treatment. The authors concluded that traditional forms of practice led to healing and did not just limit themselves to curing an illness. They argued that for healing to occur, medical care could not be in the abstract but had to be anchored in the patient's particular social and cultural contexts. That would provide the balance between "control of sickness and the provision of meaning to the experience of illness" (1979, 7–8). The universal therapeutic components of psychotherapy have been noted to be present and effective in both traditional and Western treatments.

Other studies in Thailand and Cambodia have attested to the need for and use of traditional healing systems in dealing with the mental problems of populations that have been massively traumatized by war (see, for example, Van de Put and Eisenbruch 2002). These studies present evidence showing that traditional beliefs and traditional healers of many kinds were essential in offering people at least a continuous identity in the massive turmoil that threatened their existence and culture, and that any intervention aimed at alleviating the psychological suffering of the war-traumatized people needed to be complementary to or at least be informed by the work of the traditional healers.

In Africa, Seggane Musisi and coauthors (2000) also found that many war-traumatized individuals resorted to traditional and faith healing practices to deal with their massive psychological problems. Researchers in Latin America described the beneficial role of traditional healers, including the *curanderos*, in helping the massively traumatized local indigenous Indian populations during the displacements by hurricanes, for example (Desjarlais et al. 1995). The work done in Uganda by Abbo (2003) identified several methods of work by traditional healers. The following are some of the approaches that patients felt were help-ful: talking therapies (psychotherapies and counseling); behavioral modifica-tion therapies (including rituals, drumming and dancing, and interactive group therapies); and spiritual, or faith, healing (including spirit consultations, praying, possession states, and the use of protective artifacts) and ancestor worship.

Impressive evidence exists for the important role of traditional healers in providing care for people infected with HIV/AIDS and dealing with their at-tendant psychosocial issues (Traditional and Modern Health Practitioners To-gether against AIDS 2001). In South Africa, traditional healers formally involved in community-based directly observed therapies for tuberculosis have helped achieve compliance and cure rates of 75 percent or more, which was far above the national average and better than what had been previously accomplished by many standard community-based directly observed therapy program.

In Uganda, Traditional and Modern Health Practitioners Together against AIDS (2001) and other organizations have involved thousands of African tradi-tional healers in the prevention of HIV/AIDS and other sexually transmitted dis-eases, and in care for patients with those diseases. Once equipped with adequate knowledge, skills, and support, these traditional healers have efficiently integrated biomedical information of HIV/AIDS into their practices and have performed as well, if not better than, community health workers in educating communities; promoting the use of condoms and distributing them; and counseling, treating, and referring to other health care providers people who have HIV/AIDS. These healers have reached millions of individuals infected and affected by HIV/AIDS and have remained actively engaged years after their initial involvement, a defi-nite advantage in sustainability over conventional community health workers.

Studies indicate that traditional medicine is not only the most common and accessible health care provided around the world but also that, taken as a whole, it consists of a large body of knowledge passed on for centuries, from which close to half of our modern drugs have been discovered. For example, herbs found useful in mental health problems include St. John's wort for depression, kava for anxiety, ginkgo biloba for dementia, and rauwolfia for psychosis.

CHALLENGES AND OPPORTUNITIES FOR TRADITIONAL HEALING SYSTEMS IN AFRICA

One of the many challenges facing the health care system in Africa is the need to incorporate the various strands of medicine used by Africa's diverse popu-lation. In particular, there is some resurgence of interest in traditional healing methods as practiced by indigenous Africans. Although traditional and Western health systems have operated side by side in Africa since the advent of European interventions, Western healing has enjoyed greater official acceptance by governments because it was seen to be based on scientific and rational knowledge. In contrast, traditional healing has been officially frowned upon and marginalized by governments and religious leaders because it was perceived to be based on mystical, magical, and satanic religious beliefs (Freeman 1992). Consequently, massive amounts of state and private resources have been poured into Western medicine at the expense of its traditional counterpart. This is in spite of the fact that more than 70 percent of Africans consult traditional healers (Bodibe 1992).

THE LEGAL ENVIRONMENT

Surprisingly, even though the majority of Africans use traditional medicine, it is illegal in many African nations. A survey of the legal status of traditional and complementary or alternative medicine by the World Health Organization (2001) revealed that of the forty-four African nations surveyed, 61 percent had statutes regulating traditional medicine. However, such statues have not always been enforced. Often, the responsibility for certifying practitioners is assigned to a local governmental authorities and there is no national uniformity. Seventeen nations have local and national councils to supervise the practice of traditional medicine. However, no African nation surveyed provided insurance or financial reimbursement for the use of traditional medicine.

The World Health Organization classifies collaborations between national health care and traditional medicine systems as integrative, inclusive, or tolerant. No African nation is categorized as having an integrative system, and only three countries—Ghana, Nigeria, and South Africa—have an inclusive one. The majority of other countries in Africa have tolerant systems. In this category, the national health care system is based entirely on Western medicine, and the law tolerates only some traditional practices. These laws are often ignored, and in practice traditional medicine is accepted and tolerated throughout Africa. Pressure from organized Western medicine also helps sideline traditional medicine, keeping it out of policy discussions and specifically out of strategic plans for and official systems of national health care.

Relatively few countries have developed a policy on traditional healing practices (World Health Organization 2002). Yet such a policy would provide a sound basis for defining the role of traditional practices in national health care delivery and could ensure that the necessary regulatory and legal mechanisms were created for promoting and maintaining good practices. To maximize the potential of traditional healing practices as a source of health care, a number of issues need to be tackled. The development of standards and methods for evaluating safety, efficacy, and quality is crucial.

Traditional healers are considered the most important link between the rural Africans and health care delivery. The healers use their knowledge of methods and practices that have evolved in the social, cultural, and spiritual context of the communities the healers serve. Traditional healers are entrusted with the lives of many people who otherwise would have no recourse but to suffer or to travel long distances to see Western physicians. Traditional healers continue to thrive in the modern era in a continent with numerous health problems and great poverty, and their contribution to health care deserves to be noticed. Traditional healers will continue to play a valuable role in resolving the problems related to the physical and mental anguish of illness and the associated hardships. However, policies to define the role of traditional practices in national health care systems, as well as regulatory and legal mechanisms to promote good practices and the use of standards for safety and measures to assess the effectiveness of traditional treatments, must be created. Further contextualized research is needed to understand how collaboration could occur on a local basis that would demonstrate the contributions of both forms of health care delivery.

REFERENCES

Abbo, C. 2003. "Management of Mental Health Problems by Traditional Healers as Seen in Kampala, Uganda." Master's thesis, Makerere University, Department of Psychiatry.

Beck, A. 1985. "Old and New Approaches to Medicine in Rhodesia and Zimbabwe." In *African Healing Strategies,* edited by B. M. du Toit and I. H. Abdalla, 182–89. Owerri, Nigeria: Trado-Medic Books.

Bodibe, R. 1992. "Traditional Healing: An Indigenous Approach to Mental Health Problems." In *Psychological Counselling in the South African Context,* edited by J. Uys, 149–65. Cape Town: Maskew Miller Longman.

Desjarlais, R., L. Eisenberg, B. Good, and A. Kleinman. 1995. *World Mental Health: Problems and Priorities in Low-Income Countries.* Oxford: Oxford University Press.

Frank, J. D. 1974. *Persuasion and Healing: A Comparative Study of Psychotherapy.* New York: Schocken.

Freeman, M. 1992. *Recognition and Registration of Traditional Healers: Possibilities and Problems.* Johannesburg: Centre for Health Policy, Department of Community Health, University of the Witwatersrand.

Freeman, M., and M. Motsei. 1992. "Planning Health Care in South Africa: Is There a Role for Traditional Healers?" *Social Science and Medicine* 34 (11): 1183–90.

Good, C. M. 1980. "A Comparison of Rural and Urban Ethnomedicine among the Kamba in Kenya." In *Traditional Health Care Delivery in Contemporary Africa,* edited by P. R. Ulin, M. H. Segall, and C. M. Good, 13–56. Syracuse, NY: Maxwell School of Citizenship and Public Affairs Syracuse University Press.

Green, E. C. 1999. "Engaging Indigenous African Healers in the Prevention of AIDS and STDS." In *Anthropology in Public Health: Bridging Differences in Culture and Society,* edited by R. A. Hahn, 63–83. New York: Oxford University Press.

Kale, R. 1995. "Traditional Healers in South Africa: A Parallel Health Care System: South Africa's Health." *British Medical Journal* 310 (6988): 1182–86.

Kleinman, A., and L. H. Sung. 1979. "Why Do Indigenous Practitioners Successfully Heal?" *Social Science and Medicine* 13 (1): 7–26.

Musisi, S., E. Kinyanda, E. Liebling, and K Mayengo. 2000. "Posttraumatic Torture Disorders in Uganda—A Three-Year Retrospective Study of Patient Records as Seen at a Specialized Torture Treatment Center in Kampala, Uganda." *Torture* 10 (3): 81–87.

Naur, M. 2000. "Indigenous Knowledge and HIV/AIDS: Ghana and Zambia." *IK Notes,* March 2001. www.worldbank.org/afr/ik/iknt30.pdf.

Ndege, G. 2001. *Health, State, and Society in Kenya.* Rochester, NY: University of Rochester Press.

Ndulo, J., E. Faxelid, and I. Krantz. 2001. "Traditional Healers in Zambia and Their Care for Patients with Urethral/Vaginal Discharge." *Journal of Alternative and Complementary Medicine* 7 (5): 529–36.

Nzima, D., S. Edwards, and N. Makunga. 1992. "Professionalization of Traditional Healers in South Africa: A Case Study." *University of Zululand Journal of Psychology* 88 (1), 82–91.

Okasha, A., and E. Karam. 1998. "Mental Health Services and Research in the Arab World." *Acta Psychiatrica Scandinavica* 98 (5): 406–13.

Okello, E., and S. Ekblad. 2006. "Lay Concepts of Depression among the Baganda of Uganda: A Pilot Study." *Journal of Transcultural Psychiatry* 43 (2): 287–313.

Okello, E., and S. Musisi. 2006. "Depression as a Clan Illness (eByekika): An Indigenous Model of Psychotic Depression among the Baganda of Uganda." *Journal of World Cultural Psychiatry Research Review* 1 (2): 60–67.

Okello, E., and S. Neema. 2007. "Explanatory Models and Help-Seeking Behaviour: Pathways to Psychiatric Care among Patients Admitted for Depression in Mulago Hospital, Kampala, Uganda." *Journal of Qualitative Health Research* 17 (1): 14–25.

Okello, E. S., C. Abbo, S. Musisi, and C. Tusaba. 2006. "Incorporating Traditional Healers in Primary Mental Health Care in Uganda." *Makerere University Research Journal* 001 (2): 139–48.

Ozekhome, F. 1990. *The Theory and Practice of Traditional Medicine in Nigeria.* Lagos, Nigeria: Okey Okwechime.

Pillay, A. L. 2002. "Rural and Urban South African Women's Awareness of Cancers of the Breast and Cervix." *Ethnicity and Health* 7 (2): 103–14.

Traditional and Modern Health Practitioners Together against AIDS. 2001. *Contributions of Traditional Medicine to Health Care Deliveries in Uganda.* Kampala: Uganda Ministry of Health.

Van de Put, W. A. C. M., and M. Eisenbruch. 2002. "The Cambodian Experience." In *Trauma, War and Violence: Public Mental Health in a Social-Cultural Context,* edited by J. De Jong, 93–155. New York: Kluwer Academic Publishers.

World Bank. 1998. *African Development Indicators 1998/99.* Washington: World Bank.

World Health Organization. 1978. *The Promotion and Development of Traditional Medicine.* Geneva: World Health Organization.

———. 2001. *The World Health Report: Mental Health: New Understanding, New Hope.* Geneva: World Health Organization.

———. 2002. *Traditional Medicine Strategy, 2002–2005.* Geneva: World Health Organization.

11 IMPROVING ACCESS TO PSYCHIATRIC MEDICINES IN AFRICA

SHOBA RAJA, SARAH KIPPEN WOOD,
AND MICHAEL R. REICH

THE WORLD HEALTH Organization (WHO) recommends a combined psycho-social and pharmacological approach to treating mental illness (2001). However, the limited availability of the essential medicines recommended by the WHO contributes significantly to the mental health treatment gap in most of Africa. The irregular supply of medicines seriously undermines intervention efforts, especially community-based mental health treatment initiatives. BasicNeeds is an international mental health organization that works with poor people with mental disorders in ten low-income countries in Asia and Africa. The organization does not generally provide direct treatment services, nor does it promote one form of treatment over another. BasicNeeds works through local partner organizations—often governments—to optimize the use of scarce medical treatment resources. Current governmental support for mental health interventions in Africa is limited, and it is largely allocated to pharmaceutical treatment. Limited access to psychiatric medicine therefore prevents many people in Africa from receiving any treatment for mental disorders. Accordingly, BasicNeeds has taken a considerable interest in studying the access and availability of psychiatric medicine in each country it serves. This chapter is based on four independent but simultaneous studies undertaken by BasicNeeds in 2007 in Ghana, Uganda, Kenya, and Tanzania. These studies investigated factors in government systems that contributed to shortages in psychiatric medicines as well as the perspectives of both caregivers and patients on how shortages and erratic supply of medicines affect them.

This chapter draws on these studies to examine the management of the psychiatric medicine supply in the public sector in Africa, with some reference to the situation in the private sector. The processes of selection, procurement, distribution, and use of psychiatric medicines are examined in each country. Additionally, the Kangemi Health Center, in Kenya, is examined as a case study on recent trends in the consumption of psychiatric medicines. Key issues are highlighted, including inconsistent government financing, inadequate prescribing and dispensing personnel, poor estimates of the needed volumes of drugs, and outdated lists of essential medicines. Finally, we draw on our analysis to suggest several actions that could help improve access to psychiatric medicines in Africa.

ACCESS TO ESSENTIAL MEDICINES

The WHO recommends a periodically updated list of essential medicines to satisfy high-priority health care needs in every country (World Health Organization 2007). However, in the poorest parts of Africa, over half the population lacks regular access to these essential medicines. "Access" refers to a consumer's ability to obtain and use essential medicines. When speaking of access, one must consider both "availability," defined as the supply aspects of access, and "affordability," referring both to the government's ability to procure medicines and the consumer's ability to buy them (Frost and Reich 2008).

Recent research highlights some of the issues surrounding access to essential medicines in Africa. The lack of adequate personnel to prescribe and dispense medication poses a pervasive barrier to improving access to essential medicines in health care systems, affecting both the supply and demand for essential medicines. Simply allocating increased funding to health care systems will not improve access to medical treatment without confronting this human resources crisis (Narasimhan et al. 2004).

Additionally, governments must carefully consider whether they should produce essential medicines locally or import them. In some countries, importation may prove more cost-effective than producing medicines locally. Another potential mechanism to improve access to psychiatric medicines in Africa is the development of public-private partnerships to advance mental health treatment (Reich 2000).

The informal private sector also plays an important role in providing medicine to poor people in Africa, as shown by the anthropological research by Susan Reynolds Whyte, Sjaak van der Geest, and Anita Hardon (2002). In Uganda, for example, medicines that are sold in private-sector drug shops (often near hospital pharmacies) are sometimes the only ones poor people can afford. The sources of the drugs sold in these shops and their prescribing policies, however, remain questionable and problematic (Jitta, Whyte, and Nshakira 2003). These unauthorized sellers may undermine efforts mandated by the government to provide safe and efficacious medical treatment. But at the same time, other than local traditional healers, the informal private sector often represents for many poor people their main alternative to no pharmaceutical medication at all.

UNIQUE ACCESS CHALLENGES FOR PSYCHIATRIC MEDICINES

Although access to all essential medicines in Africa is inadequate, the nature of psychiatric medicines presents some unique challenges. The *WHO Model List of Essential Medicines* categorizes psychotherapeutic medicines under psychosis; mood disorders, both depressive and bipolar; obsessive compulsive and panic disorders; generalized anxiety and sleep disorders; and substance dependence. Some overlap exists between medicines recommended for psychotherapeutics and epilepsy (World Health Organization 2007). We briefly examine three specific factors that limit the availability and affordability of psychiatric medicines: lack of knowledge about psychotropic drug treatment, drug patent law regulations, and the propensity for drug abuse.

Lack of Knowledge

Government leaders frequently cite a lack of evidence-based research on psychiatric treatment alternatives as an important reason why mental health remains a low priority on their health care agendas. Most studies of the effectiveness of psychiatric medicines are performed in high-income countries. But studies on the cost-effectiveness of these treatments in North America have little relevance to countries in Africa. As a result, decisions on budget allocations for mental health treatment are not well informed in developing countries (Knapp et al. 2006).

Recent studies in low- and middle-income countries are beginning to show that community-based mental health care through the primary health care system can be a more cost-effective and appropriate treatment alternative to long-term, institutionalized care (Patel 2007). However, community approaches to mental health intervention, although accepted in principle, are not yet widespread in practice. For example, current mental health policies in Ghana tend to be institution-based despite proclaimed government policies designed to decentralize mental health services (Appiah-Kubi, Raja, and Boyce, 2008). Older generations of essential medicines can be more cost-effective in a community-based setting than some of the newer medicines that have shown to be only slightly more efficacious (Saxena et al. 2007). However, older generic pharmaceutical treatments are sometimes overlooked in favor of more expensive brand-name pharmaceuticals. Such inefficient use of resources diminishes access to psychiatric medicines. Mental health consumers must then turn to the private sector for their treatment. Since medicines in the private sector can be both expensive and unavailable in many areas, this is not a viable alternative for many mental health consumers in Africa (Gelders et al. 2006).

Drug Patents

International efforts to expand patent protection for medicines around the world could also reduce access to new psychiatric medicines in Africa. The most important event in this field was the Agreement on Trade-Related Aspects of Intellectual Property Rights (TRIPS) in 1995, which extends patent protection to many countries and provides a minimum of twenty years' patent protection for pharmaceuticals, including psychiatric drugs. In 2001, however, the Doha Agreement extended the deadline to 2016 for the world's least developed countries to comply with TRIPS. This extension could allow some potentially affordable generic medicines (produced, for example, in India or China) to be sold in African countries that have not yet passed patent protection for new medicines. Another possible mechanism is the use of compulsory licensing, which allows a national government to exempt certain products from patent protection if they are used to treat life-threatening diseases or are necessary during a national emergency. However, psychiatric medicines are not generally considered eligible for this exemption. Pharmacological treatment and prescribing practices for psychiatric medicines have made significant progress in the past few years. These increasingly strict rules for patent protection of new medicines, therefore, could contribute to delayed access (through higher prices) of new products that might be more efficacious or have fewer side effects for poor people in Africa. Additionally, the removal of some generic pharmaceuticals produced in India or China could reduce access to new psychiatric medicines in Africa (De Silva and Hanwella 2008).

Drug Abuse

Some psychiatric medicines are addictive and thus liable to be misused. Psychotropic drug abuse at the prescriber, dispenser, and user levels has increased in recent years, particularly in Africa. Such misuse can contribute to drug shortages. This has sparked an interest in added government controls on certain psychotropic drugs (Odejide 2006). An unfortunate consequence of such regulations is that they can make it substantially more difficult to import certain psychotropic drugs on a country's list of essential medicines, further contributing to drug shortages. In Ghana, interviewees reported that psychiatric medicine is difficult to find in both the public and private sectors due to these restrictions. Clearly, the propensity for misuse must be weighed against access limitations imposed by governmental restrictions.

The WHO has recognized some of these barriers to access to psychiatric medicines in low- and middle-income countries and has provided a framework for improving access. Four factors are considered important for systematic improvement: rational selection process, affordable prices, sustainable financing, and reliable health care and supply systems (World Health Organization 2005a). Exploring each phase of the public-sector drug management cycle, as well as listening to the various (and sometimes conflicting) perspectives of key players, can inform policy and implementation decisions that will improve access to psychiatric medicine in Africa.

Through literature reviews of government policy documents, in-depth interviews with key players, and observations at service points, we identified specific challenges to access to psychotropic medicines in Uganda, Kenya, Ghana, and Tanzania (Raja et al. 2008). Our findings from these public-sector studies form the basis for the following discussion of issues related to access that occur during the selection, procurement, distribution, and use phases of the drug management cycle. This analysis leads to a number of concrete proposals to improve access to psychiatric medicines in Africa.

NATIONAL ESSENTIAL DRUG LISTS

The WHO identified a limited number of psychiatric medicines to be included in the WHO *Model List of Essential Medicines* (World Health Organization 2001, 2007). The WHO updates its list of psychiatric medicines every two years based on their relevance, efficacy, and safety, in order to represent treatment that should be available for high-priority mental health care. The list of essential psychotropic medicines is updated based on improvements in efficacy and cost and reductions of side effects. In response to WHO recommendations, many African countries have added psychiatric products to their lists of essential medicines. Nevertheless, our studies found that country-level information on psychiatric medications is updated infrequently, and items on the essential medicines list are either unavailable at the most accessible points of delivery or not available at all.

Tanzania, Uganda, Kenya, and Ghana each has an essential psychiatric medicines list modeled after the WHO list. In each country, the Ministry of Health has appointed a Pharmacy and Therapeutics Committee to select efficacious, safe, and cost-effective medicines. All of the medicines on each list are in principle reviewed every two years and the list is amended, but this does not happen in practice. As of 2007, the public mental health care sector in Uganda was operating with the 2001 list despite more recent revisions.

Table 11.1 shows which psychotropic drugs from the WHO *Model List of Essential Medicines* (World Health Organization 2007) were included in the national medicines lists of Kenya (Republic of Kenya Ministry of Health 2003), Ghana (Ghana Ministry of Health 2004), Uganda (Uganda National Drug Authority 2001), and Tanzania (United Republic of Tanzania Ministry of Health 1997) as of

Table 11.1. National and World Health Organization (WHO) Essential Drug Lists

WHO (2007)	UGANDA (2001)	KENYA (2003)	GHANA (2004)	TANZANIA (1997)
PSYCHOTHERAPEUTIC				
Psychosis				
Chlorpromazine	B*	B	B*	A
Fluphenazine	D	C	Not included	C
Haloperidol	D	C	D	B
Depressive mood disorders				
Amitryptiline	B*	C	D	C
Fluoxetine	Not included	Not included	D	Not included
Bipolar mood disorders				
Carbamazepine	Not included	C	D	Not included
Lithium carbonate	D	D	Not included	D
Valproic acid	D	Not included	Not included	Not included
Generalized anxiety and sleep disorders				
Diazepam	Not included	C	B*	Not included
Obsessive compulsive and panic disorders				
Clomipramine	Not included	Not included	Not included	D
Substance dependence				
Methadone**	Not included	Not included	Not included	Not included
ANTIEPILEPTIC/ANTICONVULSANT				
Carbamazepine	B*	C	D	D
Diazepam	B*	A	B	A
Magnesium sulphate	Not included	Not included	C	D
Phenobarbital	D	A	B*	A
Phenytoin	B*	C	B*	A
Valproic acid	D	D	Not included	D
Ethosuximide**	C	C	D	D

Note: Years indicate when each list was last updated. Letters indicate the lowest level of health care where each drug is approved to be available: A is dispensary, B is health center, C is district or subdistrict hospital, and D is regional or referral hospital. * indicates that the health center must have a qualified medical practitioner. ** indicates that a medicine is essential for priority diseases but may not be cost-effective in a particular setting.

April 2007. The table also indicates the lowest level of health care at which each medicine could be dispensed. Medicines that were not included in the 2007 WHO list were omitted from the table.

Selected medicines may be distributed only to certain health unit levels, a decision that usually depends on the availability of qualified staff members to prescribe and dispense psychiatric medication. Dispensaries represent the lowest level of health care, and very few psychiatric drugs are prescribed and distributed there. Health workers trained in mental health care are very rare in dispensaries. Health centers are usually located at the community level and may be directed by a doctor or clinical officer. In some health centers, however, qualified medical practitioners do not appear regularly. District and subdistrict hospitals are often found in urban areas. Regional and referral hospitals often have psychiatrists on staff.

What Is Missing from the National Lists

The antidepressant fluoxetine was not on any of the national lists except that of Ghana, where it was available only at regional or referral hospitals (Ghana Ministry of Health 2004). Fluoxetine (marketed as Prozac) is a member of a class of second-generation antidepressants known as serotonin-specific reuptake inhibitors (SSRIs). As the only SSRI included on the 2007 WHO list, fluoxetine has been shown to be as efficacious as, and to produce fewer side effects than, the first-generation antidepressants such as amitriptyline (Brambilla et al. 2005).

Although fluoxetine may be available on the private market in both Kenya and Uganda, it is not necessarily affordable to poor people. A 2006 comparative analysis on the affordability of chronic disease medication revealed that the lowest paid unskilled government worker in Kenya would need to work 20.2 days to pay for one month's supply of generic fluoxetine. In Uganda, 7.2 days' wages would be needed. Conversely, one month's supply of amitriptyline was available in the private sector for 1.8 days' wage in Uganda and just 0.8 day's wage in Kenya (Gelders et al. 2006).

Notably, although fluoxetine was listed on Ghana's essential medicines list, it was not found in any of the public health facilities, and in 3 percent of facilities in the private sector only the brand-name (nongeneric) form was found (Gelders et al. 2006). Promoting the public-sector use of generic fluoxetine may make this medicine more affordable to mental health patients.

Additionally, chlomipramine was the only medicine on the 2007 WHO list for obsessive compulsive and panic disorders, and it appeared only on Tanzania's national list (United Republic of Tanzania 1997). Furthermore, carbamazepine and diazepam were included on the antiepileptic/anticonvulsant portion of all four national lists, but they were listed on the psychotherapeutic portion of only two of the lists. Valproic acid was listed under antiepileptics/anticonvulsants in three countries but listed under psychotherapeutics only on Uganda's list (Uganda National Drug Authority 2001). This suggests that these medicines were primarily used to treat epilepsy, even though they were also recommended by the WHO for the treatment of mental disorders. Even in Kenya and Ghana, whose lists included carbamazepine and diazepam under psychotherapeutics, respondents cited these medicines as frequently unavailable (Republic of Kenya Ministry of Health 2003; Ghana Ministry of Health 2004).

Lack of Medicines at Lower Health Care Levels

Most of the psychotherapeutic drugs on the 2007 WHO list shown in Table 11.1 could be dispensed only at urban hospitals. In each country, only one or two of the recommended psychotherapeutics was available at health centers. Chlorpromazine, a first-generation drug for psychosis, was the only medicine available at health centers in all four countries.

Older Medicines on the Lists

Many older medicines—including imipramine, a first-generation antidepressant, and trifluoperazine, a first-generation antipsychotic drug—that were not included on the 2007 WHO list because they are less efficacious and safer than other first-generation drugs were on all four national lists. Respondents at psychiatry hospitals in Ghana described that country's national list as inadequate because it did not include several essential medicines. One government official also said that the list for psychotherapeutics was inadequate because it did not include new drugs that are much more convenient for the patient to take than older medicines. Some of the health professionals indicated that new drugs such as olanzapine are more effective but were not on the national list. This lack of inclusion compels prescribers to use drugs available only in the private sector, which adds to the consumer's cost. At the time of this research in 2007, Ghana's national list had been last revised in 2004, although few alterations were made at that time to the psychotherapeutic medicines section of the list.

Lack of Understanding about Mental Health Treatment

The lack of understanding about mental health treatment among decision makers is a serious impediment to access to medicines. For example, a few district mental health officials and health workers in Uganda felt that the government has an insufficient understanding of pharmacological treatment for mental disorders. Government officials with decision-making powers on resource allocation for psychiatric medications believe that mental illness is not very prevalent and should not compete for government funds with pharmacological treatments for HIV and malaria. There is also a lack of understanding about the chronic nature of mental disorders. Some government officials do not realize that treatment for mental disorders often requires consistent doses repeated over time. Psychiatric medicines are perceived as the specialty of a few highly trained psychiatrists and taken care of by the national mental health referral hospital, so they are not needed at local health units.

Affordability of Second-Generation Pharmaceuticals

Registration procedures for new medicines can also create barriers to access. The newest generation of psychiatric medicine is not available in Uganda, for example, because the process of registering new medicines is both expensive and bureaucratic. According to the country's National Drug Authority, all new imported medicines must be registered for an initial fee of $1,000 and a $500 retention fee (Uganda National Drug Authority 2008). Uganda must rely on importers to supply psychiatric medicines because only diazepam is manufactured locally. Some respondents indicated that pharmacies were not importing enough psychiatric medicines because of the belief that the national mental health referral hospital would provide them. Each of the countries surveyed imported a substantial portion of their psychiatric medicines.

A more regular periodic review of national lists of psychotherapeutic medicines in these countries is imperative. Efficacy, safety, and affordability must be considered when comparing second-generation and first-generation medicines. Every effort should be made to ensure that these medicines are available at the lowest possible health care level. The belief that mental health care must be provided only at referral hospitals is a major obstacle to access to treatment. Improving access to psychiatric medicine in Africa requires a careful examination of the full range of practices used to select essential medicines for national lists.

PROCUREMENT

Government procurement practices in each of the four countries are somewhat similar and represent a major barrier to access to psychiatric medicines. Tanzania lacks a domestic pharmaceutical industry for psychiatric medicines, so it imports them from India, the United Kingdom, Cyprus, and Germany. The Medical Stores Department, a para-statal organization that operates on a self-sustaining commercial basis, is paid directly by the Tanzanian government to procure, store, and distribute drugs to health centers and dispensaries at more affordable prices than private pharmaceutical companies offer. Accordingly, a standardized monthly kit containing drugs from the national list of essential medicines is provided to hospitals, health centers, and dispensaries.

Psychotropic medicine in Kenya is regulated through the Pharmacy and Poisons Board. Most psychiatric medicines are procured through the Kenya Medical Supplies Agency (KEMSA) via a tendering system with the Kenyan government.

KEMSA drug kits are then distributed to local health centers and dispensaries on a quarterly basis. Supplemental medicines may be purchased through the Nairobi City Council stores. Additionally, international nongovernmental organizations such as Mission for Essential Drugs and BasicNeeds Kenya provide some psychotropic medicines to health facilities in the Westlands Health Division.

In Ghana the Chief Director, the highest ranking official in the Ministry of Health, who reports directly to the Minister, conducts the procurement process by providing budgetary and administrative assistance. The director of procurement, another official in the ministry, oversees the management of the public-sector supply chain. Procurement planning precedes budget approval, which is designed to reduce delays and drug shortages. This involves reviewing the previous procurement plan for such drugs, selecting the appropriate procedure, and estimating the quantities of drugs that need to be procured based on rates of previous use.

In Uganda medicines are procured, stored, and distributed through the National Medical Stores. Systems by which the drugs are purchased include the Primary Health Care recurrent budget and District Medicines Credit Line System. The recurrent budget is managed at the district level, while the Credit Line system was instituted as a supplementary way for health centers to order drugs from the National Medical Stores by billing the Ministry of Health at a later date. The distribution of psychotropic medicines depends on the level of the health care facility and the qualifications of the health workers there.

Drug Shortages

Shortages of psychiatric medicine occur frequently in the public procurement system, according to respondents in each country. A health administrator from Ghana reported that the community psychiatry nurses receive only 60 percent of the drugs they require.

Likewise, Kenya's tender system does not always meet the demand for these medicines. One official admitted: "For the year just ended, no one responded to our advertisement for chlorpromazine injection, so we could not buy it, and the whole year we did not have it."

Limited Budgets for Psychotropic Drugs

Fluctuations in government budgets for psychotropic drugs also contribute to the frequent shortages experienced by the central medical stores in each country. Late government payments lead to drugs being on back order and delays in shipments. As noted above, some countries have alternative ways of purchasing drugs when usual government funds are scarce. However, these alternate plans are not always effective. In the event of a shortage in Tanzania, hospitals may purchase supplementary drugs from private pharmacies, but this must be done through patients' cost sharing or with funds from donors rather than regular government funding. Often, health facilities do not have the funds available to make such needed purchases. Similarly, respondents from Uganda claimed that the District Medicines Credit Line System is inadequate for purchasing needed drugs.

Concerning the low priority given to mental health care during the budget and planning stages, a district mental health coordinator in Tanzania stated: "Every department is asked to prepare a list of requirements but our mental health budget is reduced by the budget committee at the municipal/district level and later on by the Ministry of Health as compared to other diseases. Therefore, we end up with a very small amount of money, which is not enough to buy psychotropic drugs." Without the provision of adequate government funding, the procurement process is irregular and problematic, reducing access to psychiatric medicines.

Push System or Pull System

Psychiatric drug procurement in Tanzania, Kenya, and Uganda operates under what is called a push system, in which standardized kits of medicine are distributed from a national warehouse on a monthly or quarterly basis to each facility, as described above. Many respondents felt that the push system contributes to psychotropic drug shortages. A high-ranking official in Kenya explained: "You can't expect that kit to be effective in all those areas, because you find the workloads and disease patterns vary as you move from one part of the country to another."

In a pull system, in contrast, individual health units place estimates and orders based on actual use. Supply elasticity in the procurement system is crucial to reducing drug shortages. As of 2007, these countries were making some efforts to adopt a pull system for drug supply management, although this practice was not widespread or effective on a national basis.

Private-Sector Support Is Not Adequate

Ghana relies on donor support for all imported medicines; consequently, access to psychiatric medicines often depends on the availability of donor funds. Late payments reduce suppliers' willingness to provide products, further limiting access to psychiatric medicines.

When medicine is unavailable in the public sector, prescribers, dispensers, and users turn to the private sector for needed psychiatric drugs. Unfortunately,

Table 11.2. Medicines Commonly Prescribed in Ghana
but Unavailable in the Public Sector

NOT ON THE NATIONAL LIST OF ESSENTIAL MEDICINES	ON THE LIST BUT FREQUENTLY UNAVAILABLE
Benzhezole (tab.)	Amitriptyline (25mg and 50mg tab.)
Carbamazepine (tab.)	Chlorpromazine (25mg, 50mg, and 100mg tab.; inj.)
Cogentin	Diazepam (5mg and 10mg tab.; inj.)
Emipremin	Haloperidol (5mg and 10mg tab.; inj.)
Fluphenazine (tab.; inj.)	Risperidone
Modicate	Trifluperazine (tab.)
Olanzapine (inj.)	
Phenobarbitone (30mg and 60mg tab.)	
Phenytoin (tab.)	
Tonocebrine	

Source: Ghana interview respondents.
Note: Tab. is tablet. Inj. is injection.

respondents in each country reported that psychiatric drugs are also frequently unavailable in the private sector, or very expensive. Pharmacies in the private sector are also not easily reached by most of the population. For example, 68 percent of the pharmacies in Uganda are in the Kampala District, which has only 5 percent of the country's population.

Table 11.2 shows the medicines that are commonly prescribed in Ghana but that are either not included on the national list of essential medicines or are on the list but are frequently unavailable. These medicines must be purchased through the private sector, often at high prices that many consumers cannot afford. Reliance on the private sector for so many commonly prescribed medications is less than ideal. In such situations, a public-private partnership might benefit both sectors and improve access to needed psychiatric medication.

Bureaucratic Procurement Process

General bureaucratic inefficiencies plague the procurement system for all kinds of medicines in Africa, including psychiatric drugs. The procurement process can be lengthy, and delays are common. Respondents in Uganda, for example, indicated that the National Medical Stores does not currently have the resources required to operate effectively. On average, it takes eight months from the time when an order is placed before the supply is received in Uganda.

DISTRIBUTION

Personnel

An inadequate number of trained mental health personnel in these countries greatly reduces access to psychiatric medication. In Kenya the psychotropic drug registration process through the Pharmacy and Poisons Board is a lengthy one. In addition, certain types of poisons (including many psychotropic drugs) are strictly controlled, requiring a qualified medical practitioner to dispense them. This means that local health centers in the Westlands Division lack the staff necessary to appropriately prescribe and dispense psychotropic drugs. In this division, only two of the ten facilities examined have mental health units. As a result, many local health centers do not dispense psychotropic drugs at all.

In each country many psychotropic drugs are not distributed to primary health centers because there are too few psychiatrists to prescribe them. Patients must travel to district hospitals that have psychiatrists on staff in order to receive psychotropic drugs. This presents a challenge for many people who do not live near a district hospital and cannot afford the travel expenses required on a regular basis.

Quantification

Insufficient training for health workers in recording consumption data and making appropriate estimates for needed drugs presents another significant challenge. Respondents in Kenya stated that their consumption data are not very reliable due to poor recording techniques. Since estimated drug requirements for the coming year are based on consumption data, accurate recording is very important. One Kenyan respondent indicated that some psychiatric nurses do not submit estimations by appointed deadlines, resulting in the underestimation of the psychotropic medication needed. Psychiatric nurses, however, reported that the estimation protocols are often difficult to understand. Increased training in these protocols could help improve the management of the supply chain and access to medicines.

USE

Consumption Trends in Kangemi Health Center

The mental health clinic at Kangemi Health Center is the only public health facility providing mental health services in the entire Westlands District of Nairobi, representing 308,000 people. Facilitated by BasicNeeds Kenya, the mental health program started operations there in May 2006. As part of the study reported in this chapter, the trends in psychotropic drug volumes were examined at this facility for the period of May 2006 to April 2007.

Table 11.3. Number of Psychiatric Drug Prescriptions at
Kangemi Health Center, May 2006 to April 2007

DRUG	NUMBER OF PRESCRIPTIONS	% TOTAL PRESCRIPTIONS
Carbamazepine	667	32
Amitryptiline	323	15
Chlorpromazine	302	14
Phenobarbitone	299	14
Benzhexol	296	14
Diazepam	96	5
Haloperidol	93	4
Fluphenazine (injection)	10	0.5
Other rarely prescribed psychotropics	26	1.5

Table 11.4. Medicines Prescribed and Dispensed at
Kangemi Clinic, May 2006 to April 2007

	NUMBER OF PRESCRIPTIONS	NUMBER OF PRESCRIPTIONS DISPENSED	DEFICIT	% DRUG NEEDS SATISFIED
Carbamazepine	34,431	26,214	-8,217	76
Chlorpromazine	14,089	12,025	-2,064	85
Phenobarbitone	12,862	10,690	-2,172	83
Amitryptiline	10,858	7,185	-3,673	66
Benzhexol	8,775	5,908	-2,867	67
Diazepam	2,557	1,267	-1,290	50
Other rarely prescribed psychotropic drugs	782	555	-227	71

Table 11.3 shows the most prescribed psychiatric medicines at the clinic during that period. Carbamazepine, a drug used to treat both epilepsy and bipolar disorder, was by far the most commonly prescribed medicine. It is also the only psychiatric medicine permitted to be dispensed at most local health centers in Kenya. The discrepancy between prescribed and dispensed medication is shown in table 11.4. The clinic did not entirely meet the prescribed demand for each medicine, with deficiencies ranging from 15 percent for chlorpromazine to 50 percent for diazepam.

The inadequate availability of specific psychiatric medicines at the Kangemi Health Center in Kenya is similar to the frequently unavailable medicines cited by respondents in Ghana (see Table 11.2). Prescribing practices may be influenced by the known limited availability of these medicines, further widening the treatment gap. Because medicines are supposed to be provided to the Kangemi Health Center based on staff estimations of use, psychiatric medicine deficiencies are likely to be even greater in health units that rely solely on the push system than in those that use the pull system.

Consumers' Perspectives on Access, Availability, and Affordability

Access

Access to psychotropic drugs poses a challenge to people with mental disorders and their families in each country studied. According to patient exit interviews conducted in Kenya, six out of ten patients who attended mental health clinics returned home without all of their prescriptions filled, and in some cases with none of the medication prescribed to them. Common reasons included long lines, limited availability of clinic services, distance from the facility, high cost of medications, and drug shortages. In Ghana, 32 percent of the focus group participants reported being unable to obtain their prescribed medication after visits to clinics and hospitals in June and July 2007.

Availability

When respondents were able to visit health centers that prescribe and dispense psychotropic medication, many of them had to deal with limited drug availability. One caregiver in Kenya lamented: "One thing I don't like about the clinic is the lack of drugs. Sometimes two drugs have been prescribed but one is unavailable. Then you are told to come back on a later date to check. Additionally, sometimes we do not get enough drugs. You see he [a patient] sometimes is supposed to take four tablets but he is given only three."

A caregiver in Tanzania stated: "Our patients have been taking drugs without getting relief. This is because they do not get the full dose due to drugs shortage in health centers." A patient in Ghana reported: "Sometimes we go to the hospital and do not get our required drugs. The nurses usually change to other drugs for us, which are not very effective for our treatment." When medicines are unavailable, nurses adjust doses or give different medicines than the ones originally prescribed. These alternative medicines can be ineffective; if they are wrongly dispensed, they may be harmful.

Affordability

Ghana's cash-and-carry system, in which patients must pay for their medication through copayments, also disrupts access to essential psychiatric medicines.

Originally instituted to provide an additional source of funds for essential medicines, the system poses a challenge for people who cannot afford the copayments (Smith 2004). Many patients cited the high cost of medication as a reason for returning home without treatment. One caregiver explained: "The drug they prescribed for me cost ¢275,000 ($29.57). Since I could not afford all this amount of money, I bought only ¢35,000 ($3.76) worth. One tablet costs ¢5,000 ($0.54). I was to buy sixty tablets, but I only succeeded in buying ten tablets."

When psychiatric medicines are available only in the private sector, high prices keep some consumers from purchasing the full regimen and in some cases prevent the purchase of any of the prescribed medication. Prescribers and patients compensate for the scarcity and high price of medicines by using available medications and affordable doses (Petryna, Lakoff, and Kleinman 2006). When prescribers are unable to dispense the appropriate medication due to a lack of availability and patients are unable to buy the appropriate amount of medicine due to costs the patient may not recover. In the case of schizophrenia, nonadherence to prescribed doses of medication is a strong predictor of relapse (Schooler 2006). Inadequate access to prescribed medication undermines treatment efforts and can reduce patients' confidence in mental health treatment.

IMPROVING MENTAL HEALTH TREATMENT
IN AFRICAN HEALTH SYSTEMS

Because other treatment options for mental disorders are not currently promoted by government policy in African countries, pharmaceutical treatment—even with all of its aforementioned shortcomings—remains the most accessible option for people with mental disorders, especially patients from poor families. Therefore, improving the limited access to psychiatric medicine is vital to reducing the burden of mental illness in Africa. Overcoming key challenges requires both strengthening the existing primary health care system from the ground up and increasing top-down governmental support of specific treatment measures for mental disorders (Reich et al. 2008).

Some of the problems in selection, procurement, and distribution that reduce access to psychiatric medicine in Africa reflect more general deficiencies in the health care system (Roberts and Reich 2011). Inadequate personnel for prescribing and dispensing medicine, the commonly used push system for distributing medicine kits, and overall inefficiencies in the procurement process are issues that are not unique to mental health care in Africa. Organizational and managerial improvements to the entire drug management process will make the supply chain run more smoothly and decrease medicine shortages. Estimation protocols can be revised to ensure more accurate quantification. Personnel can be better trained to understand and implement these protocols. These improvements would strengthen the health system from the bottom up by improving the capacity to deliver mental health care through the primary health care system. Thus, strengthening the existing primary health care infrastructure is crucial to increasing access to psychiatric medicine in Africa. There is growing recognition in the global health community of the need to strengthen health systems, especially in Africa.

However, some problems in access to psychiatric medication discussed in this chapter reveal the need for top-down solutions, requiring greater governmental attention and priority to mental health treatment initiatives. As mental health care becomes a higher priority for governments, appropriate and sustainable financing will be needed to improve the quantity and quality of psychiatric medicines available to people in Africa. Having a national mental health policy and including psychiatric medicines on the national list of essential medicines are a start, but they are far from enough. Funds are needed to implement mental health policies. Furthermore, these policies must be updated and revised according to the changing needs of the population. Increased government funding for safe and efficacious psychiatric pharmaceuticals is vital to addressing the currently inadequate availability of both first- and second-generation psychiatric medicines. Finally, effective strategies for implementation must be designed and applied so that available funds are effectively used.

Government health priorities also must be reconsidered and adjusted. Psychiatric medicine has not been prioritized alongside treatment for HIV/AIDS and malaria.

The relatively low priority that mental health care has been given by African governments is, in part, due to a lack of knowledge about effective treatment options. This is why further evidence-based study in Africa on the efficacy, safety, and cost-effectiveness of psychiatric medicine (as well as alternative treatments) is so necessary to African countries. Furthermore, increasing the transparency of government supply sources (both domestic and imported) and pricing for pharmaceuticals would help African countries make more informed policy decisions about improving public-sector access to psychiatric medicine. In the four countries studied, the existing primary health care system thus far has been unable to effectively treat people with mental disorders; thus, new government policies in this area are needed.

The following are specific recommendations based on our findings from Uganda, Tanzania, Kenya, and Ghana. These recommendations can help inform health care policy makers in Africa about measures that could improve access to psychiatric medication and treatment in their countries.

1. More effective use of national lists of essential medicines. National lists need to be reviewed more frequently and carefully to determine if any more efficacious treatment options are available that would be cost-effective considering the government's resources. If such options exist, steps should be taken to ensure that these medications are available at points where the most people are accessing mental health care (usually the primary health care units) (Saraceno et al. 2007).

2. Better estimation of medicine needs. The improvement of psychiatric medicine estimation in practice is vital to helping governments understand the nature of the treatment gap, thus encouraging them to allocate adequate resources to meet the need. Estimation protocols must be reviewed, keeping in mind the best way to obtain accurate estimations in practice, given personnel constraints. Health care staff can be helped to effectively implement these protocols through proper supervision and training.

3. Better management of procurement processes. Given that a large portion of psychiatric medicines in the four countries studied are imported, improved coordination between the public and private sectors on the selection, procurement, and distribution of psychiatric medicines could increase access to them. This has proven to be an effective means of increasing access to HIV/AIDS medication in Botswana (Dreesch et al. 2007).

4. Better evidence for mental health treatment in Africa. Finally, enhanced local research efforts are needed to examine and evaluate the most efficacious, safe, and cost-effective mental health treatment options for countries in Africa. Evidence-based support for appropriate alternative pharmaceutical treatments would assist African governments in designing more appropriate and effective policies and practices to promote mental health.

REFERENCES

Appiah-Kubi, K., S. Raja, and W. Boyce. 2008. "Mental Health: Access to Treatment and Macroeconomics in Ghana." Unpublished manuscript.

Brambilla, P., A. Cipriani, M. Hotopf, and C. Barbui. 2005. "Side-Effect Profile of Fluoxetine in Comparison with Other SSRIs, Tricyclic and Newer Antidepressants: A Meta-Analysis of Clinical Trial Data," *Pharmacopsychiatry* 38 (2): 69–77.

De Silva, V., and R. Hanwella. 2008. "Pharmaceutical Patents and the Quality of Mental Healthcare in Low- and Middle-Income Countries." *Psychiatric Bulletin* 32 (4): 121–23.

Dreesch, N., J. Nyoni, O. Mokopakgosi, K. Seipone, J. A. Kalilani, O. Kaluwa, and V. Musowe. 2007. "Public-Private Options for Expanding Access to Human Resources for HIV/AIDS in Botswana." *Human Resources for Health* 5 (25).

Frost, L. J., and M. R. Reich. 2008. *Access: How Do Good Health Technologies Get to Poor People in Poor Countries.* Cambridge, MA: Harvard University Press.

Gelders, S., M. Ewen, N. Noguchi, and R. O. Laing. 2006. *Price, Availability and Affordability: An International Comparison of Chronic Disease Medicines.* Geneva: World Health Organization.

Ghana Ministry of Health. 2004. *Ghana Essential Medicines List.* 5th ed. Accra: Ghana Ministry of Health.

Jitta, J., S. R. Whyte, and N. Nshakira. 2003. "The Availability of Drugs: What Does It Mean in Ugandan Primary Care." *Health Policy* 65 (2): 167–79.

Knapp, M., M. Funk, C. Curran, M. Prince, M. Grigg, and D. McDaid. 2006. "Economic Barriers to Better Mental Health Practice and Policy." *Health Policy and Planning* 21 (3): 157–70.

Narasimhan, V., H. Brown, A. Pablos-Mendez, O. Adams, G. Dussault, G, Elzinga, A. Nordstrom, et al. 2004. "Responding to the Global Human Resources Crisis." *Lancet* 363 (9419): 1469–72.

Odejide, A. O. 2006. "Status of Drug Use/Abuse in Africa." *International Journal of Mental Health and Addiction* 4 (2): 87–105.

Patel, V. 2007. "Mental Health in Low- and Middle-Income Countries." *British Medical Bulletin* 81–82 (1): 81–96.

Petryna, A., A. Lakoff, and A. Kleinman, eds. 2006. *Global Pharmaceuticals: Ethics, Markets, Practices.* Durham, NC: Duke University Press.

Raja, S., S. K. Wood, S. Robert, D. Deme-Der, K. Higini, and A. Oginga. 2008. "Public Sector Access to Psychiatric Medication in Four African Countries." Unpublished manuscript.

Reich, M. R. 2000. "The Global Drug Gap." *Science* 287 (5460): 1979–81.

Reich, M. R., K. Takemi, M. J. Roberts, and W. C. Hsiao. 2008. "Global Action on Health Systems: A Proposal for the Tokayo G8 Summit." *Lancet* 371 (615): 865–69.

Republic of Kenya Ministry of Health. 2003. *Kenya Essential Drugs List.* 3rd ed. Nairobi: Ministry of Health.

Roberts, M. J., and M. R. Reich. 2011. *Pharmaceutical Reform: A Guide to Improved Performance and Equity.* Washington: World Bank.

Saraceno, B., M. van Ommeren, R. Batniji, A. Cohen, O. Gureje, J. Mahoney, D. Sridhar, and C. Underhill. 2007. "Barriers to Improvement of Mental Health Services in Low-Income and Middle-Income Countries." *Lancet* 370 (9593): 1164–74.

Saxena, S., G. Thornicroft, M. Knapp, and H. Whiteford. 2007. "Resources for Mental Health: Scarcity, Inequity, and Inefficiency." *Lancet* 370 (9590): 878–89.

Schooler, N. R. 2006. "Relapse Prevention and Recovery in the Treatment of Schizophrenia." *Journal of Clinical Psychiatry* 67 (Supplement 5): 19–23.

Smith, F. 2004. "Community Pharmacy in Ghana: Enhancing the Contribution to Primary Care." *Health Policy and Planning* 19 (4): 234–41.

Uganda National Drug Authority. 2001. *Essential Drugs List for Uganda.* 3rd ed. Kampala: National Drug Authority.

Uganda National Drug Authority. 2008. *Drug Registration.* Kampala: National Drug Authority.

United Republic of Tanzania Ministry of Health. 1997. *Standard Treatment Guidelines and the National Essential Drugs List for Tanzania.* 2nd ed. Dar es Salaam: Ministry of Health.

Whyte, S. R., S. van der Geest, and A. Hardon. 2002. *Social Lives of Medicines.* Cambridge: Cambridge University Press.

World Health Organization. 2001. *The World Health Report: Mental Health: New Under-standing, New Hope. Geneva: World Health Organization.*

———. 2005a. *Improving Access and Use of Psychotropic Medicines.* Geneva: World Health Organization.

———. 2005b. *Mental Health Atlas: 2005. Geneva: World Health Organization.* http://www.who.int/mental_health/evidence/mhatlas05/en/index.html.

———. 2007. *WHO Model List of Essential Medicines: 15th list, March 2007.* http://whqlibdoc.who.int/hq/2007/a95075_eng.pdf.

12 CHILD SOLDIERS AND COMMUNITY RECONCILIATION IN POSTWAR SIERRA LEONE

African Psychiatry in the Twenty-First Century

WILLIAM P. MURPHY

Reconciling former child soldiers with their communities has become a central problem in contemporary African psychiatry. It is a dramatic problem because the goal is to heal the traumas of children who were victims and/or perpetrators of violence during a civil war, and to enable them to live peacefully and productively in postconflict communities. It is also a problem of scale. Since 1975 Africa has become "the epicenter of the problem, providing the largest concentration of both [civil] conflicts and child soldiers," with estimates suggesting that "120,000 children, 40 percent of all child soldiers, were soldiering in Africa at the beginning of the twenty-first century" (Achvarina and Reich 2006, 130–31). In postconflict situations in Africa and elsewhere, rehabilitating former child soldiers is a central task of reconstituted governments and societies (see, for example, Boyden and de Berry 2004; Brett and Sprecht 2004, 129–36; Cohn and Goodwin-Gil 1994, chap. 5; Rosen 2005, chap. 10). In postwar Sierra Leone, a nation whose civil war ended in 2002 after more than a decade, this challenge is referred to as the "youth question," a phrase often used by government officials throughout the rest of Africa to refer to the demography of a bulging youth population, leading to large pools of unemployed, disenfranchised youth vulnerable to the economic and psychological attractions of violent projects. In this government discourse, youth are viewed as a threat to society as well as an opportunity for national development. All the problems and possibilities attached to the "youth question"—such as urban youth, street children, HIV/AIDS orphans, and child labor—are condensed into the image of the child soldier. This image, however, creates a misleading equation of "youth" with "violent and dangerous," an idea that overlooks the majority of youth during the civil war (and during postconflict rebuilding) who were not combatants (see Hoffman 2011).

The challenge of rehabilitating former child soldiers has also generated re-newed and urgent interest in community-based modes of therapeutic interven-tion, the signature style of African psychiatric approaches. Reincorporating the individual into the community, with the help of traditional healing modalities, is viewed as a key step in healing the psychic traumas of individuals. This form of social healing characterizes the adaptation of African therapeutic styles to psychiatric problems, (Chavunduka 1978; Feierman and Janzen 1992; Last and Chavunduka 1986). In recent scholarship on the mass traumas of war, collective violence, and forced migration, the psychosocial and mental health problems are conceived as intricately connected to the historical, political, and sociocultural context of conflict and postconflict (see, for example, De Jong 2002; for the case of Liberia, see also Abramowitz 2012).

In the debate about how to rehabilitate former child soldiers, techniques based on the healing benefits of reconciliation with family and community are often viewed as preferable to standard, Western psychotherapies which focus on the individual. Alcinda Honwana, who carried out extensive ethnographic re-search on child soldiers and their rehabilitation in Angola and Mozambique, has emphasized this difference. She characterizes the "dominant Western psycho-therapeutic models" as locating "the causes of psychosocial distress within the individual" and, therefore, producing "responses which are primarily based on individual therapy" (Honwana 2006, 150). In contrast, "community-based sup-port, the family, and especially traditional approaches to healing [in Mozam-bique and Angola] play a crucial and constructive role in the rehabilitation of war-affected young people," and "these institutions are the fundamental means through which healing occurs and order can be reestablished" (ibid.). Honwana (2006) argues that the "talk therapy" of Western approaches to post-traumatic patients such as war veterans and the goal of getting individuals to talk about and integrate traumatic memories of being a perpetrator or victim of violence (or both) "are not necessarily applicable in non-Western contexts or cultures" (152). Instead, the challenges are to mobilize the beliefs, values, and practices of local institutions as resources in the healing modalities for former child combatants, and to protect children from participation in future armed conflicts (162).

Another challenge arises from a different issue. Are the institutional struc-tures of the community detrimental rather than helpful to the process of healing former child soldiers and reconciling them to the community? This chapter ad-dresses that question. It does not seek to evaluate the contrast between individual and community-based modalities of psychological healing. But it does argue that community structures may replicate social conditions and organization—for ex-ample, patriarchy, gerontocracy, and lineage hierarchies (see, for example, Mur-phy 1980)—that contribute to the subordination and marginalization of young people and thus increase their social and psychological alienation rather than their reintegration into society after a conflict has ended.

The chapter, therefore, treats "community" as an anthropological problematic rather than as a benign psychological resource. On the one hand, it interprets the patriarchal imagery that justifies the subordination of youth during a civil war (for example, the language used by military commanders) and postconflict rehabilitation (for the case of Mozambique, see Schafer 2004) as representing the ideology of a "big man" patron of youth labor and services rather than that of a benign father. On the other hand, it argues that the connotations of the word "community" can be analytically misleading because these meanings often idealize notions of common, cooperative, shared life and overlook harsher institutional aspects of community life, such as the sociopolitical hierarchies, economic privileges, and ritual power that youth often find restrictive or even oppressive. Other scholars have made similar arguments about the social structural problem of reintegrating former child soldiers in postconflict Sierra Leone (see, for example, Coulter 2009; Denov 2010; Fithen and Richards 2005; Peters 2004, 2006, and 2011; Shepler 2014) as well as in Liberia (see, for example, Utas 2005a and 2005b). Krijn Peters's excellent analysis of the complexities of the Disarmament, Demobilization, and Reintegration program of rehabilitating former child soldiers in postconflict Sierra Leone will be discussed further below. A major challenge facing these reintegration programs, however, is summarized in a formulation used by Mats Utas (2005b) for the case of youth in postconflict Liberia: namely, youth marginalization before the civil war easily becomes remarginalization after the civil war. This challenge is further complicated by the special social structural and psychological problems of girls and women who experienced sexual violence during civil war (Utas 2009; see also Abramowitz and Moran 2012). Such gender problems create constraints on women's "voice" in post-conflict reconstruction (for the dramatic case of the silences in women's testimony in truth and reconciliation hearings in South Africa, see Ross 2010).

This challenge is analyzed here in the context of the psychiatric project of community-based therapies for former child soldiers. The analytical groundwork, outlined in the next section, is constructed from a theory of youth and selfhood derived from anthropology, social psychology, and semiotics, and from a social theory of "big man" authority structures in political communities with which youth are asked to be reconciled.

THEORETICAL BACKGROUND

Defining youth by structural location in society is one method of avoiding the error of equating youth violence with the naturalized emotions and attributes of childhood. Such an approach is characteristic of recent studies in the anthropology of youth (Cole and Durham 2007) and African youth specifically (Honwana and De Boeck 2005), including a special focus on youth in postcolonial structures (see, for example, Diouf 2003; Comaroff and Comaroff 2005) and youth identity and practices (including violence) within religious structures and cosmologies of power (Ashforth 2005; Ellis 1999; Ferme 2001; Shaw 2002). The broad analytical principle is that youth is a relational social category, not a natural state. Youth is defined by social relations with other categories in the community, such as elders, and is constituted as a social category by particular experiences, such as marriage, labor, and violence. The "youth" question is thus not just about asking what is wrong with youth psychology, which causes society so many problems. Rather, the question concerns the kind of social relations (for example, political and economic) that constitute the social reality and subjectivity of being a youth—such as relations with elders, chiefs, lineage heads, ritual leaders, national government leaders, rebel commanders, and global institutions.

One paradox of the "youth question" is that governments' rhetorical preoccupation with the issue in contemporary Africa, when not translated into practical results, produces a contradiction between public promises of government officials and their failure to provide tangible benefits for post-conflict youth, as the Sierra Leone Truth and Reconciliation Commission (TRC) noted. The TRC was commissioned in 2002, at the end of the civil war, by the Sierra Leonean government and finished its work in March 2004. The TRC held extensive hearings in each of the country's fourteen districts, as well as in Freetown, the capital city, that enabled victims and the perpetrators of violence during the civil war to give testimony, including written statements collected by interviewers. The TRC's mandate was to produce a truthful record of the conflict as well as to facilitate community healing and reconciliation. The TRC report concluded that failure of government youth policy "is symptomatic of the continued marginalization of youth" (Sierra Leone Truth and Reconciliation Commission Report 2004, 3B:358).

The method of analyzing youth within a structure of social relations entails the further step of analyzing youth as constituted by communicative practices. The core principle, derived from George Herbert Mead's (1934) social psychology, is that the self emerges in social relations with others, but those relations are constituted by communicative practices. As Steve Caton summarizes Mead's argument, human beings are not born with selves. Rather, the "the self has to develop, to emerge in a distinct process of action . . . and this process is a social one, an interaction between the individual and some other or others in its environment" (Caton 1993, 321). The individual becomes an object to himself or herself—and thus a self—through reflecting on the attitudes and standpoints of others, which are made available to the individual through linguistic communication (as well as gestures). Mead wrote: "I know of no other form of behavior than the linguistic in which the individual is an object to himself, and, so far as I can see, the individual is not a self in a reflexive sense unless he is an object to himself. It is this fact that gives critical importance to communication, since this is a type of behavior in which the individual does so respond to himself" (quoted in Caton 1993, 321).

The self is a social construction because the self is constituted through communication in social interaction, as well as a semiotic construction because communication is the transmission of signs in those interactions. This notion of the self was developed by Mead's fellow American pragmatist, Charles Sanders Peirce, who saw the thought and the mind of a person as a composite of signs: "The word or sign that man uses is the man himself. . . . Thus my language is the sum total of myself; for the man is the thought [and] . . . all thought . . . must necessarily be in signs . . . that thought-sign . . . is myself" (quoted in Innis 1985, 2–3; see also Agha 1995; Colapietro 1989; Lee and Urban 1989; Mertz 1989; Skagested 2004). Signs are learned in communication, so the self emerges through the semiotic reflexivity of communication. Innis summarizes Peirce's position this way: "Self-knowledge comes not from introspection . . . but from reflection on the field of expressions in which one finds oneself, individually and socially. The self is 'semiotically' defined as well as semiotically accessible" (Innis 1985, 2).

The fact that all thought must be in signs means that all thought is social. This semiotic theory of the self is a theory of socialization as well as a theory of mind. It is also a theory of personality change, which is conditioned by processes of social change involving communication. The self in Mead's social psychology "is at the same time flexible and open to communication with more and more partners" (Joas 1993, 213), and, therefore, open to different internalizations of self-evaluation and orientations to action because communication with different social partners generates different expectations as well as different—in Peirce's sense—signs of the self. In this Peircean model, the unitary nature of the psychological self becomes a plasticity of the self constructed through the communicative and semiotic processes of social life.

This semiotic and communicative theory of the self shifts the question from what is wrong with youth's psychological dispositions to what is the structural location of youth as instantiated in the communicative and semiotic practices of social worlds of war and peace, as well as to how these practices shape the meanings (and emotions) of the selves that youth become. In this anthropological approach to the self, as derived from Mead, "psychology can attempt to study 'inner' mental processes only insofar as these can be modeled from the same kind of data from which 'outer,' publicly observable events are modeled," namely, events of "public . . . semiotic behavior" (Agha 1995, 131–32).

Wars and postconflict periods are embodied in the public, communicative practices that define subjectivity in varying social contexts of violence or reconciliation. A good example of this type of semiotic behavior is the rituals of reconciliation in postconflict situations, in which the ritual signs of youths' selves may index social dependency and exclusion as much as reconciliation. Social dependency and exclusion, in turn, can reinforce youths' alienation and hopelessness during postconflict reconstruction.

RITUALS OF RECONCILIATION

Rituals of cleansing and reconciliation based on traditional healing techniques are common modalities in community-based therapies, but one sobering question is whether the rituals as embodiments of the sociopolitical structure of the community may legitimate social conditions detrimental to the rehabilitation and psychological healing of former child soldiers. One message in the semiotics of such rituals, for example, is the dependency of youth on the authority of the elders in mediating relations with the spiritual world. Elders perform important spiritual and therapeutic services for the community, but this institutional mediation includes the potential use of ritual power to threaten youth with spiritual punishments (see, for example, Murphy 1980). Participating in these rituals indexes youths' vulnerability to this power, a vulnerability also signified by elders' and ritual specialists' privileged control of the language register of spiritual mediation and social reconciliation (on register socialization, see Agha 2007, 155–57).

Consider a typical example of a ritual of reconciliation from Honwana's discussion of traditional healing in Angola. The case concerns Pitango, a boy who served for three years in the government forces during the civil war and, at the age of eighteen, returned to his family, who organized a ritual for him. The ritual took place the day Pitango arrived, before he was allowed to socialize with relatives and friends. His body was washed with cassava meal. A chicken was killed during the proceedings and its blood was placed on his forehead. Then his mother took some palm oil and rubbed it on Pitango's hands and feet. During this ritual, the ancestral spirits of the family were repeatedly called in to protect the young man who was back from war and had to start a new life. The prayers were offered by his elder relatives whose generational position brought them closest to the ancestors. Pitango mentioned that the elders of his family explained to him that the performance of this ritual was necessary so that the spirits of those killed in the war would not harm him (Honwana 2006, 110). This case is typical of the iconography of rituals of cleansing in postconflict periods, such as the washing of the body (or sometimes the burning of objects associated with the past violence), drinking potions of purification, praying to the ancestors, and the spiritual mediation of elders.

On the one hand, the ritual is a sign of healing. On the other hand, it indexes the authority of family elders who intercede with the ancestral world, as well as indexing the authority of other community ritual leaders who mediate between the youth and spirit forces, including those of Christianity and Islam. It is a sign of the dependency of those who need that mediation. Young former combatants are sometimes uncomfortable immersing themselves in these cultural and religious traditions and acceding to the social dependency represented by the practices. Honwana notes that some of these youths "see such actions as a return to the old ways—a world of tradition and gerontocracy—and aspire to a more modern outlook on life" (2006, 119). This pattern is just not a rejection of traditional ways of doing things because they are not modern. It is also a rejection of the social dependencies and vulnerabilities represented by such rituals. For example, it rejects the power of the elder who cures through mediation with the ancestors and who can use this same power to curse or punish, and thereby control.

Refusing to participate in such rituals often marks a rejection of family and community authority. Honwana mentions such a case. One young man, Zita, refused the attempts of his mother and grandmother in Mozambique to have him undergo "a cleansing treatment with a healer or in a Zionist church" and "also refused to accept the authority of his stepfather . . . and rejected the authority of the elders" (2006, 119–20). Such refusal is not simply youthful intransigence; it is also a sign of changed intergenerational community relations, with former combatants being reluctant to return to the sociopolitical structures—and the rituals supporting them—that many youths before the war saw as oppressive.

Rituals of reconciliation are further compromised because their leaders are sometimes seen an instruments of secular political power, used by community leaders as a means of socially controlling the young. Child soldiers experienced this political manipulation of ritual authority during the civil war in Mozambique. The same institution of local healers and diviners called on to produce healing in the postwar situation was often used by rebel commanders to initiate young recruits into violence and organize their violent services. Honwana gives an example from the Angolan civil war: "Herbal medicines were sometimes given to recruits in order to enable them to fight courageously and protect them from death during combat. Local healers, called *kimbandas,* treated soldiers in the Angolan camps. Commanders often sought the aid of healers to win battles and shield them from injury" (2006, 62).

In addition, local healers were used during the war to treat young soldiers when they became upset with the required ritualized killings during training. After such a killing, those "who cried in the evening . . . were treated by the *kim-*

bandas" (Honwana 2006, 62). The postwar context is characterized by a contradiction: the same ritual healers who were used by rebel leaders to initiate children into a life of violence in the civil war are now used to reincorporate former child soldiers into their community after the war. In either context, the common message is one of the community's social control of youth through ritual practices.

These contradictions in reconciliation programs were highlighted in the report of Sierra Leone's TRC (2004). The culmination of each TRC hearing was usually a ritual of apologizing and asking for forgiveness, with individual victims and the community accepting apologies from perpetrators. A ceremony of community reconciliation, involving local ritual and secular leaders, often brought a hearing to a close. The TRC realized that this approach meant that community leaders did not ask for forgiveness, nor were they required to express remorse for their role during the civil war. This was a problem:

> The Commission was surprised by the number of complaints about the violations committed by many of the Chiefs during the conflict, for which they neither as a group nor individually expressed remorse or offered any explanation to their communities. In reality, while the Commission had to rely on the Chiefs as leaders of their communities and had to work closely with them, the Commission was cognizant of the fact that many chiefs have been discredited by their failure to explain the roles they played during the war. It is for this reason that the Commission has not felt entirely comfortable relying on traditional structures to help foster reconciliation. The reconciliation process must continue and traditional leadership will play an important role in this process. However, the Commission has recommended that the role of Chiefs and the manner in which they have been manipulated by successive governments must be placed on the national agenda for discussion, as it has huge potential for future conflict in the future. (Sierra Leone's Truth and Reconciliation Commission 2004, 3B:438)

The TRC report foregrounds the problem of requiring those subordinate in the sociopolitical structure to express remorse and ask for forgiveness, while allowing community and national authorities, who were not blameless during the civil war, to perform the superior role of granting forgiveness without asking for it. This problem led some participants—to borrow a phrase from a participant in the more recent proceedings of the Truth and Reconciliation Commission of Liberia (Republic of Liberia Truth and Reconciliation Commission. 2008–2009)— to view the whole process as a "reconciliation fiasco."[1]

A preoccupation with rehabilitating former child soldiers can lead to the overlooking of structural injustices that marginalized and exploited youth, such as by forcing them to perform labor. Such forms of injustice become erased in the process of youths' asking adults for forgiveness. To make this institutional forgetting more visible, consider a different scenario: imagine an alternative social universe in which chiefs and ritual leaders (as well as officials in a new national government, who include former rebel leaders) apologize to the youth for their role in creating the injustices leading up to and carried out during the war.

POLITICS OF RECONCILIATION

Whether psychosocial healing in the aftermath of war succeeds or fails depends on the social structures and political economy of the postconflict period. Reconciliation and rehabilitation programs for former youth combatants in African civil wars seek to replace the symbolic, ritual, and social universe of meanings and obligations created in a world of violent civil strife with a renewed symbolic, ritual, social universe of community reconciliation and reassimilation. Honwana's (2006, especially chapters 5 and 6) work in Angola and Mozambique exemplifies this approach. She argues that reconciliation must be located in the context of local cultural notions of pollution and contamination of the social body caused by violence. Those who perpetrated violence as well as those who were victims to or witnesses of it are, in the view of the community, socially contaminated. Programs for their resocialization in the community replace the socialization practices and initiation rituals that military groups used to indoctrinate youth into their violent projects.

The resocialization of youth, however, may become renewed socialization into subordination when the sociopolitical structures of the communities marginalize youth. The case of Sierra Leone illustrates this dilemma. One of the best studies of reintegration and reconciliation of child soldiers in postwar Sierra Leone is Peters's *Footpaths to Reintegration* (2006; see also Peters 2011) because it analyzes community structural problems that compromise such programs. Peters's ethnography and analysis add support to the theoretical theme developed in this chapter, as brief selections below demonstrate.

The civil war in Sierra Leone was started in March 1991 by the Revolutionary United Front (RUF) led by Foday Sankoh, an ally of Charles Taylor. Taylor began the Liberian civil war in December 1989 (and was convicted in April 2012 of war crimes by the Special Court for Sierra Leone in The Hague). Many villages and communities in Sierra Leone suffered extensive destruction during the war. In "the decade long war more than half the country was displaced," and community social institutions stopped functioning (Peters 2006, 135). To rebuild the communities after the war was a challenge because "roads had to be safe and repaired to allow transport to resume," "legal institutions" had to be restarted, "local authorities" reelected or reappointed, and "schools and clinics had to be rebuilt" (ibid.).

Reconstituting social institutions is more difficult than rebuilding the physical infrastructure because institutional "rehabilitation is as much a fight as the war"; when people returned to rebuild their communities, there was the inevitable new "fight in which contested claims concerning rights and positions surface" (Peters 2006, 135). Community receptions of former child soldiers varied depending on the war experiences of the soldier; and whether the former combatant was male or female and affiliated with the RUF rebel group, the government army, or a local militia (civil defense force) organized to protect communities (Shepler 2014). Contested claims in the rebuilding process were often justified by actions during the war: for example, people who had remained in their village during the war as well as those who had been leaders in civil defense forces expected more farming privileges and more authority in community life (Peters 2006, 235). Such claims inevitably led to conflicts with traditional local authorities, such as chiefs, elders, and lineage leaders, who expected that the sociopolitical life of the community would return to the "business as usual" of respecting their rights, privileges, and authority. Many former combatants in postconflict Liberia, for example, had problems securing a livelihood because of their exclusion and lack of legitimacy in the traditional order of rights and claims to land tenure (Rincon 2010, 21).

This is the crux of the issue of reconciling former child soldiers to their communities. In Peters's words, "there is more at stake than only the physical reconstruction of war-torn villages," and the reconciling of former combatants to the people in those villages, because "one realizes that the causes of the conflict must be sought in the marginalization of young people" through traditional institutions controlled by elders and chiefs, who often allied themselves with national elites to control local resources and labor (2006, 136). Chiefs and elders traditionally controlled access to land, women, dispute resolution, and ritual power—and this authority over basic social functions provided a strong, and often harsh, means of controlling youth, including keeping youth in debt or debt servitude through heavy court fines. After the war former combatants, especially those who held leadership positions during it, challenged any excessive and exploitative use of traditional authority. Many of them felt emancipated from the use of "customary" authority "to sanction or exploit young people" (ibid.). In addition, the strategies of former combatants repositioning themselves in civil society and local communities were shaped by the lessons and values learned during the civil war (Fithen and Richards 2005; Peters 2006).

For youth returning home, community authority structures may be the problem rather than the solution. One of the fundamental grievances in the Sierra Leonean civil war was the patriarchal and gerontocratic repression of youth in the community, as well as the patrimonial national government's failures, through the use of "big man" politics, to provide employment and educational opportunities for youth. The "legitimacy of African political elites . . . derives from their ability to nourish the clientele on which their power rests," and therefore it requires them "to exploit government resources for patrimonial purposes"—that is, to maintain their personal power by rewarding clients' dependence on them (Chabal and Daloz 1999, 15; see also Utas 2012). There is thus a fundamental instability to patrimonial power because rival patrons are tempted to challenge each other, and those left out of the benefits of the clientalist network are tempted to seek other avenues—including violence—for capturing their piece of the patrimonial pie. This unstable political logic was first clarified in Max Weber's foundational study of patrimonialism (Weber 1978, chapter 12). One implication of this logic that is pertinent to the argument here about youth and postconflict psychosocial rehabilitation is that young people's social and economic insecurity is a product of being caught in the middle of these patrimonial struggles (Murphy 2003 and 2010). Civil war itself and the use of child soldiers by rival factions are often violent manifestations of such struggles. And the testimony of former combatants in postconflict periods often shows—through reporting the language of military leaders during the conflict—that the patronage logic of violent domination was the key legitimating mechanism during the civil war. In a postconflict political economy of dire economic need and extreme social dependency, the logic of patronage is reproduced in a wide variety of structural domains, such as former combatants' turning to motorcycle taxi driving (see Menzel 2011a).

The above summary of "big men" social structures and political economy underscores the dilemma of community-based therapies: in reconciling individuals, especially youth, in postwar situations, the therapist cannot assume the existence of a benign and supportive community. The vulnerable position of youth within "big man" authority structures needs to be factored into the therapeutic equation. The history of Sierra Leone confirms the role of these structures—namely, the deprivations and sufferings of youth under the duress of local and national patrimonialism—as a contributing factor to the civil war (see, for example Richards 1996; Peters 2006 and 2011; see also Abdullah 2004; Gberie 2005; Murphy 2003; Reno 1998), and, as argued here, a potential impediment to community-based therapies in the aftermath of the war.

Psychological and social dilemmas are even more complex in postconflict situations because the deprivations and sufferings of youth under the rebel regime, with its use of widespread forced conscription and violence against civilians, undermined young people's faith not only in the local and national patrimonial and gerontocratic system that was in place before the war but also in the rebel regime, which was noted for an even more violent form of patrimonialism. Prewar and wartime social conditions shared a patrimonial logic of controlling youth (Murphy 2003). One conclusion to be drawn from this analysis is that a major challenge for postconflict rehabilitation is avoiding the reproduction of social subordination and alienation of youth in community psychosocial healing programs that overlook this political logic of youth dependency on patronage in a patrimonial organization.

REBEL DISCOURSE ON YOUTH EMOTIONS

A related challenge facing community reconciliation programs is to understand the violence of youth as conditioned by social structural factors and, thereby, to avoid the error of essentializing young people's emotions as a natural cause of violence. Anthropology has tried to avoid the interpretive trap of naturalizing emotions by shifting attention to the social reality of emotions, especially by considering "the many ways emotion gets its meaning and force from its location and performance in the public realm of discourse" (Abu-Lughod and Lutz 1990, 7). Equating emotional dispositions with gender identity exemplifies the pervasive logic and social history of treating cultural phenomena as natural and using this naturalization to legitimate social control. Analogously, naturalizing young people's emotions, especially as wild and uncontrollable, provides a language for naturalizing youth violence.

Media representations of child soldiers fall into these traps, using stereotypical language and imagery of gun-toting, drug-crazed, bizarrely dressed teenagers as a way to make sense of the violence as something inherent to adolescent psychology. Even distinguished Africanist scholars can slip into such stereotypes. For example, Paul Collier, in his excellent book on poverty and civil conflict, recognizes that young men, "who are the recruits for rebel armies, come pretty cheap in an environment of hopeless poverty . . . and joining a rebel movement gives these young men a small chance of riches," but he ends up blaming much of the violence against civilians in the civil war in Sierra Leone on "teenage drug addicts . . . not excessively inhibited by moral scruples" (2007, 25). What is overlooked in the rhetoric of youth blame is the organized project of terror and control in the military campaigns of the civil war that used child soldiers to carry out what commanders saw as a rational policy of violence, such as punishing civilians who were disloyal to the rebel project.

The stereotype of youth emotions and lack of moral scruples provides a rhetorical trope of spontaneous, uncontrollable youth violence that is strategically invoked by military leaders to deflect blame from organized projects of violence. Outsiders and media commentaries often "buy into" this language, which resonates with the common—and ancient—view of youth as the cause of society's problems. The case below exemplifies the exploitation of this image of "wild youth" as a language for covering up organized projects of collective violence in the civil war.

There was extensive local and world criticism of the RUF for the practice of civilian limb amputations. In response to this criticism, the RUF released an official statement exonerating itself for this form of violence. The statement was dated June 15, 1999, and designated as a statement of the "RUF Political Leadership" issued by its legal representative, Omrie Michael Golley, and signed by the "RUF Political Leadership–Kailahun District." The four-page statement is titled "RUF Calls for Independent Investigations." The statement does not deny that "untold atrocities" and civilian limb amputations were committed by RUF fighters, but its major purpose is to explain civilian limb amputations by constructing a theory of war atrocities (and a theory of war, more broadly) out of a repertoire of psychological assumptions about young people's emotions, and those of rebel soldiers generally (for the full text, available on the Sierra Leone civil war document website, see Revolutionary United Front 1999).

The following excerpts, taken from this official document, emphasize a causative link between the youthful emotions of rebel fighters and the atrocities committed. The document begins with a theory of war and emotions: "As stated earlier, in war, pent up rage and the breakdown of law and order leads to untold atrocities." In addition, this rage was related to the calling of national elections to which the RUF objected, so the amputations became both a threat and a punishment for civilians: "A few RUF fighters in the bush went on the rampage and as their own way of stating their objection to the planned elections, they proceeded on a campaign to cut off the hands of innocent villagers as a message that no voting should occur. This was how amputations started in Sierra Leone by desperate RUF men." The desperate RUF men on a rampage are identified in the next two statements as out-of-control youth: "Our leader [Foday Sankoh] is aware that in war, atrocities occur especially when young disenfranchised men are revolting against an oppressive system." This theory of war identifies the volatile mixture of youth and angry emotions: "Many fighters tend to be harboring huge negative pent up emotions during warfare. Generally, War results in a breakdown of civil law and order. Fighters tend to use this breakdown in law and order to unleash their angry negative emotions by committing untold atrocities. It is very difficult to control fighters in a war situation."

In the RUF theory of war, emotions are causative, leading to violent excesses such as the atrocities of civilian limb amputations. This causative formula exonerates RUF leaders from blame for atrocities because the "pent up" and "angry negative emotions" make it "difficult to control fighters." Those carrying out these atrocities were "young" and "difficult to control" because of their age and "angry negative emotions." This theory of war naturalizes violence by blaming atrocities on the spontaneous, angry emotions of young rebels. The rhetoric, of course, has efficacy in the global media, a main audience of the RUF document, because the media generally make similar assumptions about young people's emotions.

Testimonies from victims of this violence as well as from former child soldiers abducted to carry out the violence, however, blame the rebels' organizational structure more than uncontrollable emotional outbursts of youth, and thereby point to a contradiction between the "blame the youth" language of political leaders and the youth's "bottom up" critique of these leaders' organizational projects of war-making. This contradiction is considered in the next section.

YOUTH TESTIMONIES

The previous section identifies one "discursive formation"—using Michel Foucault's (1972, 31) term for the underlying principles organizing the statements and reasoning in a particular institutional domain. As articulated in the official discourse of the RUF leadership, this reasoning encodes ideas about youth and violence in the civil war, reasoning as a set of statements that presuppose, in Foucault's terminology, a "way of looking at things" (1972, 33). In this way of looking at things, young people's anger against an oppressive government spilled over into atrocities against civilians. This official RUF view exonerates the organization from strategically planning violence.

In contrast, much of the testimony by youth about the civil war offers another "discursive formation" about the meaning of youth violence. This testimony is the outcome of a shift in the social context of speaking. In one context, represented in the previous section, adults explain youth violence. In another context, considered in this section, youth talk about the violence and commands of adults, especially the role of military commanders in organizing violence.

The following testimonies were collected by the Sierra Leone TRC, whose mandate was to include the voices of children in the testimonies of victims and perpetrators.[2] The parliamentary act commissioning the TRC specified that special attention should be given to "the experiences of children in the armed conflict" (Sierra Leone Truth and Reconciliation Commission 2004, 1:141). Although the TRC sought to protect children by limiting their testimony to closed hearings, offering children an opportunity to speak and testify is not typical in most Sierra Leonean communities. The TRC report explains that typically "in Sierra Leone children are not allowed to speak for themselves before the elders and chiefs" (ibid., 3B:241). There are, of course, exceptions to such cultural prohibitions, but this norm is significant because it is supported by a set of beliefs about knowledge and truth, the cognitive unreliability of children, and the role of age in measuring reliability. Such beliefs rest on cultural premises that, in turn, are the foundation of gerontocratic structures in which important knowledge (and power) is reserved for the elders.

The act of giving testimony is itself a communicative practice of constructing a self. This is an important principle in Peirce's semiotic theory of the self: "For Peirce, the very moment at which testimony comes to play a role marks the origin of the self" (de Waal 2001, 80). The concept of testimony means that the individual understands the difference between a fact directly perceived and a fact learned from the testimony of others. In one of Peirce's examples, a child may learn that a stove is hot by touching it, or he may learn by being told that it is hot (ibid.). In understanding the concept of testimony, the child, in Peirce's words, "becomes aware of ignorance" as well as "an ego in whom this ignorance can inhere" (quoted in ibid.). "The dawning of the conception of testimony is the dawning of self-consciousness," because that conception entails the discovery of error and ignorance and "a self that is fallible" (ibid.). Thus, the idea of testimony connotes a search to understand the world in the context of the potentially fallible testimony of self and others. For Peirce, this understanding is an important step in beginning the social construction of the self.

Peirce's argument about testimony and the semiotics of the self has important implications for understanding the voices of youth (and women) in postwar Sierra Leone, and the construction of postconflict selves through those voices. The concept of "testimony" is a social category as well as a cognitive category because some categories of people—such as women, children, and people of low status—may be socially excluded, or limited in their rights and opportunities to speak in the public sphere, and thus unable to contribute testimony to public debate. In addition, there is a tension between public testimony as individual psychological catharsis and such testimony as collective social catharsis (for a discussion of a dramatic case of this tension, women's testimony in truth and reconciliation hearings in South Africa, see Ross 2010). The institutional structuring of discourse about youth violence defines who has the authority to speak about this topic and what can be said, such as emphasizing young people's essential and natural qualities as causes of violence. However, the TRC procedures challenged those restrictions by allocating public space for testimony from segments of society, such as youth, who seldom have a voice in society's public sphere.[3]

The extensive violence of this civil war, which often focused on civilians rather than rival combatants, gave urgency to the TRC's mandate to hear from all the voices in the community. Shared suffering bestows legitimacy on everyone's testimony of pain. The excerpts below from the TRC report illustrate this link between suffering and testimony—in this instance, the suffering of children and youth. These voices contribute to an archive of statements about violence, adding another discursive formation to the official discourse of the rebel group (or community authorities). The production of such archives, however, involves the difficulty—social, political, and psychological—of transforming the pain of violence into language and memory without erasing, obscuring, or intentionally forgetting aspects of that experience. This difficulty has been analyzed by anthropologists studying the South African Truth and Reconciliation Commission (Ross and Reynolds 1999) and in the specific case of women's voices in testimonies to that commission (Ross 2003 and 2005). Despite constraints in the public process of remembering violence, the goal of privileging youth voices in the Sierra Leone TRC proceedings created an archival record that at least avoided representing youth experience solely through adult voices.

The first example of such testimony comes from a youth who was ten years old when he was captured to join the RUF. In addition to describing the physical means of threatening violence during his abduction—for example, a gun was placed against his head—he reports what was said during his abduction, the threats made by the military commander of the group, and the name of the commander:

> My mother and I were on the farm. Six armed men entered the farm and hid themselves in the hut. We entered . . . and were captured and detained with their guns against our heads. . . . The commander of the group was Colonel Mohammed Sesay . . . he said to me that I should join them or they will kill my mother and myself. I choose to join them since I had no option. . . . On our way to Kailahun I was given a weapon called AK-47 and taught how to shoot on sight. We attacked so many villages I could not remember their names, until we reached Kailahun, which was the headquarter town of the RUF. (Sierra Leone Truth and Reconciliation Commission 2004, 3B:260)

This testimony supports the conclusion of the TRC report that most of the child soldiers and child laborers in the rebel group were forcefully conscripted. Many of those who joined voluntarily often had little real choice—their other alternatives were often starvation or remaining vulnerable to the predations of rival militias. The testimony above exemplifies the harsh choices children faced: either join or you (and perhaps your mother or father) will be killed. Choices were also constrained when family members became destitute or were killed in the civil war. The military organization became the child's new family. An eloquent memoir of being a child soldier in Sierra Leone, written by Ishmael Beah, sums up these existential pressures: "My squad was my family, my gun was my provider and protector, and my rule was to kill or be killed" (2007, 126).

The next testimony describes the economic use of children as porters and domestic servants, often called "manpower" by the rebels (Sierra Leone Truth and Reconciliation Commission 2004, 3B:267). Manpower problems meant not having enough soldiers for fighting or laborers for logistical needs (carrying ammunition, food, and supplies; cooking food; and so on). The following case illustrates the rebel group's solution to manpower problems: abducting children (as well as adults) as laborers. The phrase "small boy" in the excerpt below is an idiom the speaker used to identify himself as prepubescent—not yet a strong, fully grown boy—when this abduction took place.

> I was caught, tied and given a big bag of things to carry to Pujehun. . . . As a small boy, I suffered under the load from Tarinahun to Pujehun. . . . At Pujehun . . . they used to beat me every morning, I had barely enough food to eat. . . . I used to launder for them and their girlfriends. I was taken to almost all of the nearby villages to get food and fowls for them. I was punished if I failed. (Sierra Leone Truth and Reconciliation Commission 2004, 3B:268).

The command to get "food and fowls" refers to looting nearby villages and farms. Stealing food and farm products from civilians was the main means of feeding the rebel army. Civilian resistance to this looting often resulted in severe punishment or death. In addition, child soldiers and child servants were themselves harshly punished for failing to collect these food products and other valuables from civilians.

Testimony about commands and punishments provides an important window into the organizational structure and political logic of sanctions in the rebel group. In the previous testimony, the child had to respond diligently to many commands, such as laundering clothes and collecting food from nearby villagers. Failure was met with punishment. Such testimony—supported by numerous other such testimonies from many different sources (such as Human Rights Watch, Amnesty International, and Doctors without Borders)—provides extensive evidence that child soldiers as well as child laborers lived in a highly structured rebel social order, or a strict world of command and obedience, as well as punishment and violence.

Civilian limb amputations were also part of that military regime of social control. The RUF was not the only military group in the civil war that carried out civilian limb amputations. Regardless of which military group was involved, testimonies indicate that this violence was not the random, spontaneous actions of a few angry young soldiers. In one testimony to the TRC, for example, several victims who had had their limbs amputated wanted a sergeant in the Sierra Leone Armed Forces to admit that it was not just a few wayward soldiers who carried out this violence. The sergeant agreed that the violence was organized: "I gave the orders to my boys to carry out the amputation" (Sierra Leone Truth and Reconciliation Commission 2004, 3B:453).

There is ample evidence in the voluminous testimony of victims and witnesses from a variety of sources, such as the sergeant's statement above, that amputations were an important part of an organized plan. The language of orders and planning was often communicated in the military vocabulary of a "mission." One survivor of a massacre at a mosque reports the rebel use of the word "mission" to describe their project of amputating limbs: "One of the [rebel soldiers] raised his machete and screamed, Our mission is to kill you and cut your hands."[4] Much of such testimony takes the form of youth reporting the language of command and legitimacy used by military leaders and soldiers in exercising violent domination (on the evidence of organizational authority indexed in reports of the speech surrounding sexual violence, see Murphy 2009).

The words of young people (and other victims) about the communicative practices—such as the commands and justifications for punishments in this violent social world—exemplified in the TRC testimonies above add a perspective missing from the official rebel discourse about youth violence. The theory of emotions in this latter discourse can seem persuasive, reflecting the natural relationship between childhood and emotions, but it fails to locate youths' emotions as social constructs in the organized violent projects of the rebel group. A broader sociological approach to young people's experience—as embedded in military organizations during the war as well as in community organizations before the war—is necessary if psychosocial therapeutic practice in postconflict conditions is to avoid becoming an accomplice to the structural injustices experienced by youth before and during the war.

CONCLUSION AND THEORETICAL IMPLICATIONS

The social identity and subjectivity of youth vary according to the discursive formations in a society that constitute the different institutional sites of statements (and signs) that are enunciated, logically related and presupposing a "way of looking at things," such as "looking" at the social object called "youth"—as well as the object called "youth violence." A social-psychological method of analyzing such institutional formations of the self might be called "archeological," but not in Freud's sense of excavating the levels of experience and meaning that make up the stratigraphy of the individual's psychic landscape—that is, unearthing buried, and disturbing, objects of feeling, which Freud compares to "priceless though mutilated relics of antiquity" (quoted in Schnapp, Shanks, and Tiews 2004, 6). Rather, it would be archeological in Foucault's sense of excavating the self from the layers of meaning articulated in the discursive domains of social classifications, exclusions, and restrictions. Archeological analysis, in this sociological sense, "does not imply a search for beginnings . . . but describes discourses as practices" and "individualizes . . . discursive formations" (1972, 131, 157).[5] The layers of meaning that are unearthed are built up chronologically as well as separated synchronically by the various institutional contexts of discursive formations. For Foucault, the archeology of the self is an institutional analysis of these separate discursive domains of speaking and reasoning about the self—or, in Peirce's methodology, different logical domains of signs of the self communicated in a social context.

Four different institutional domains of discourse were "individualized" in this essay: postwar communities carrying out reconciliation programs for former child soldiers; rebels' public explanations of youth emotions and violence during the civil war; youths' testimonies about the organizational order of violent projects in civil war, as collected by the TRC; and witnesses' testimonies about violence against civilians collected by Human Rights Watch. These different institutional sites are defined by different goals in speaking and reasoning about violence, and thus they comprise different discursive formations. Together they present a more comprehensive picture than each presents alone of the social reality of youth violence in this civil war. The RUF's discourse about violence against civilians, for example, was a response to national and global criticism of atrocities committed, and a strategy for deflecting responsibility for the atrocities from the organization. This interpretation of the discourse is supported by numerous testimonies confirming that civilian limb amputations, for example, were—on particular occasions, at least—part of a policy of punishment by the rebels (Carey 2006).

Reconciliation presupposes that a child learns the discursive formation of violence in a kind of apprenticeship to the signs and their meanings that constitute the social world he or she inhabits. The self is constructed through this apprenticeship.[6] When that world is violently disrupted through civil strife, this apprenticeship becomes one to the signs and meanings of violence—a semiotic turn that is central to survival, because interpreting signs incorrectly in a civil war can mean death. Rebuilding social worlds in the aftermath of civil strife is another form of apprenticeship. "Community healing," as Veena Das and Arthur Kleinman argue, "means repair but it also means transformation—transformation to a different moral state" (2001, 23). This transformation is also a semiotic transformation, in which the social creativity of everyday life as well as the creativity of culture consists in rebuilding the signs and meanings of social relations, especially in the aftermath of violence and civil unrest (on violence and the everyday, see also Nordstrom and Robben 1995).

The TRC testimonies discussed above represent, to borrow a felicitous phrase from Das and Kleinman, a "retrieval of voice" (2001, 20) in the sense that the voices of victims and youth add important insights often excluded from the discursive formations of official discourse by chiefs, elders, officials in the national government, and rebel commanders (while recognizing, of course, that the voices of victims are also structured by genres of suffering). In addition, the retrieval of voices reframes the social-psychological task of rehabilitating former child soldiers by incorporating knowledge of how the social and political structures of communities work in the context of war and peace-building from the perspective of those most vulnerable to the suffering caused by those structures.[7] The psychological technique of allowing war-affected youth to take photographs of their postconflict social world and then explain that world through the photographs—a technique known as photovoice—is another way of retrieving the voices of youth (for the case of Sierra Leone, see Denov, Doucet, and Kamara 2012).

Therapies built on understanding the social worlds of young people and the semiotics of youth subjectivity, however, also confront the realities of young people's predicaments in Africa that arise from national political economies. Postconflict youth programs are affected by the political economy of youth opportunities for education, employment, and political participation—and community social services in general. The Ugandan psychiatrist Seggane Musisi highlights such community infrastructural problems in postconflict situations: what the individual needs, beside therapeutic intervention, is community rehabilitation "through the construction of infrastructure, roads, clean water, power, health centers, housing, schools and viable small economic projects and vocational skills training" (2004, 81).[8]

To dramatize these pressures of everyday postconflict life, consider a quote from a Sierra Leonean man in 2009 (seven years after the civil war was declared over) that was used as the title of a recent article: "We don't even have toilets! How can the country have peace?" (Menzel 2011b). Anne Menzel quotes another Sierra Leonean young man around the same time who sounds like Musisi in outlining the dire problems of everyday postconflict life: "The peace we are fighting for today . . . the problem is, people don't have enough money, and this is what makes them all disgruntled. . . . There is not enough work for people in Sierra Leone. This is the only problem. If the people have jobs, there will be peace, but as the poor man has not job, it will not be easy to make peace in this country" (Menzel 2011a, 107).

These testimonies support Musisi's basic point that the task of psychosocial healing is inextricably linked to the fundamental challenge of alleviating extreme impoverishment in a postconflict society. Much of the social-scientific literature on postconflict Sierra Leone—as well as on the related, and similar, case of postconflict Liberia—have addressed these structural problems of dire need by identifying the specific constraints, incentives, difficulties, and opportunities of the postconflict political economy in which people, especially youth, have to rebuild their social lives and psychological well-being (see, for example, Christensen 2012; Christensen and Utas 2008; Coulter 2009; Denov 2010 and 2011; Hoffman 2011; Ibrahim and Shepler 2011; MacKenzie 2012; Menzel 2011a and 2011b; Munive 2010; Munive and Jakobsen 2012; Persson 2012; Peters 2006 and 2011; Peters and Richards 2011; Schroven 2011; Shepler 2014; Utas 2005a and 2005b).

In addition, the political economy of youth in Africa is regional as well as national: the end of civil war in one country often frees impoverished youth to take advantage of the civil strife in a neighboring country to prey on people there. Former youth combatants in the Liberian civil war, for example, sold their services to parties in the civil conflict in the Côte d'Ivoire. Thus, a further challenge to community-based healing practices in the aftermath of civil strife is coping with the regional as well as the local dimension of a political economy of child soldiering.

Moreover, therapeutic practices of resocializing youth in the aftermath of violent conflict, as formulated in the theoretical model of communication and semiotics discussed above, involve a new social apprenticeship in both interpreting past signs of violence and reconstituting present signs of community solidarity, reconciliation, peace, and equity. However, postconflict signs of reconciliation may also be signs of the subordination, dependency, and marginalization of youth in the community. The focus on forgiving former child soldiers in the semiotics of community reconciliation ceremonies, for example, erases the recognition of community authority structures that alienate youth politically and economically. Reproducing youth subordination through the communicative practices and semiotics of reconciliation in the postwar community (notably, rituals of reconciliation are also rituals of sociopolitical hierarchy) contributes to renewed alienation of young people rather than their rehabilitation.

The great lesson of African psychiatric practice, as it was formulated in the middle part of the twentieth century, was that the individual's psychic healing involves the cultural resources of reconciliation with family and community. Such reconciliation is also shaped by the mechanisms of transitional justice, which can enhance or inhibit both individual and collective healing (Shaw 2010; Kelsall 2009). For the contemporary challenge of coping with mass trauma arising from widespread violent civil conflicts, new lessons (for the twenty-first century) have emerged about the complex sociopolitical structure called "community" and the broader social scope of individual psychological problems in the context of community social dynamics. As Musisi has emphasized, psychiatry's response to mass trauma requires a far more complex conceptualization that locates individual mental health within the wider infrastructural context of the community's social structure and political economy. People in postconflict situations need community-based psychiatric interventions, but rehabilitating their mental health also requires building a community with clean water, good schools, health services, employment opportunities, and so forth.[9] Similarly, the work of Theresa Betancourt and her colleagues (2008 and 2010) in postconflict Sierra Leone has emphasized the importance of the infrastructure for education and social services, in addition to mental health services, for war-affected youth. The general methodological principle from such studies is clear: understanding postconflict psychological healing requires profound interdisciplinary insights into the intricate relationships between individual and collective trauma, neurobiology and the social structure of violent trauma, community and culture as constituted by power, and the social reproduction of the personal suffering of war in the structural violence of postconflict peace (Abramowitz 2005, 2010, and 2014; Abramowitz and Kleinman 2008).

The African cases, of course, should not be exoticized as unique: mental health in all countries is conditioned by political and economic factors that can create feelings of hopelessness, alienation, depression, and anxiety. Moreover, the idea that the mind exists within a social world is fundamental to modern psychology (see, for example, Bateson 1972) as well as African psychiatry. Nevertheless, the crises of mass trauma in war and civil conflict create a special, intense research interest in the relationship of psychological healing to the social ecology of the mind.

In conclusion, psychosocial therapeutic practice is a vital part of civil society's broader task of ameliorating oppressive structures of social domination and subordination that lead, in the first place, to violent conflict and mass trauma and, later, to conditions that—in the aftermath of war—create harsh epidemiological consequences (both social and psychological) when those structures are reproduced. Finally, the vulnerability of youth in civil war and in postconflict peacemaking provides an emblematic image of the general research problem of understanding the relationship between community sociopolitical structures and psychological trauma or healing.

NOTES

I am grateful to the editors of the volume for organizing a conference where I could begin to address and discuss the research puzzle worked through in this chapter. I want to thank my daily anthropological interlocutor at Northwestern University, Robert Launay, for comments on an earlier version of this essay, and Karrie Stewart for introducing me to the work of the Ugandan-born psychiatrist, Seggane Musisi. To my exercise companions, Souleymane Bachir Diagne and Kenneth Vaux, I express my appreciation for their guidance in all things philosophical. I am also grateful to Asif Agha for suggesting important additional works about the semiotics of the self. Finally, Sharon Abramowitz offered very helpful suggestions for refining the conceptual and ethnographic problematic of psychiatry and culture in postconflict societies, and for rounding out the bibliography. Any remaining analytical and ethnographic infelicities are my own.

1. Quoted in Barry (2007). The Liberian Truth and Reconciliation Commission was established by an act of the Liberian National Transitional Legislature on May 12, 2005. The commission's work was officially launched at a ceremony in Monrovia on June 22, 2006. A unique feature of the work of this commission was a program that collected testimonies from the Liberians living outside the country's borders. The quote in the text, for example, came from a session held in New York City on September 8, 2007.

2. The TRC report makes a distinction between "child" and "youth" and assigns different chapters to these categories: "Every Sierra Leonean between the ages of 18 and 35 years old is considered to be youth" (Sierra Leone Truth and Reconciliation Commission 2004, 3B:343). Children are defined as under eighteen, which is also the definition used by international conventions. In this essay, the distinction is not critical for the argument, so the terms are used interchangeably. But when the reference is to children under eighteen, the ages are usually specified in the essay. The TRC is clear, however, about the social construction of the category "youth": the "word 'youth' [in Sierra Leone] itself became a synonym for the unemployed young person who was vulnerable to manipulation. Youths were considered to be auxiliary troops for political parties" (ibid., 346).

3. On the "politics of age" in the TRC's approach to children in the context of a discourse of forgiveness and responsibility, see Rosen (2005, 146–53).

4. This quote comes from the case of Ibrahim described in section IV ("Human Rights Abuses Committed by RUF Rebels") of Human Rights Watch (1999), http://www.hrw.org/legacy/reports/1999/sierra/SIERLE99-03.htm#P667_117336.

5. Foucault's formulation shifts between the idea of discourse as an event and a concrete enunciation of statements and the idea of discursive formation as underlying institutional rules that make statements possible, including making social classifications and exclusions possible through enunciations. This essay interrelates the two notions by emphasizing the purposive dimensions of a rhetoric and politics of reasoning—in this case, about youth violence.

6. I borrow the concept of apprenticeship to signs from Deleuze, who uses it in his study of memory in Proust's narrative art (2000).

7. To correct a weakness in the theory of socialization—in which the child is viewed as a passive recipient of adult instruction—much of the recent work in the anthropology of youth has emphasized the agency of youth (see, for example, Cole and Durham 2007), including the agency of child soldiers (see, for example, Honwana 2005; Utas 2005a). In this essay, the structural constraints on youth agency—in the context of the great coercive resources of adults in civil wars—are emphasized. In addition, the role of a violent semiotics in indoctrinating youth is foregrounded. Nevertheless, the focus on youths' voices and the retrieval of those voices in postconflict situations privileges the expression of youth agency through language and other semiotic forms. This latter form of agency includes children's creativity in expressing their suffering caused by political conflict (see Reynolds 2005).

8. As an anthropologist, I share Musisi's focus on the sociopolitical context and the political economy of personal and community rehabilitation after the mass trauma of civil conflict.

9. Besides a focus on the effect of the political economy and civil conflict on mental health, another dimension of twenty-first-century African psychiatry, also exemplified in Musisi's work, is a greater use of pharmacological interventions—such as drugs for anxiety and depression—as part of a complete package of psychiatric interventions.

REFERENCES

Abdullah, I., ed. 2004. *Between Democracy and Terror: The Sierra Leone Civil War.* Dakar: Council for the Development of Social Science Research in Africa.

Abramowitz, S. 2005. "The Poor Have Become Rich, and the Rich Have Become Poor: Collective Trauma in the Guinean Languette." *Social Science and Medicine* 61 (10): 2106–18.

———. 2010. "Trauma and Humanitarian Translation in Liberia: The Tale of Open Mole." *Culture, Medicine, and Psychiatry* 34 (2): 353–79.

———. 2012. "Producing Peace Subjectivities: Psychosocial Interventions in Liberia's Post-Conflict Recovery." Paper presented at Transcending Traditional Tropes: Conceptualizing Politics and Policies in 21st Century Upper Guinea Coast conference, Halle/Saale, Germany, September 26.

———. 2014. *Searching for Normal in the Wake of the Liberian War.* Philadelphia: University of Pennsylvania Press.

Abramowitz, S., and A. Kleinman. 2008. "Humanitarian Intervention and Cultural Translation: IASC Guidelines on Mental Health and Psychosocial Support in Emergency Settings." *Intervention* 6 (3–4): 219–27.

Abramowitz, S., and M. H. Moran. 2012. "International Human Rights, Gender-Based Violence, and Local Discourses of Abuse in Postconflict Liberia: A Problem of 'Culture'?" *African Studies Review* 55 (2): 119–46.

Abu-Lughod, L., and C. A. Lutz. 1990. "Introduction: Emotion, Discourse, and the Politics of Everyday Life." In *The Language and Politics of Emotion,* edited by C. A. Lutz and L. Abu-Lughod, 1–23. Cambridge: Cambridge University Press.

Achvarina, V., and S. F. Reich. 2006. "No Place to Hide: Refugees, Displaced Persons, and the Recruitment of Child Soldiers." *International Security* 31 (1): 127–64.

Agha, A. 1995. "Process and Personality." *Semiotica* 107 (1–2): 125–46.

———. 2007. *Language and Social Relations.* Cambridge: Cambridge University Press.

Ashforth, A. 2005. *Witchcraft, Violence, and Democracy in South Africa.* Chicago: University of Chicago Press.

Barry, E. 2007. "From Staten Island Haven, Liberians Reveal War's Scars." New York Times, September 18, A16. http://www.nytimes.com/2007/09/18/nyregion/18liberians.html?pagewanted=all&module=Search&mabReward=relbias%3Ar%2C{%222%22%3A%22RI%3A12%22}&_r=0.

Bateson, G. 1972. *Steps to an Ecology of the Mind: Collected Essays in Anthropology, Psychiatry, Evolution, and Epistemology.* San Francisco: Chandler.

Beah, I. 2007. *A Long Way Gone: Memoirs of a Boy Soldier.* New York: Farrar, Straus and Giroux.

Betancourt, T. S., I. I. Borisova, T. P. Williams, T. H. Whitfield, M. de la Soudiere, J. Williamson, and S. E. Gilman. 2010. "Sierra Leone's Former Child Soldiers: A Follow-Up Study of Psychosocial Adjustment and Community Reintegration." *Child Development* 81 (4): 1077–95.

Betancourt, T. S., S. Simmons, I. Borisova, S. E. Brewer, U. Iweala, and M. de la Soudiere. 2008. "High Hopes, Grim Reality: Reintegration and the Education of Former Child Soldiers in Sierra Leone." *Comparative Education Review* 52 (4): 565–87.

Boyden, J., and J. de Berry, eds. 2004. *Children and Youth on the Front Line: Ethnography, Armed Conflict and Displacement.* New York: Berghahn.

Brett, R., and I. Specht. 2004. *Young Soldiers: Why They Choose to Fight.* Boulder, CO: Lynne Rienner.

Carey, M. 2006. "'Survival Is Political': History, Violence and the Contemporary Power Struggle in Sierra Leone." In *States of Violence: Politics, Youth and Memory in Contemporary Africa,* edited by E. G. Bay and D. L. Donham, 97–126. Charlottesville, VA: University of Virginia Press.

Caton, S. C. 1993. "The Importance of Reflexive Language in George H. Mead's Theory of Self and Communication." In *Reflexive Language: Reported Speech and Metapragmatics,* edited by J. A. Lucy, 315–38. Cambridge: Cambridge University Press.

Chabal, P., and J.-P. Daloz. 1999. *Africa Works: Disorder as Political Instrument.* Oxford: James Currey.

Chavunduka, G. 1978. *Traditional Healers and the Shona Patient.* Gwelo, Zimbabwe: Mambo.

Christensen, M. M. 2012. "Big Man Business in the Borderland of Sierra Leone." In *African Conflicts and Informal Power: Big Men and Networks,* edited by M. Utas, 60–77. London: Zed.

Christensen, M. M., and M. Utas. 2008. "Mercenaries of Democracy: The 'Politricks' of Remobilized Combatants in the 2007 General Elections, Sierra Leone." *African Affairs* 107 (429): 515–39.

Cohn, I., and G. S. Goodwin-Gil. 1994. *Child Soldiers: The Role of Children in Armed Conflict.* Oxford: Oxford University.

Colapietro, V. M. 1989. *Peirce's Approach to the Self: A Semiotic Perspective on Human Subjectivity.* Albany: State University of New York Press.

Cole, J., and D. Durham, eds. 2007. *Generations and Globalizations: Youth, Age, and Family in the New World Economy.* Bloomington: Indiana University Press.

Collier, P. 2007. *The Bottom Billion: Why the Poorest Countries Are Failing and What Can Be Done About It.* Oxford: Oxford University Press.

Comaroff, J., and J. L. Comaroff. 2005. "Reflections on Youth: From the Past to the Postcolony." In *Makers and Breakers: Children and Youth in Postcolonial Africa,* edited by A. Honwana and F. De Boeck 19–30. Trenton, NJ: Africa World.

Coulter, C. 2009. *Bush Wives and Girl Soldiers: Women's Lives through War and Peace in Sierra Leone.* Ithaca, NY: Cornell University Press.

Das, V., and A. Kleinman. 2001. Introduction to *Remaking a World: Violence, Social Suffering, and Recovery,* edited by V. Das, A. Kleinman, M. Lock, M. Ramphele, and P. Reynolds, 1–30. Berkeley: University of California Press.

De Jong, J., ed. 2002. *Trauma, War, and Violence: Public Mental Health in Socio-Cultural Context.* Hingham, MA: Kluwer Academic.

De Waal, C. 2001. *On Peirce.* Belmont, CA: Wadsworth.

Deleuze, G. 2000. *Proust and Signs.* Translated by Richard Howard. Minneapolis: University of Minnesota Press.

Denov, M. 2010. *Child Soldiers: Sierra Leone's Revolutionary United Front.* Cambridge: Cambridge University Press.

———. 2011. "Social Navigation and Power in Post-Conflict Sierra Leone: Reflections from a Former Child Soldier Turned Bike Rider." In *Child Soldiers: From Recruitment to Reintegration,* edited by A. Ozerdem and S. Podder, 191–212. New York: Palgrave Macmillan.

Denov, M., D. Doucet, and A. Kamara. 2012. "Engaging War-Affected Youth through Photography: Photovoice with Former Child Soldiers in Sierra Leone." *Intervention* 10 (2): 117–33.

Diouf, M. 2003. "Engaging Postcolonial Cultures: African Youth and Public Space." *African Studies Review* 46 (1): 1–12.

Ellis, S. 1999. *The Mask of Anarchy: The Destruction of Liberia and the Religious Dimension of an African Civil War.* New York: New York University Press.

Feierman, S., and J. M. Janzen, eds. 1992. *The Social Basis of Health and Healing in Africa.* Berkeley: University of California Press.

Ferme, M. 2001. *The Underneath of Things: Violence, History, and the Everyday in Sierra Leone.* Berkeley: University of California Press.

Fithen, C., and P. Richards. 2005. "Making War, Crafting Peace: Militia Solidarities and Demobilization in Sierra Leone." In *No Peace No War: An Anthropology of Contemporary Armed Conflicts,* edited by P. Richards, 117–36. Athens: Ohio University Press.

Foucault, M. 1972. *The Archeology of Knowledge and the Discourse on Language.* Translated by Rupert Swyer. New York: Pantheon.

Gberie, L. 2005. *A Dirty War in West Africa: The RUF and the Destruction of Sierra Leone.* Bloomington: Indiana University Press.

Hoffman, D. 2011. *The War Machines: Young Men and Violence in Sierra Leone and Liberia.* Durham, NC: Duke University.

Honwana, A. 2005. "Innocent and Guilty: Child-Soldiers as Interstitial and Tactical Agents." In *Makers and Breakers: Children and Youth in Postcolonial Africa,* edited by A. Honwana and F. De Boeck, 31–52. Trenton, NJ: Africa World.

———. 2006. *Child Soldiers in Africa.* Philadelphia: University of Pennsylvania Press.

Honwana, A., and F. De Boeck, eds. 2005. *Makers and Breakers: Children and Youth in Postcolonial Africa.* Trenton, NJ: Africa World.

Human Rights Watch. 1999. "Sierra Leone: Getting Away with Murder, Mutilation, Rape. New Testimony from Sierra Leone, July 1999, Vol 11 No 3(A)." http://www.hrw.org/reports/1999/sierra/.

Ibrahim, A. F., and S. Shepler. 2011. "Introduction: Everyday Life in Postwar Sierra Leone." *Africa Today* 58 (2): v–xii.

Innis, R. E. 1985. "Charles S. Pierce." In *Semiotics: An Introductory Anthology,* edited by R. E. Innis, 1–4. Bloomington: Indiana University Press.

Joas, H. 1993. *Pragmatism and Social Theory.* Chicago: University of Chicago Press.

Kelsall, Tim. 2009. *Culture under Cross-Examination: International Justice and the Special Court for Sierra Leone.* Cambridge: Cambridge University Press.

Last, M., and G. L. Chavunduka, eds. 1986. *The Professionalization of African Medicine.* Manchester, UK: Manchester University Press.

Lee, B., and G. Urban, eds. 1989. *Semiotics, Self, and Society.* Berlin: Mouton de Gruyter.

MacKenzie, M. H. 2012. *Female Soldiers in Sierra Leone: Sex, Security, and Post-Conflict Development.* New York: New York University Press.

Mead, G. H. 1934. *Mind, Self, and Society.* Chicago: University of Chicago Press.

Menzel, A. 2011a. "Between Ex-Combatization and Opportunities for Peace: The Double-Edged Qualities of Motorcycle-Taxi Driving in Urban Postwar Sierra Leone." *Africa Today* 58 (2): 97–127.

———. 2011b. "'We Don't Even Have Toilets! How Can the Country Have Peace?': *Obwohl Armut kein Krieg ist, fühlt sie sich im Sierra Leonischen 'Frieden' so an.*" *Powision: Neue Räume für Politik.* http://www.uni-leipzig.de/~powision/wordpress/magazin/anne-menzel/.

Mertz, E. 1989. "Steps toward a Social Semiotic of Selves." *Semiotica* 90 (3–4): 295–309.

Munive, J. 2010. "The Army of 'Unemployed' Young People." *Young* 18 (3): 321–38.

Munive, J., and S. F. Jakobsen. 2012. "Revisiting DDR in Liberia: Exploring the Power, Agency and Interests of Local and International Actors in the 'Making' and 'Unmaking' of Combatants." *Conflict, Security, and Development* 12 (4): 359–85.

Murphy, W. P. 1980. "Secret Knowledge as Property and Power in Kpelle Society: Elders versus Youth." *Africa* 50 (2): 193–207.

———. 2003. "Military Patrimonialism and Child Soldier Clientalism in the Liberian and Sierra Leonean Civil Wars." *African Studies Review* 46 (2): 61–87.

———. 2009. "Rape and Reported Speech: Patronage Model of Sexual Violence in the Sierra Leonean Civil War." Paper presented at the Semiotics Workshop: Culture in Context, University of Chicago, IL, October 9.

———. 2010. "Patrimonial Logic of Centrifugal Forces in the Political History of the Upper Guinea Coast." In *The Powerful Presence of the Past: Integration and Conflict along the Upper Guinea Coast,* edited by J. Knorr and W. T. Filho, 27–53. Leiden, the Netherlands: Brill.

Musisi, S. 2004. "Editorial: Mass Trauma and Mental Health in Africa." *African Health Sciences* 4 (2): 80–82.

Nordstrom, C., and A. C. G. M. Robben, eds. 1995. *Fieldwork under Fire: Contemporary Studies of Violence and Survival.* Berkeley: University of California Press.

Persson, M. 2012. "Demobilized or Remobilized? Lingering Rebel Structures in Post-War Liberia." In *African Conflicts and Informal Power: Big Men and Networks,* edited by M. Utas, 101–18. London: Zed.

Peters, K. 2004. "Reintegrating Young Ex-Combatants in Sierra Leone: Accommodating Indigenous and Wartime Value Systems." In *Vanguard or Vandals: Youth, Politics and Conflict in Africa,* edited by J. Abbink and I. van Kessel, 267–98. Leiden, the Netherlands: Brill.

———. 2006. "Footpaths to Reintegration: Armed Conflict, Youth and the Rural Crisis in Sierra Leone." PhD diss. Wageningen University.

———. 2011. *War and the Crisis of Youth in Sierra Leone.* Cambridge: Cambridge University Press.

Peters, K., and P. Richards. 2011. "Rebellion and Agrarian Tensions in Sierra Leone." *Journal of Agrarian Change* 11 (3): 377–95.

Reno, W. 1998. *Warlord Politics and African States.* Boulder, CO: Lynne Rienner.

Republic of Liberia Truth and Reconciliation Commission. 2008–2009. *Final Report of the Truth and Reconciliation Commission of Liberia.* http://trcofliberia.org/reports/final-report).

Reynolds, P. 2005. "Forming Identities: Conceptions of Pain and Children's Expressions of It in South Africa." In *Makers and Breakers: Children and Youth in Postcolonial Africa,* edited by A. Honwana and F. De Boeck, 81–101. Trenton, NJ: Africa World.

Revolutionary United Front. 1999. "RUF Calls for Independent Investigations." The Sierra Leone Web. http://www.sierra-leone.org/AFRC-RUF/RUF-011599.html).

Richards, P. 1996. *Fighting for the Rain Forest: War, Youth and Resources in Sierra Leone.* London: James Currey.

Rincon, J. M. 2010. "Ex-Combatants, Returnees, Land and Conflict in Liberia." Copenhagen, Denmark: Danish Institute for International Studies. Working Paper No. 5.

Rosen, D. M. 2005. *Armies of the Young: Child Soldiers in War and Terrorism.* New Brunswick, NJ: Rutgers University Press.

Ross, F. 2003. *Bearing Witness: Women and the Truth and Reconciliation Commission in South Africa.* London: Pluto.

———. 2005. "Women and the Politics of Identity: Voices in the South African Truth and Reconciliation Commission." In *Violence and Belonging: The Quest for Identity in Post-Colonial Africa,* edited by V. Broch-Due., 214–35. London: Routledge.

———. 2010. "An Acknowledged Failure: Women, Voice, and the South African Truth and Reconciliation Commission." In *Localizing Transitional Justice: Interventions and Priorities after Mass Violence,* edited by R. Shaw and L. Waldorf, with P. Hazan, 69–91. Stanford: Stanford University Press.

Ross, F., and P. Reynolds. 1999. "Wrapped in Pain: Moral Economies and the South African Truth and Reconciliation Commission." *Context* 3: 1–9.

Schafer, J. 2004. "The Use of Patriarchal Imagery in the Civil War in Mozambique and Its Implications for the Reintegration of Child Soldiers." In *Children and Youth on the Front Line: Ethnography, Armed Conflict and Displacement,* edited by J. Boyden and J. de Berry, 87–104. New York: Berghahn.

Schnapp, J., M. Shanks, and M. Tiews. 2004. "Archeology, Modernism, Modernity: Editor's Introduction." *Modernism/Modernity* 11 (1): 1–16.

Schroven, A. 2011. "The (Re-) Conceptualization of Women in Gendered International Interventions: Examples from Post-War Sierra Leone." *Max Planck Institute for Social Anthropology Working Papers,* Halle/Saale, Germany, no. 130.

Shaw, R. 2002. *Memories of the Slave Trade: Ritual and the Historical Imagination in Sierra Leone.* Chicago: University of Chicago Press.

———. 2010. "Linking Justice with Reintegration? Ex-Combatants and the Sierra Leone Experiment." In *Localizing Transitional Justice: Interventions and Priorities after Mass Violence,* edited by R. Shaw and L. Waldorf, with P. Hazan, 111–32. Stanford, CA: Stanford University Press.

Shepler, S. A. 2014. *Childhood Deployed: Remaking Child Soldiers in Sierra Leone.* New York: New York University Press.

Sierra Leone Truth and Reconciliation Commission. 2004. *Witness to Truth: Report of the Sierra Leone Truth and Reconciliation Commission.* http://www.sierra-leone.org /TRCDocuments.html.

Skagested, P. 2004. "Peirce's Semeiotic Model of the Mind." In *The Cambridge Companion to Peirce,* edited by C. Misak, 241–56. Cambridge: Cambridge University Press.

Utas, M. 2005a. "Agency of Victims: Young Women in the Liberian Civil War." In *Makers and Breakers: Children and Youth in Postcolonial Africa,* edited by A. Honwana and F. De Boeck, 53–80. Trenton, NJ: Africa World.

———. 2005b. "Building a Future? The Reintegration and Remarginalisation of Youth in Liberia." In *No Peace No War: An Anthropology of Contemporary Armed Conflicts,* edited by P. Richards, 137–54. Athens: Ohio University Press.

————. 2009. *Sexual Abuse Survivors and the Complex of Traditional Healing: (G)local Prospects in the Aftermath of an African War.* Uppsala, Sweden: Nordic Africa Institute.

————, ed. 2012. *African Conflicts and Informal Power: Big Men and Networks.* London: Zed.

Weber, M. 1978. *Economy and Society.* Edited by G. Roth and C. Wittich. Translated by E. Fischoff, H. Gerth, C. Wright Mills, F. Kolegar, A. M. Henderson, T. Parsons, E. Shills, and M. Rheinstein. Berkeley: University of California Press.

13 USING MIXED METHODS TO PLAN AND EVALUATE MENTAL HEALTH PROGRAMS FOR WAR-AFFECTED CHILDREN IN SUB-SAHARAN AFRICA

THERESA BETANCOURT

Few child and adolescent mental health interventions have been proved effective in addressing the needs of war-affected children in sub-Saharan Africa. Such interventions are difficult to develop because of the absence of appropriate and valid measures of mental health problems and related constructs, as well as the practical problems of working in settings with few trained mental health professionals. Ethical issues also complicate research on children's mental health in resource-poor settings. Research addressing these ethical, logistical, and methodological challenges is sorely needed. There is little empirical work that identifies the key ingredients needed to develop interventions or assesses which interventions are the most effective for addressing children's mental health problems across the diverse settings in which children suffer extraordinary stress (Betancourt and Beardslee 2012). Yet there is a growing awareness in the field that new approaches must be developed for use in low-resource settings. This chapter argues for the application of a qualitative and quantitative "mixed methodology" approach as a way to more completely understand the mental health issues facing war-affected children and families. A mixed-methods model is presented for use in planning and evaluating mental health services in diverse cultural settings. Such integrated approaches can help address some of the challenges that have stymied progress in the field. Core issues are illustrated drawing from field research with war-affected children and families in Sierra Leone, Ethiopia, and northern Uganda.

CHILDREN AND WAR

Wars dramatically alter the lives of children everywhere. UNICEF reports that conflicts in the last decade have killed an estimated two million children and have left another six million disabled and twenty million homeless. Of the twenty million homeless children, over one million are separated from their parents (UNICEF 2009). The changing tactics and technology of warfare today have magnified the hazards for children. Wars are increasingly fought within states and involve nonstate actors, such as rebel or terrorist groups, whose members are less likely than formal military groups to be aware of or abide by humanitarian laws providing for the protection of civilians in conflict (Stichick and Bruderlein 2001). In addition, child combatants are common in wars from Afghanistan to northern Uganda. The proliferation of newer and deadlier technologies of warfare such as land mines and small arms has also had dramatic consequences on morbidity and mortality among children. By some estimates, for every child who dies from armed attacks, another three are left severely wounded or disabled. The effects of the loss and violence that children have experienced in wartime are catastrophic (Machel 1996). Estimates of psychological trauma or distress due to war are high for war-affected youth around the globe, including sub-Saharan Africa (Bayer, Klasen, and Adam 2007; Betancourt et al. 2010a, 2010b; Derluyn et al. 2004), Asia (Kinzie et al. 1986; Kohrt 2007), and the Middle East (Ahmad 2008; Macksoud and Aber 1996; Razokhi et al. 2006).

The scourge of war has disproportionately compounded the already sizable baseline threats to child health and development in many African countries. Health and developmental risks to children are particularly high in regions where conflict is intermingled with the HIV/AIDS pandemic, extreme poverty, or both, as is the case in many parts of sub-Saharan Africa (Black, Morris, and Bryce 2003).

The Challenge of Measurement

Mental health screening and assessment instruments are needed to assess the burden of mental health disorders associated with war. To rely on Western-based diagnostic systems in diverse cultural settings without a critical examination of those systems runs the risk of missing or incorrectly diagnosing clinically significant indicators of distress as well as protective factors among populations where standard Western criteria are inappropriate (Guarnaccia, Lewis-Fernandez, and Marano 2003; Lewis-Fernandez et al. 2002). When applied to developing country settings with no adaptations, many of the standard assessments used to screen children in the West for mental health problems can present problems (Stichick 2001). The literature on refugee trauma and mental health frequently reports quantitative data using measures with unproven validity and reliability in culturally diverse refugee populations (Hollifield et al. 2002). These challenges bring the issue of the validity and cultural relevance of assessment and screening tools to the forefront of research on the mental health of war-affected children.

In most cases, war-affected populations in developing countries, particularly in sub-Saharan Africa, have life experiences as well as cultural and political contexts that differ dramatically from those of populations in the West, where most standard mental health measures were developed (for an extended discussion of the anthropological context, see Murphy, this volume).

LIMITATIONS OF THE "STANDARD APPROACH" TO MENTAL HEALTH ASSESSMENT

Currently, most mental health assessments in war zones begin with the design of a questionnaire or standard survey. These are intended to measure mental health constructs in the affected population but routinely use existing Western measures that may have little relation to the setting of interest. In the best-case scenario, these measures are adapted to new settings by altering or modifying questions to reflect local terminology and translated backward and forward—in some cases employing more advanced translation methods (Matías-Carrelo et al. 2003)—before they are used in the new cultural setting. In this manner, constructs to be studied are often developed outside the local culture or context. Despite high-quality translation methods, very few attempts are made to assess the validity of the constructs being assessed in much of the research on the mental health of war-affected children. When such approaches are used in baseline assessments to determine the problems to be targeted by interventions, need is determined by the frequency of responses on items intended to measure certain mental health conditions. The choice of these conditions and therefore the related intervention is thus based on quantitative results. After the delivery of an intervention informed by such a baseline assessment, the same measures are then repeated to assess a program's impact. Although this is a perfectly legitimate approach and one that many of us (including me) have used in several cultural settings, as anyone who has conducted research of this type realizes, there are a number of problems with this "standard approach."

Its first limitation has to do with the question of cultural validity. We cannot be sure how closely concepts in a questionnaire developed outside of the context match local concepts. Second, there may be important local issues or concepts that are not assessed because we do not know to ask about them. This is an inherent problem in using closed-ended survey items on questionnaires in any research, but it is particularly precarious in cross-cultural work. By establishing the constructs in advance, without consulting local stakeholders, we may shine a strong light on a preordained area of interest while overlooking central issues of local importance. A third challenge returns us again to issues of translation. What sorts of people typically serve as translators? Working in low-resource settings, we often strive to hire local staff who speak English and the local dialect. The fact that such individuals are educated enough to speak English and apply for a translation job distinguishes them as being more educated and often having had a very different set of life experiences (and possibly vocabulary) than the larger, often very poor community that is usually the target of intervention. Even using forward and backward translation can result in semantic equivalence but real-world insignificance. An interesting example of such an effect can be found in my experience using the Achenbach Youth Self-Report (YSR) and Child Behavior Checklist (CBCL) in war-affected settings (Achenbach 1991). The YSR and the checklist have enjoyed wide cross-cultural use as tools for evaluating emotional and behavioral problems in children and adolescents. They have been translated into more than thirty-six languages and used in various impoverished settings, from South Africa to Indonesia. I have used the measures in several war-affected settings, including camps for internally displaced persons (IDP) in Ingushetia, Russia, and a refugee camp on the Ethiopia-Eritrea border.

In assessing the immediate face validity of these measures in diverse war-affected settings (that is, determining how well they appear to be a good fit with the local context), it becomes apparent that for use with certain cultural or religious groups or in settings with very few resources, a number of items may need to be dropped or modified. For example, in some Muslim cultures, items about sexual behavior and suicide can be offensive or inappropriate (for example, items about "acting like the opposite sex"). In refugee camps, some of the items can be misleading or irrelevant (such as items about "bowel movements outside of the toilet" in a setting where there are no toilets). In fact, many items on common assessments of children's mental health such as the Child Behavior Checklist and the YSR can yield misleading results even if translated perfectly. Items on "lighting fires," for instance, can easily be translated, but the meaning of this behavior can be very different in a refugee camp than in typical city or town in the West. In developed countries, such an item might detect a child with aggression or conduct problems. In many of the refugee camps where I have worked, lighting fires is a daily chore of many young people to assist with the preparation of meals and is hardly an indication of psychopathology. Certainly, with good translation, such an item could be clarified along the lines of "lighting fires for destructive reasons," but in many African countries where I have worked, this behavior would likely be seen as very rare and would not be considered a salient item for capturing conduct problems in the local population, whereas other important indicators of psychopathology do exist. For instance, in many collective cultures, not exchanging greetings upon meeting others, particularly elders, may be seen as offensive. Indeed, our qualitative work to develop an Acholi language youth psychosocial assessment from qualitative data (Betancourt et al. 2009a, 2009b) included an item on "not greeting others" as an important indicator of possible psychopathology.

Without careful attention to locally relevant indicators of distress, current "standard approaches" to measurement can easily specify constructs that are culturally irrelevant or miss highly relevant symptoms that have cultural and contextual significance. The serious risk of these measurement errors is that evaluations using standard methods may fail to accurately measure the impact of an intervention. They may indicate that a program is successful when it truly is not; equally, a very effective program may be dismissed because measurement errors led to a misrepresentation of its true success.

THE CASE FOR A MIXED-METHODS APPROACH TO ASSESSMENT

Researchers with experience in cross-cultural mental health assessment have argued for using qualitative measures as the starting point for developing context-appropriate quantitative assessment measures (Betancourt and Bolton 2005; Bolton 2001; Mollica et al. 2004). By combining qualitative and quantitative methodologies, a mixed-methods approach can go a long way toward addressing some of the concerns raised above. The value of qualitative methods is that they begin from the emic or local perspective (Geertz 1973). They are extremely useful for generating hypotheses and answering questions such as how or what. They involve smaller, focused samples often collected using purposive or maximum-variation sampling techniques (S. Maxwell and Delaney 2000). A real value of qualitative methods for use in field settings in diverse cultures is the ability to go back repeatedly to investigate concepts in depth as they arise across multiple informants. Quantitative methods, in contrast, can be used to confirm a hypothesis and can address classic epidemiological questions such as determining the prevalence of a given disorder in a community or assess the statistical strength of a relationship between quantitative variables. Samples for these purposes are normally collected using probabilistic sampling aimed at representing the underlying population (J. Maxwell 2005; Creswell 2003). Calculations can be performed on larger numbers and allow the researcher to make statistical inferences. Certainly there are strengths and weaknesses to either approach. The greatest benefit is in using qualitative and quantitative methods in combination. In fact, qualitative and quantitative methods are not fundamentally at odds with each other. Applying them in a complementary fashion can result in much more insightful and accurate scientific understanding of issues as complex as the mental health of children affected by armed conflict. The growing field of mixed-methods research discusses clear approaches for sequencing qualitative and quantitative data, depending on the research questions at hand, and utilizing methods for synthesizing, comparing, or integrating the two types of results (Creswell et al. 2011).

A MODEL FOR PLANNING AND EVALUATING MENTAL HEALTH SERVICES

Figure 13.1 presents a model grounded in the power of mixed methods for advancing cross-cultural mental health research and drawing on methods used in prior research in low-resource settings. This sequential exploratory approach to mixed methods research can be used to develop appropriate assessments for identifying mental health problems and sources of resilience in war-affected children, to develop mental health interventions based on this information, and to use the refined assessment tools to evaluate intervention effectiveness. In such designs, investigators first begin with qualitative research to discover local constructs of importance to child mental health (both indicators of psychopathology and protective factors) as demonstrated by the first circle in figure 13.1. Then, in a second phase (the second circle), these findings are used to adapt or select quantitative measures and to subject them to as many efforts to examine their validity as time and budgets will allow. This attention to the validity of measures pertains to evaluating assessments of mental health problems and functional limitations as well as measures of protective processes like social support or coping, which are thought to be the active ingredients of many interventions. Validation efforts are most robust when they use multiple assessments of validity (Goldstein and Simpson 1995), including face validity (the degree to which the measurement appears relevant to the construct of interest), construct validity (the degree to which the measure actually assesses what it purports to measure per some objective external standard), predictive validity (documentation of the measure's ability to predict something it should theoretically be able to predict), concurrent validity (the degree to which the measure correlates with other measures of similar constructs), and criterion validity (the degree to which the measure agrees with an outside "gold standard" for measuring the same construct). As measures validation proceeds, parallel lines of qualitative research can continue to identify issues of importance in the community and enrich understanding of protective processes that can be harnessed in intervention (figure 13.1, top arrow). In the last phase of such an exploratory sequential design, the assessments and intervention models, informed by this qualitative data, can be used to evaluate the impact of the intervention model (the third circle). Lessons learned in applying this approach (as represented in figure 13.1 by the arrow moving back to the beginning) can then be fed back to new settings and the approach can be refined and built upon in an iterative manner across different service populations. Infor-

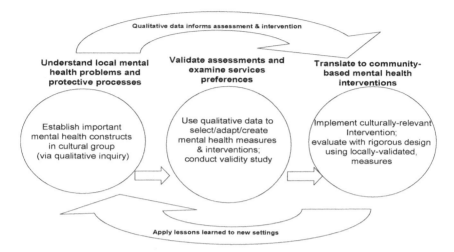

Figure 13.1. A Mixed-Methods Model for Planning and Evaluating
Mental Health Services in Diverse Cultural Settings

mation gathered on the effectiveness of the intervention and lessons learned in
the process of service delivery can thus form the basis for adapting procedures,
assessments, and interventions in new settings.

Field Examples

The concepts presented in the model above and related ethical and methodological lessons learned will be discussed next, together with relevant field research experiences in three African settings: Ethiopia, Sierra Leone, and northern Uganda.

Ethiopia

My research in Ethiopia began in 2001 in collaboration with the International
Rescue Committee (IRC), an international humanitarian nongovernmental organization (NGO) with headquarters in New York City. The study used multiple
methods for data collection, including surveys and focus group interviews with
youth respondents and their caregivers and interviews with key informants
(leaders from a refugee camp). In the planning period for the study, focus group
discussions were held with community members and small groups of Kunama
(the main ethnic group originating in Eritrea) children and adolescents aged ten
through seventeen. The aim of this qualitative data collection via focus group discussions and key informant interviews was to examine the cultural appropriateness of the concepts being investigated and the measures being either created or

adapted for this population. Qualitative interviews were also used to ensure that locally relevant constructs were well reflected in the measures chosen, and that locally important terms, idioms, and concepts were integrated into the translation of the final measures (including several standard Western mental health measures such as the YSR and Child Behavior Checklist [Achenbach 1991]). Kunama camp representatives, health workers, and local members of the IRC staff helped develop the instrument and plan the study. Baseline measures were collected in 2001, at the start of an education program based in the refugee camp. A follow-up survey of youth participants in the education program and their caregivers was conducted one year later (Betancourt et al. 2012b).

Sierra Leone

My research in Sierra Leone began in 2002, again in collaboration with the International Rescue Committee, with funding support from the US Agency for International Development's Displaced Children and Orphans Fund. The specific aim of the research was to assess the factors that contributed to risk and resilience in a cohort of former child soldiers (children formerly affiliated with the fighting forces, or ex-CAFF for short) over time. The original survey sample consisted of 259 ex-CAFF, 88 percent males and 12 percent females, formerly held by the Revolutionary United Front (RUF). All respondents were served by the IRC's interim care centers between June 2001 and February 2002 following formal disarmament and demobilization by the government and UN agencies. The average age of the ex-CAFF sample at baseline was 15.12 years. At baseline we also surveyed a comparison group of 136 youth randomly selected from the same communities where the ex-CAFF in the sample had been resettled, allowing us to make some comparisons between RUF-involved and non-RUF involved youth. The two groups were of similar age and gender composition. A follow-up study of the original cohort was conducted in 2004. The 2004 survey added a comparison sample of 127 ex-CAFF from the Makeni region who had reintegrated themselves into their communities without organized services from an NGO. Our follow-up research also included a series of interviews with thirty key informants, ex-CAFF, and their caregivers selected from those who had participated at baseline. Focus group interviews were conducted with community members to learn about community responses to reintegrated ex-CAFF.

Northern Uganda

My research in northern Uganda began in 2004 as part of a collaboration between the Boston University Applied Mental Health Research Group, Columbia University, and World Vision Uganda and War Child Holland, two international

NGOs that were developing mental health services for children living in the IDP (internally displaced person) camps of Gulu District in northern Uganda. World Vision Uganda and War Child Holland funded the research, and Paul Bolton and I served as co–principal investigators. Our goal was to investigate local perceptions of mental health problems affecting children living in IDP camps and to plan and test appropriate mental health interventions. Over the course of two years, the research moved through three main phases of work: a qualitative study, a validity study, and a randomized controlled trial of mental health interventions. The process of this project will be discussed more fully at the end of this chapter, as it represents a full application of the conceptual model presented above.

Lessons Learned in Mixed-Methods Research with African War-Affected Youth

Through field experience in conducting research with war-affected youth in sub-Saharan Africa, I have directly experienced the value of integrating qualitative and quantitative methodologies at all phases of the research. Across these three field experiences, a number of general themes arose that merit consideration when conducting mixed-methods research among youth affected by violence or war in other low-resource settings.

ETHICAL CONSIDERATIONS

Research ethics must take center stage at all phases of research. Particularly close attention must be given to research ethics in low-resource settings, given the major power disparities between researchers and affected populations. Evaluating the relative value of research is extremely important when operating in a context in which resources are extremely limited. Particularly in situations of complex humanitarian emergencies, securing the funding to carry out the delivery of basic health, nutrition, and shelter programs is challenging, let alone finding support for research. For research to be ethical, it must be valuable. Researchers must ask whether data collection could contribute to improvements in the safety or well-being of the target population on a larger scale, or whether it will be possible to derive methods of enhancing health (well-being) or some other beneficial knowledge from the research. Because resources are so limited, the costs versus benefits of research must be weighed carefully, and there must be a solid rationale for investing in data collection.

In many parts of the world, the conduct of researchers or the involvement of participants in research has proved damaging to the population being studied. For example, one of our NGO collaborators recounted the story of a community in Rwanda where a foreign university had conducted surveys on trauma and children's mental health. As a part of the data collection, researchers had engaged children and adolescents in very detailed interviews about past traumas, including the violence they had experienced and witnessed. The research group spent several weeks in the field, were hosted by people in the community, and were never heard from again after their departure. The data were eventually published, but the findings were never disseminated in the community, nor were they used to help establish or improve programs for children and families. As a result, leaders in the community were very angry and later were reluctant to allow other outside agencies to establish humanitarian programs in the region. This reluctance affected not only future research (a minor issue for members of the community) but also future efforts at intervention (a major issue for them). This example underscores the importance that researchers must place on collecting data from vulnerable populations in an ethical manner.

One of the central ethical challenges in working in low-resource settings is the difficulty of securing real informed consent. Such consent requires that participants be informed about the general purpose and procedures of the research, understand any potential risks and benefits of the research, and be able to provide voluntary consent, free of coercion. It also requires that the participants have access to proper channels of communication with the research staff and feel safe and free to discontinue participation throughout the study. Approaches to informed consent differ according to the context of the research. In some war-affected settings in sub-Saharan Africa, signing a formal document can be a source of anxiety for participants worried about persecution. In our research in northern Uganda (discussed below), we requested verbal consent in the presence of a witness, because there was a high rate of illiteracy in the population and because a written consent document would be the only form linking the participant to the research. In collective settings, options for group consent or consent from designated authorities such as community leaders or village chiefs and sector leaders is often of additional importance. Local community support and collaboration can be vital to the success of the research: it may help engage local participants while reducing the risk of mistrust and misunderstanding, because local leaders can help explain the purposes and procedures of the study. Just as important, village elders and chiefs may serve as a resource for others in the community who have concerns or questions about the research and may intervene in cases where the risk of harm exists or in cases of challenges to the research. That said, it is extremely important for investigators and research staff to work closely with, and earn the trust of, community elders and chiefs to ensure that their endorsement does not coerce people who remain uncomfortable with the research to participate in it.

THE IMPORTANCE OF LOCAL PARTICIPATION

Research with war-affected populations cannot achieve the goal of local relevance and appropriateness without the meaningful participation of people from the target population. Research that includes a strong element of collaboration with the community in its design (Trickett and Espino 2004) can be an effective means of developing and integrating sustainable interventions to improve mental health outcomes. It allows us to establish more equitable partnerships between communities and researchers and to develop services of importance to the community, thus combining knowledge with practical action (Israel et al. 1998; Israel et al. 2003). People with an intimate understanding of the local context and culture must carefully review the meaning of the constructs being measured and the manner in which procedures are administered for the local population. Finally, respect for a community-based participatory approach should also be reflected in a true commitment to sharing the findings of research with members of the community, particularly those who are the focus of the research (Wells et al. 2004).

Integrating Qualitative Participatory Methods into Survey Designs

I argued above that the use of inappropriate or poorly conceived methods in cross-cultural research goes beyond bad science; it is also an ethical issue that may generate invalid results, thus wasting time and resources and potentially jeopardizing future intervention efforts in the region. In this light, a mixed methodology can be seen as a way of ensuring that locally derived data are both relevant and valid. Qualitative methods, particularly those drawn from the perspective of community-based participatory research (Minkler and Wallerstein 2005), may help outside researchers avoid misunderstandings while reducing the risk of relying on poorly translated or adapted measures.

In our studies of African youth, our work with local research assistants and other community participants yielded important and eye-opening insights. In addition, designing a study through a participatory process with a local research team can ensure that the local researchers are invested in the quality of the study and can help improve the cultural accurateness of questions and highlight the differences between local meaning and outside assumptions.

In Ethiopia, for example, linguistic challenges had a great impact on our research. The Kunama refugees who were the focus of this research are traditional agropastoralists who have cultivated the land along the Ethiopian-Eritrean border for centuries. The history of the Kunama in the region is scarred by a litany of human rights abuses that include their exclusion from educational opportunities, the forced recruitment of their young men into the Eritrean military, and cases of enslavement. As a result of such abuses, a series of brutal wars, forced displacement, and poor economic opportunities, the Kunama people are dwindling in numbers. Their language, Kunamenga, is also struggling to survive. Although many of the Kunama speak Tigrinya, the regional language of northern Ethiopia, in order to show respect and engage participants, it was important that the surveys be conducted in Kunamenga. Due to the high illiteracy rate in the population, very few Kunama know how to read or write Kunamenga. Furthermore, a single word in Kunamenga is often used to represent a construct that may be described by several terms of varying shades of meaning in English. Such realities are particularly challenging when many assessments of mental health symptoms may come at a construct such as depression from many different angles and across multiple symptoms. For example, the YSR, which we used in this setting because it had been translated into Ethiopian Amharic, contains as one symptom of depression the item "I am unhappy, sad, or depressed." In Kunamenga, it was difficult to make these subtle distinctions because the language has just one word for sadness; distinguishing between "unhappy" and "depressed" was next to impossible. This example is indicative of problems that may be encountered in some settings when researchers begin with symptom items and terms from an existing measure.

We observed other differences between our assumptions and local meanings when we began to work with local staff members at the refugee camp and at the International Rescue Committee to investigate the circumstances of these war-affected youth. For example, we wanted to include on one scale questions about sexual violence, and we had crafted an initial scale mainly with the help of foreign staff members based in Ethiopia. We had included an item that said: "It's not safe for women and girls to walk in the camp after dark." As researchers, we felt that this item represented one point along a gradient of perceived risk of sexual violence. When we began reviewing this draft scale with local staff members, however, we quickly learned that such an item could just as easily be interpreted as referring to the risk women and girls might face of tripping on tree roots or stepping on a snake. In this local setting, this item could be seen as not referring to the construct of interest—interpersonal aspects of safety—but to a common experience, which could greatly distort our findings.

As this example demonstrates, when working in low-resource settings, it is very important to consider the degree of abstractness inherent in a survey item or scale. This dynamic is particularly important in groups where illiteracy is high and respondents have not had a lot of exposure to questionnaires, particularly multiple-choice tests. Yet much survey research involves the use of multiple-choice questions, with many measures relying on Likert scales to express degrees of variation in the construct being assessed. It is not safe to assume that an understanding of such abstract gradients of opinion will come naturally to populations characterized by low rates of literacy. Youth—particularly those who have had some exposure to schooling—usually quickly understand such scales. However, careful pilot testing and warm-up questions at the start of the scale can help a great deal.

One successful approach we have used in field research is to employ a pictorial representation of the scale gradient to allow the participant to use a visual aid to identify their degree of agreement with a statement being made. For example, in Ethiopia, we showed participants the Likert scale of the YSR with a visual aid representing the option of "a little bit," "somewhat," and "a lot" with a picture of one small pebble, a few pebbles, and a lot of pebbles. We used a practice statement such as "I like to sing" and ask people to give the answer that fit best for them—"a little bit," "somewhat," or "a lot"—by pointing to the visual aid with the pebbles in varying amounts. Some participants used this aid for the whole survey, while others found it useful for a time but then came to understand the scale and would finish the 112 items without the aid once they had gotten comfortable with the multiple-choice format.

In addition, central constructs such as "age" can have very different meanings across cultural settings. In some parts of the world, particularly where illiteracy is common, very few people may know their age or precise date of birth. This is true of many of the war-affected countries where we have conducted research. It is common for massive population flight or displacement to result in the loss of identification documents and paperwork that would normally provide a source of such information. In some countries, birth certificates or identification documents are uncommon. In this light, relying too heavily on self-reported age can quickly become a problem. That was the case in our follow-up study of ex-CAFF in Sierra Leone. From the outset, the research was designed to be longitudinal, meaning that we would endeavor to re-contact the boys and girls in the cohort sample over the course of several years. One of the big issues in ensuring that we were truly following up with the same individual was to check the name of the respondent against other descriptors such as age, gender, tribe, and religious affiliation. Between the baseline assessments and a follow-up two years later, age proved to be the most vexing of all the indicators measured. It was not uncommon to have a participant report being "sixteen" in 2002, only to say "fifteen" when we returned in 2003 or 2004. In discussing this issue with local staff members and youth, we quickly learned that very few young people in this war-affected rural setting knew their true date of birth or age. Very few people had formal identification documents. Our data demonstrated that most ex-CAFF in the sample had been with the rebels in the bush for many years (Betancourt et al. 2010a, 2010b, 2013). Keeping track of their birthdays and actual ages became nearly impossible for many of these youth during their time in the bush. As a result, it was very common in our sample to find that participants gave an approximate age rather than an exact age when responding to the survey question "How old are you?" In conducting research containing variables such as time, these items may be better represented by locally relevant markers such as the passage of seasons or harvest times rather than by actual dates.

Working in low-literacy settings, it is important to keep survey items as concrete as possible. Many measures of emotions or behaviors used with children in Western populations rely on euphemisms or sayings that do not translate well in cross-cultural research. Some good examples can be found in measures of social support, self-esteem, and temperament, which require just as much attention to culture and contextual relevance as indicators of psychopathology. For instance, phrases often seen in measures of social support such as "I can count on my friends when things go wrong" can easily be mistranslated or misinterpreted in translation. After extensive discussions with many of the African refugees we have worked with, we often found that there is a phrase akin to being able to rely or "to count on someone," but starting with the Western term rather than learning about important local terms and constructs can waste a lot of time and not properly represent local priorities. Exploratory qualitative work in mixed methods sequences such as those laid out by Creswell et al. (2011) might help identify how constructs like social support or similar aspects of social relatedness and connection are manifested in cultural settings new to the researcher. Our experience in conducting field research with refugees in a number of settings has demonstrated many ceiling effects (universally high ratings) for social support when using standard measures that had been translated forward and backward. Such findings may reflect problems in measurement that arise because there is insufficient variability in the responses. It is also possible that such ceiling effects may be driven by investigator influences (such as a desire to appear polite or give responses thought to be what the investigator wants) or a reporting bias grounded in the desire to not dishonor one's family or community in one's responses. These ratings may also be accurate. They may be a true expression of the sort of banding together that can be fostered by surviving in the face of a common threat such as war. In cross-cultural research, varieties of ethnographic and anthropological approaches are needed to understand these protective processes and how they operate in order to arrive at appropriate measurement.

Again, working with local staff members and engaging local people in the process of learning about the constructs central to the research from a local perspective are critical. This feedback loop can improve the quality of data collection, including respondents' comprehension of survey items and the valid representation of complex constructs or questions. Qualitative work can be important for documenting the process of doing research and the lessons learned, as well as for determining the most salient outcomes and intervention models.

As these examples demonstrate, ethically and scientifically sound humanitarian research cannot be rushed. Hurried data collection and analysis can yield invalid data and run the risk of damaging important relationships with potential community collaborators. As shown in figure 13.1, researchers need to first spend time learning and understanding a culture in order to identify locally relevant service needs, as well as local conceptualizations of mental health and healing. With such knowledge, one may also explore typical local responses to identified mental health needs, which can also inform the adaptation of interventions. Priority should also be given to establishing the local validity and reliability of measures. And ultimately, priority should be given to measures designed in a participatory, locally relevant way. Certainly, standard approaches to translation are important, such as using group translation and ensuring that forward and backward translation are completed where possible. As demonstrated in the examples above, however, the value of qualitative understanding of a culture and its context reaches far beyond conducting good translation. In planning cross-cultural research according to the mixed methods conceptual model presented in this chapter, it is important to ensure that adequate time and resources are available to invest in ethnographic or qualitative investigation of mental health issues in a new setting or culture. This is particularly important when very little information on mental health services needs and preferences are available.

Moving through the Full Conceptual Model: Northern Uganda

Research that I co-led in northern Uganda represents a full movement through each phase of the model presented in figure 13.1 for integrating qualitative and quantitative cross-cultural mental health research in an explanatory sequential design. As mentioned above, the purpose of this research was to investigate local perceptions of mental health problems affecting children living in IDP (internally displaced persons) camps and to plan and test appropriate mental health interventions. This research was funded by two international NGOs, World Vision Uganda and War Child Holland, who were developing mental health services for children living in the IDP camps of Gulu District, northern Uganda. Over a course of two years, the research moved through three main phases of work: a qualitative study, validity study, and randomized controlled trial of mental health interventions. The process of this project will be discussed more fully at the end of this chapter as it represents a full application of the conceptual model presented above. As in the sequential exploratory design illustrated in figure 13.1, findings from each phase of the work informed the subsequent phase over the course of two years of field research. The final result was a randomized controlled trial of interventions for the treatment of symptoms of depression in war-affected youth (Bolton et al. 2007).

As in the mixed methods model described previously, the first phase of the research involved a qualitative study. Given the time constraints inherent in working during a complex humanitarian emergency, techniques were based on rapid ethnographic assessment methods that had been used in previous cross-cultural mental health research (Bolton et al. 2003). In our qualitative study (Betancourt et al. 2009a, 2009b), we interviewed children aged ten to seventeen and their caretakers using free listing and key informant methods. The qualitative study was intended to identify and define common mental health syndromes affecting children and adolescents and their associated symptoms. This information was intended to help adapt or develop locally relevant mental health assessments for use with children and adolescents and to inform appropriate interventions. What emerged from these interviews were several categories of locally defined syndromes indicative of the mental health needs of children in this setting: *two tam* or *par* or *kumu* (depression and dysthymia-like syndromes), *ma lwor* (a mixed anxiety and depression-like syndrome), and a category of conduct problems referred to as *kwo maraco*. The symptoms of these local syndromes are similar to many described in the fourth edition of the American Psychiatric Association's *Diagnostic and Statistical Manual of Mental Disorders* (American Psychiatric Association 2000), especially the criteria for mood, anxiety, and conduct disorders. Several culturally specific symptoms also emerged. For example, "sitting *kumu*" (sitting while holding one's cheek in one's hand) was described as hallmark symptom of the local mood disorder *kumu*, and, as described previously, "not greeting people" was an important symptom of the disorders *par* and *ma lwor.*

Symptoms of these local syndromes were used to create the Acholi Psychosocial Assessment Instrument (APAI). The APAI was developed to assess symptoms along a continuum, relying on a mean score for each subscale rather than sorting children into a specific diagnostic category. Functional limitation scales were also created using additional items derived from free-list exercises that investigated the young person's difficulties doing chores, going to school, and engaging in family and community roles.

In the next phase of the research, we conducted a brief validity study among a sample of 667 young people aged fourteen to seventeen, roughly 42 percent of the estimated 1,600 people in that age group in the two camps, who were interviewed as part of an effort to screen adolescents into the randomized controlled trial. Again, the design of the validity study was based on a process previously used among adults (Bolton et al. 2003), with the present research intended to adapt this approach for use among children. A survey measure was created containing the locally derived measure, the APAI; a standard Western measure, the Strengths and Difficulties Questionnaire (Goodman 1997), and questions on functional limitations and demographics. This survey was administered to 667 adolescents and one primary caregiver for each of them. We considered using a local psychiatrist as a gold standard or as another point of triangulation in this study. However, given how rare mental health professionals were in the region at the time (and in many war-affected settings), we decided against this strategy so we could focus more narrowly on refining an approach that could easily be replicated in other low-resource contexts. Thus, to examine the validity of mental health measures, we used the self-reports of local syndromes by local people (both youth and caregivers) as an alternate gold standard. These self-reports were the answers to yes/no questions at the end of the survey, which asked the youths if they believed they had each of the five local syndromes of interest. Caregivers were asked if they believed that their child had each of the five syndromes. Findings indicated that the APAI demonstrated good psychometric properties in this population. Reliability was examined using standard test-retest and interrater methods, which indicated that the APAI performed adequately. Cronbach's alpha analyses obtained for the children's self-reports on the APAI yielded satisfactory internal reliability estimates. Significant correlation between the APAI and the Strengths and Difficulties Questionnaire demonstrated that the APAI had good convergent validity. Because our prior qualitative study had provided us with local terms for locally relevant mental health syndromes, we were able to demonstrate that the self-reports of local people using locally derived syndrome terms can serve as an alternate gold standard for determining the validity of such measures. This emic perspective is rare, yet it is very important for cross-cultural mental health work (Kleinman 1987). By using local terms, interventions can also be presented as responding to locally recognized disorders. Such an approach has the potential to increase local people's engagement and retention in mental health interventions (Bernal 2006). Once we had established the local appropriateness and validity of our measures, we were ready for the third phase of the research: a randomized controlled trial of interventions for the identified mental health needs.

In this final phase of this project, the validated APAI was used to screen and randomize adolescents (aged fourteen to seventeen) with locally described, depression-like symptoms into a three-arm Randomized Controlled Trial: one group participated in Adapted Group Interpersonal Psychotherapy (known as IPT-G); a second group participated in a recreation-based intervention called Creative Play; and a control group consisted of youths who were on the waiting list for intervention. Our findings indicated that the IPT-G was more effective than the other two arms with war-affected adolescents in northern Uganda, particularly for treating symptoms of depression-like problems in young women (for a full description of the intervention trial findings see Bolton et al. 2007). Overall, this trial provided evidence that IPT-G was a feasible and effective intervention for addressing the symptoms of locally relevant mood disorders in this setting. Following what in mixed methods research is often called a sequential explanatory design (Creswell et al. 2011), qualitative exit interviews were also conducted with individual child or adolescent participants in the interventions, their caregivers, and the members of the project staff who delivered the interventions, so we could contextualize the trial outcomes and identify any additional domains of analysis important for understanding the differential effects of the intervention. Our differential effects analyses to date indicate that IPT-G was particularly effective in girls without a history of abduction. The opposite appears to be the case for boys, with IPT-G possibly being more effective for boys with a history of abduction (Betancourt et al. 2012a). These findings reveal the need for further mixed-methods studies to be implemented in this setting, to round out the evidence base on effective mental health services for war-affected children and youth. We suggest that future impact studies take into account possible treatment effects related to gender. To do this work well will require strong anthropological and qualitative research in these settings, which could unpack the influence of gender on trauma and healing. These qualitative data will also help inform the development of appropriate measures that capture constructs that may be the active ingredients of a change in treatment—that is, coping, social support, and improved problem-solving abilities. Future quantitative studies can then examine both the treatment's efficacy and how it operates on these theorized key ingredients by gender.

CONCLUSION

This chapter has argued for the importance of using mixed-methods research to design and evaluate mental health interventions for war-affected youth and has presented core issues and the application of such approaches, using examples from my fieldwork in several sub-Saharan African countries. Both ethical and technical issues are central to conducting high-quality research in such settings, which can be strengthened by the application of mixed methods research. The chapter has emphasized a sequential exploratory mixed methods research process that begins by using qualitative methods to examine relevant mental health constructs (local idioms of distress and impairment) and to determine potential protective processes and preferences for intervention. The resulting qualitative data are essential for informing the selection or creation of appropriate assessment measures, as well as adapting existing interventions or developing new ones.

It is important that validation exercises address assessments of emotional distress (where relevant), measures of impairment, and measures of protective processes or mechanisms of change that are seen as essential to the intervention model. Multiple forms of validity must be considered. Once the validity of the assessment measures has been established, they may be used in baseline assessments of interventions tailored to the problem areas defined in the qualitative study. Following the intervention period, these validated assessment measures can be used to conduct post-intervention assessments of the effectiveness of the intervention in the target population. Blended or hybrid mixed methods designs can also be used whereby, in an exploratory sequential fashion, qualitative exit interviews are also recommended for use with not only individual child and adolescent participants in the intervention, but also with their caregivers and the project staff members who delivered the interventions. Information gathered on the effectiveness of the intervention and lessons learned in the process of delivering services can then form the basis for adapting this procedure to other settings. This approach to mental health services research on violence-affected youth may be replicated and refined in many other cultural settings and situations of adversity.

REFERENCES

Achenbach, T. M. 1991. *Manual for the Youth Self-Report and 1991 Profile.* Burlington, VT: University of Vermont Department of Psychiatry.

Ahmad, A. 2008. "Posttraumatic Stress among Children in Kurdistan." *Acta Paediatrica.* 97 (7): 884–88.

American Psychiatric Association. 2000. *Diagnostic and Statistical Manual of Mental Disorders.* 4th ed., text revision. Washington, D.C.: American Psychiatric Association.

Bayer C. P., F. Klasen, and H. Adam. 2007. "Association of Trauma and PTSD Symptoms with Openness to Reconciliation and Feelings of Revenge among Former Ugandan and Congolese Child Soldiers." *Journal of the American Medical Association* 298 (5): 555–59.

Bernal, G. 2006. "Intervention Development and Cultural Adaptation Research with Diverse Families." *Family Process* 45 (2): 143–51.

Betancourt T. S., J. Bass, I. Borisova, R. Neugebauer, L. Speelman, G. Onyango, and P. Bolton. 2009a. "Assessing Local Instrument Validity and Reliability: A Field-Based Example from Northern Uganda." *Social Psychiatry and Psychiatric Epidemiology* 44 (8): 685–92.

Betancourt, T. S., and W. R. Beardslee. 2012. "The Consequences of Concentrated Adversity on Child and Adolescent Mental Health." In *The Oxford Handbook of Poverty and Child Development,* edited by V. Maholmes and R. King, 622–39. New York: Oxford University Press.

Betancourt, T. S., and P. Bolton. 2005. *Using Qualitative Methods to Develop a Locally-Derived Measure of Psychosocial Problems in Acholi War-Affected Children.* Unpublished report to World Vision Uganda.

Betancourt, T. S., I. I. Borisova, T. P. Williams, T. H. Whitfield, M. de la Soudiere, J. Williamson, and S. E. Gilman. 2010a. "Sierra Leone's Former Child Soldiers: A Follow-Up Study of Psychosocial Adjustment and Community Reintegration." *Child Development* 81 (4), 1077–95.

Betancourt, T. S., R. T. Brennan, J. Rubin-Smith, G. M. Fitzmaurice, and S. E. Gilman. 2010b. "Sierra Leone's Former Child Soldiers: A Longitudinal Study of Risk, Protective Factors, and Mental Health." *Journal of the American Academy of Child and Adolescent Psychiatry* 49 (6): 606–15.

Betancourt, T. S., R. McBain, E. A. Newnham, and R. T. Brennan. 2013. "Trajectories of Internalizing Problems in War-Affected Sierra Leonean Youth: Examining Conflict and Postconflict Factors." *Child Development* 84 (2): 455–70.

Betancourt, T. S., E. A. Newnham, R. T. Brennan, H. Verdeli, I. Borisova, R. Neugebauer, J. Bass, and P. Bolton. 2012a. "Moderators of Treatment Effectiveness for War-Affected Youth with Depression in Northern Uganda." *Journal of Adolescent Health* 51 (6): 544–50.

Betancourt T. S., L. Speelman, G. Onyango, and P. Bolton. 2009b. "A qualitative study of mental health problems among children displaced by war in northern Uganda." *Transcultural Psychiatry* 46 (2): 238–56.

Betancourt, T. S., M. Yudron, W. Wheaton, and M. C. Smith-Fawzi, M. C. 2012b. "Caregiver and Adolescent Mental Health in Ethiopian Kunama Refugees Participating in an Emergency Education Program." *The Journal of Adolescent Health: Official Publication of the Society for Adolescent Medicine* 51 (4): 357–65.

Black, R. E., S. S. Morris, and J. Bryce. 2003. "Where and Why Are 10 Million Children Dying Every Year?" *Lancet* 361 (9376): 2226–34.

Bolton, P. 2001. "Cross-Cultural Validity and Reliability Testing of a Standard Psychiatric Assessment Instrument without a Gold Standard." *Journal of Nervous and Mental Disease* 189 (4): 238–42.

Bolton, P., J. Bass, T. Betancourt, L. Speelman, G. Onyango, K. Clougherty, R. Neugebauer, H. Verdeli, and L. Murray. 2007. "Interventions for Depression Symptoms among Adolescent Survivors of War and Displacement in Northern Uganda: A Randomized Controlled Trial." *Journal of the American Medical Association* 298 (5): 519–27.

Bolton, P., J. Bass, R. Neugebauer, H. Verdeli, K. F. Clougherty, P. Wickramaratne, L. Speelman, L. Ndogoni, and M. Weissman. 2003. "Group Interpersonal Psychotherapy for Depression in Rural Uganda: A Randomized Controlled Trial." *Journal of the American Medical Association* 289 (23): 3117–24.

Creswell, J. W. 2003. *Research Design: Qualitative, Quantitative, and Mixed Methods Approaches.* 2nd ed. Thousand Oaks, CA: Sage.

Creswell, J. W., A. C. Klassen, V. L. Plano Clark, and K. C. Smith. 2011. "Best Practices for Mixed Methods Research in the Health Sciences." National Institutes of Health. Accessed April 1, 2013. http://obssr.od.nih.gov/mixed_methods_research.

Derluyn, I., E. Broekaert, G. Schuyten, and E. De Temmerman. 2004. "Post-traumatic Stress in Former Ugandan Child Soldiers." *Lancet* 363 (9412): 861–63.

Geertz, C. 1973. *The Interpretation of Cultures.* New York: Basic Books.

Goldstein, J. M., and J. C. Simpson. 1995. "Validity: Definitions and Applications to Psychiatric Research." In *Textbook in Psychiatric Epidemiology,* edited by M. T. Tsuang, M. Cohen, and G. E. P. Zahner, 229–42. New York: Wiley-Liss.

Goodman, R. 1997. "The Strengths and Difficulties Questionnaire: A Research Note." *Journal of Child Psychology and Psychiatry* 38 (5): 581–86.

Guarnaccia, P. J., R. Lewis-Fernandez, and M. R. Marano. 2003. "Toward a Puerto Rican Popular Nosology: Nervios and Ataque de Nervios," *Culture, Medicine and Psychiatry* 27 (3): 339–66.

Hollifield, M., T. D. Warner, N. Lian, B. Krakow, J. H. Jenkins, J. Kesler, and J. Westermeyer. 2002. "Measuring Trauma and Health Status in Refugees: A Critical Review." *Journal of the American Medical Association* 288 (5): 611–21.

Israel, B. A., A. J. Schulz, E. A. Parker, and A. B. Becker. 1998. "Review of Community-Based Research: Assessing Partnership Approaches to Improve Public Health." *Annual Review of Public Health* 19: 173–202.

Israel, B. A., A. J. Schulz, E. A. Parker, A. B. Becker, A. J. Allen 3rd, and R. Guzman. 2003. "Critical Issues in Developing and Following Community Based Participatory Research Principles." In *Community-Based Participatory Research for Health,* edited by M. Minkler and N. Wallerstein, 53–76. San Francisco: Jossey-Bass.

Kinzie, J. D., W. H. Sack, R. H. Angell, S. Manson, and B. Rath. 1986. "The Psychiatric Effects of Massive Trauma on Cambodian Children: I. The Children." *Journal of the American Academy of Child and Adolescent Psychiatry* 25 (3): 370–76.

Kleinman, A. 1987. "Anthropology and Psychiatry: The Role of Culture in Cross-Cultural Research on Illness." *British Journal of Psychiatry* 151 (4): 447–54.

Kohrt, B. A. 2007. *Recommendations to Promote Psychosocial Well-Being of Children Associated with Armed Forces and Armed Groups (CAAFAG) in Nepal.* Kathmandu, Nepal: UNICEF.

Lewis-Fernandez, R., P. J. Guarnaccia, I. E. Martinez, E. Salman, A. Schmidt, and M. Liebowitz. 2002. "Comparative Phenomenology of Ataques de Nervios, Panic Attacks, and Panic Disorder." *Culture, Medicine, and Psychiatry* (26): 199–223.

Machel, G. 1996. *Promotion and Protection of the Rights of Children: Impact of Armed Conflict on Children.* Report of the expert of the Secretary-General, submitted pursuant to UN General Assembly resolution 48/157. New York: United Nations.

Macksoud, M. S., and J. L. Aber. 1996. "The War Experiences and Psychosocial Development of Children in Lebanon." *Child Development* 67 (1): 70–88.

Matías-Carrelo, L. E., L. M. Chávez, G. Negrón, G. Canino, S. Aguilar-Gaxiola, and S. Hoppe. 2003. "The Spanish Translation and Cultural Adaptation of Five Mental Health Outcome Measures." *Culture, Medicine and Psychiatry* 27 (3): 291–313.

Maxwell, J. A. 2005. *Qualitative Research Design: An Interactive Approach.* Thousand Oaks, CA: Sage.

Maxwell, S. E., and H. D. Delaney. 2000. *Designing Experiments and Analyzing Data.* Mahwah, NJ: Lawrence Erlbaum.

Minkler, M., and N. Wallerstein, eds. 2005. *Community-Based Participatory Research for Health.* San Francisco: Jossey-Bass.

Mollica, R., B. Lopez Cardoza, H. J. Osofsky, A. Ager, and P. Salama. 2004. "Mental Health in Complex Emergencies." *Lancet* 364 (9450): 2058–67.

Razokhi, A. H., I. K. Taha, N. I. Taib, S. Sadik, and N. A. Gasseer. 2006. Mental Health of Iraqi Children. *The Lancet* 368 (9538): 838–39.

Stichick, T. 2001. "The Psychosocial Impact of Armed Conflict on Children: Rethinking Traditional Paradigms in Research and Intervention." *Child and Adolescent Psychiatric Clinics of North America* 10 (4): 797–814.

Stichick, T, and C. Bruderlein. "Children Facing Insecurity: New Strategies for Survival in a Global Era." Policy paper produced for the Canadian Department of Foreign Affairs and International Trade, The Human Security Network, 3rd Ministerial Meeting, Petra, Jordan, May 11–12, 2001.

Trickett, E. J., and S. Espino. 2004. "Collaboration and Social Inquiry: Multiple Meanings of a Construct and Its Role in Creating Useful and Valid Knowledge." *American Journal of Community Psychology* 34 (1–2): 1–69.

UNICEF. 2009. "Machel Study 10-Year Strategic Review: Children and Conflict in a Changing World." New York: UNICEF. http://www.unicef.org/publications/files /Machel_Study_10_Year_Strategic_Review_EN_030909.pdf.

Wells, K., J. Miranda, J., A. Bruce, and N. Wallerstein. 2004. "Bridging Community Intervention and Mental Health Services Research." *American Journal of Psychiatry* 161 (6): 955–63.

CONTRIBUTORS

EMMANUEL AKYEAMPONG is Professor of History and of African and African American studies at Harvard University. His publications include *Between the Sea and the Lagoon: An Eco-Social History of the Anlo of Southeastern Ghana* (2001) and *The Dictionary of African Biography,* a six-volume work edited with Henry Louis Gates Jr. (2012).

THERESA BETANCOURT is Associate Professor of Child Health and Human Rights in the Department of Global Health and Population at the Harvard School of Public Health. She directs the Research Program on Children and Global Adversity at the François-Xavier Bagnoud Center for Health and Human Rights, also at the Harvard School of Public Health.

RENÉ COLLIGNON studied psychology and clinical psychology at the University of Louvain. He is editor of the journal *Psychopathologie africaine* and author of numerous publications. He served as part of the psychiatric team with Henri Collomb at Fann Hospital, Dakar, between 1972 and 1982.

PAMELA Y. COLLINS is Director of the Office for Research on Disparities and Global Mental Health and of the Office of Rural Mental Health Research at the U.S. National Institute of Mental Health. She was coeditor of a 2011 *Lancet* series on global mental health, and is currently a leader of the Grand Challenges in Global Mental Health initiative.

ANDREW DAWES is currently Research Advisor to the Ilifa Labantwana Early Childhood Development Program. He is Emeritus Professor of Psychology at the University of Cape Town.

VICTORIA DE MENIL is a PhD student at the London School of Economics, researching the capacity of private providers to address the mental health treatment gap in Kenya, and the economic impact of those providers' efforts.

AMA DE-GRAFT AIKINS is Associate Professor of Social Psychology at the Regional Institute for Population Studies at the University of Ghana.

VICTOR C. K. DOKU is a UK-trained psychiatrist and epidemiologist. He has worked as a subinvestigator on international trials on first-episode psychosis.

ALAN FLISHER passed away at the age of 53 during the writing of his contribution to this volume. At the time he held the Streungmann Chair of Child and Adolescent Psychiatry and Mental Health in the Department of Psychiatry and Mental Health at the University of Cape Town.

ALLAN G. HILL has been the Andelot Professor of Demography at Harvard University since 1991 and is the director of the Education Office of the Department of Population and International Health in the Harvard School of Public Health.

ZUHAYR KAFAAR has been a lecturer in the Department of Psychology at Stellenbosch University, in South Africa, since 2007. He teaches research methods, lectures on psychological measurement, and supervises postgraduate research.

SARAH KIPPEN WOOD holds a master of public health degree from Boston University, with an emphasis in international public health. As International Research Manager for BasicNeeds, Wood is responsible for managing research initiatives at affiliated sites throughout Africa, South Asia, and Southeast Asia. Her interests include assessing impacts of community mental health programs in low-income countries.

ARTHUR KLEINMAN is a physician and anthropologist at Harvard University. The author of numerous books and articles, he is the recipient of the Distinguished Faculty Award, given by the Harvard Foundation.

CRICK LUND is Associate Professor and Director of the Alan J. Flisher Centre for Public Mental Health, Department of Psychiatry and Mental Health, University of Cape Town, South Africa.

WILLIAM P. MURPHY teaches anthropology and African studies at Northwestern University.

SEGGANE MUSISI is Professor and Chair of the Department of Psychiatry in the School of Medicine, College of Health Sciences, at Makerere University, in Uganda.

BRONWYN MYERS is Chief Specialist Scientist in the Alcohol and Drug Abuse Research Unit of the South African Medical Research Council and is an honorary associate professor in the Department of Psychiatry and Mental Health at the University of Cape Town, South Africa.

ELIALILIA OKELLO is a faculty member in the Department of Psychiatry at Makerere University, in Uganda.

VIKRAM PATEL is Joint Director of the Centre for Global Mental Health at the London School of Hygiene and Tropical Medicine.

SHOBA RAJA has a graduate degree in psychology from Mumbai University and a postgraduate degree in medical and psychiatric social work from the Tata Institute of Social Sciences, also in Mumbai. Raja joined BasicNeeds in 2001 and has been instrumental in developing the organisation's research, policy and knowledge work.

GIUSEPPE RAVIOLA is Assistant Professor of Psychiatry and Global Health and Social Medicine at Harvard Medical School.

URSULA M. READ has a doctorate degree in medical anthropology from University College London. She is now a career development fellow in the UK Medical Research Council's Social and Public Health Sciences Unit.

MICHAEL R. REICH is Taro Takemi Professor of International Health Policy at the Harvard School of Public Health. His recent books include *Pharmaceutical Reform: A Guide to Improving Performance and Equity,* with Marc J. Roberts, and *Access: How Do Good Health Technologies Get to Poor People in Poor Countries?* with Laura J. Frost.

SORAYA SEEDAT is Professor and Executive Head of Department of Psychiatry at the University of Stellenbosch, South African Research Chair in Posttraumatic Stress Disorder, and Codirector of the Medical Research Council Unit on Anxiety and Stress Disorders.

KATHERINE SORSDAHL is Brain and Behavior Initiatives (BBI) Project Manager in the Department of Psychiatry and Mental Health at the University of Cape Town, South Africa.

DAN J. STEIN is Professor and Chair of the Department of Psychiatry and Mental Health at the University of Cape Town, South Africa.

RITA THOM is the founder and a current member of the HIV Special Interest Group of the South African Society of Psychiatrists and serves on the Human Research Ethics Committee at the University of the Witwatersrand, in South Africa, where she is an honorary adjunct professor in the Division of Psychiatry.

INDEX

Abas, Melanie, 60

Abbo, Catherine, 252, 257–258

Accra, Ghana, 112–113, 125–126. *See also* women's mental health

Accra Psychiatric Hospital, 12, 14, 76, 102n3, 124; cannabis-related admissions, *41;* diagnoses, 78, 128, *129;* living conditions, 128, 132; long-stay patients, 127–131; marketing of, 126

Accra Survey, 112–113

acculturation (deculturation), 4, 79, 173

Achenbach Youth Self-Report (YSR), 314

Acholi language youth psychosocial assessment, 314–315

Acholi Psychosocial Assessment Instrument (APAI), 326–327

Acquah, Ione, 112–113, 139n6

acute transient psychoses, 81–82, 84, 91

Adapted Group Interpersonal Psychotherapy (IPT-G), 327–328

Addis Ababa, Ethiopia, 113

Adomi village settlement (Ghana), 132

Adverse Childhood Experiences studies, 145

advocacy, 135, 220

affective disorders, 74, 81, 91. *See also* depression

African Poor, The (Iliffe), 113

African psyche, colonial view, 9–10, 24–25, 78, 163

African psychiatrists, 3–6, 25–27, 36–37, 77, 79, 87, 93. *See also* Lambo, Thomas

Africanization, 3, 5, 13–14, 169–174

age, identifying, 323–324

aging, 190–191, 192; women, 118, 135, 192, 193–194, *194,* 197

Agossou, Thérèse, 36–37, 174, 178n28

Agreement on Trade-Related Aspects of Intellectual Property Rights (TRIPS), 265

Agyepong, I., 236

Ahyi, René Gualbert, 36–37, 174

Ainsworth, James, 230

Akan culture, 122

Akyeampong, Emmanuel, 122

Algeria, 10, 30, 31, 32

aliénés indigènes (indigenous aliens), 75

amafufunyane (possession by evil spirits), 55, 157

American Medical Association, 225

amorphous endogenous psychosis, 80

Anambra State Psychiatric Hospital (Nigeria), 32

ancestral spirits, 24, 97, 157; *rab,* 165, 167, 168; rituals of reconciliation and, 287–288; traditional healers and, 250, 253, 258

Angola, 6, 7, 8, 29; community reconciliation and child soldiers, 283, 287–288, 290

anthropology, 3–4, 131, 173–174, 293, 297; self, approach to, 285–286; studies of schizophrenia and psychosis, 73, 77–78, 83; of youth, 285, 304n7

antipsychotic prescriptions, 94–95

anxiety: depression co-occurring with, 50; *ma lwor* (mixed anxiety and depression-like syndrome), 326; sub-Saharan Africa, 50–72

apprenticeship to signs, 300, 302, 304n6

"archeological" method, 299–300

Armah, Ayi Kwei, 102n5

Aro Village experiment (Nigeria), 5–6, 10, 25, 27, 29, 32, 104n16

Aro-Cornell project, 79

assessment instruments, 19, 85, 312, 326–327; limitations of, 313–315

Association des Chercheurs Sénégalais, 171

Asuni, Tolani, 34

asylums/psychiatric hospitals, 97; abandonment in, 84, 100, 119, 123, 127, 130–131, 134, 136, 138; colonial period, 26–32, 75; custodial role, 26–27, 28, 76, 121–122; evictions from, 130; France, 30, 75; political process

—

CPSIA information can be obtained
at www.ICGtesting.com
Printed in the USA
BVOW08s0850031116

466739BV00041B/309/P

9 780253 012937